Diagnosis and Treatment Planning in Counseling

Third Edition

Diagnosis and Treatment Planning in Counseling

Third Edition

Linda Seligman

Faculty, Walden University Clinical Psychology and Health Psychology
and
Director, Center for Counseling and Consultation
Bethesda, Maryland and Fairfax, Virginia

Kluwer Academic Publishers
New York, Boston, Dordrecht

Library of Congress Cataloging-in-Publication Data

Diagnosis and treatment planning in counseling / Linda Seligman.—3rd ed.
       p. cm.
    Includes bibliographic references and index.
    ISBN 0-306-48472-2 (hardbound); 0-306-48514-1 (paperback)
       1. Mental health counseling. 2. Counseling. 3. Psychiatry—Case formulation.
    4. Psychiatry—Differential therapeutics.

RC466.S45 2004
616.89—dc22   2004044178

ISBN 0-306-48472-2 (hardbound)
ISBN 0-306-48514-1 (paperback)

© 2004 by Kluwer Academic/Plenum Publishers, New York
233 Spring Street, New York, New York 10013

http://www.kluweronline.com

10 9 8 7 6 5 4 3 2 1

A C.I.P. record for this book is available from the Library of Congress.

Permissions for books published in Europe: permissions@wkap.nl
Permissions for books published in the United States of America: permissions@wkap.com

Printed in the United States of America

Preface

The scope of the counseling profession, as well as the importance of diagnosis and treatment planning, has grown enormously since the 1986 publication of the first edition of this book. Credentialing for mental health counselors is now available in nearly all states. Training in diagnosis and treatment planning is provided by nearly all graduate programs in Counselor Education. New professional organizations, new opportunities, and new challenges are available to counselors.

The purpose of the third edition of this book is to help counselors and other mental health professionals to acquire up-to-date information on their field, to develop sound knowledge of diagnosis and treatment planning, and to acquire relevant clinical knowledge and skills that are essential to their effectiveness. Diagnosis and treatment planning are core skills for counselors, skills that permeate all counseling roles and functions. Consequently, this book takes a broad look at that process, reviewing tools and competencies associated with diagnosis and treatment planning in individual counseling, group counseling, family counseling, career counseling, and organizational development.

In addition to providing essential knowledge and skills that will enhance counseling practice, this book should be very helpful to counselors preparing to take examinations for licensure and certification in counseling. Knowledge of the material presented in this book on diagnosis, treatment planning, mental status examinations, and ethical standards will be particularly useful to people taking the National Clinical Mental Health Counseling Examination, which focuses heavily on these areas.

The following are brief descriptions of the 13 chapters in this book.

Chapter 1, The Evolving Role of the Counselor, reviews efforts to develop a definition of mental health counseling. An overview of the history of the counseling profession is provided, as well as information on the expanding role of the counselor, professional associations, credentialing for both counselors and counselor education programs, and the current impact of managed care on the profession. This chapter concludes with a review of important counselor competencies.

New roles for mental health counselors are the focus of Chapter 2, Opportunities for the Mental Health Counselor. This chapter looks at new and growing client groups, employment settings, and problem areas of relevance to the mental health counselor. The chapter also discusses the types of mental health professionals and the mental health treatment team.

The *Diagnostic and Statistical Manual of Mental Disorders* (*DSM*) is the focus of Chapter 3, Diagnostic Systems and Their Use. This chapter reviews the benefits and pitfalls of diagnosis as well as the history of diagnosis. The chapter then explains the essential features of each of the diagnoses in the current edition of the *DSM*.

The Use of Assessment in Diagnosis and Treatment Planning, Chapter 4, discusses tools and inventories for qualitative and quantitative assessment that can enhance the process of diagnosis and treatment planning. The chapter also provides information on planning an assessment and on interpreting client information.

Intake Interviews and Their Role in Diagnosis and Treatment Planning are the focus of Chapter 5. The nature and importance of the intake interview are reviewed, and an outline for an extended intake interview is provided. Also included in this chapter are a transcript of an intake interview and written reports of both brief and lengthy intake interviews. In addition, a format for a mental status examination is presented, along with an example.

Chapter 6 addresses The Nature and Importance of Treatment Planning. The DO A CLIENT MAP, a structured format for treatment planning, is presented.

In Chapter 7, Theories and Strategies of Individual Counseling are discussed. Information on the major approaches to individual counseling is presented, including important concepts, key interventions, and appropriate use. Examples of treatment plans are provided.

Diagnosis and Treatment Planning for Families is the topic of Chapter 8. Guidelines and tools are provided for assessing family functioning. Important approaches to family counseling are discussed, including their appropriate use. An example of an assessment and treatment plan for a family is provided, as well as cases for discussion.

Chapter 9 focuses on Assessment and Treatment of Groups. This chapter encompasses ways to describe and diagnose the needs of groups, counselor roles in group treatment, and important approaches to group counseling. An example of the assessment and treatment planning for a counseling group is provided.

Counseling for Career and Organizational Development is the topic of Chapter 10, written in collaboration with Shannon Peters and Brian Peters. Although formal diagnoses of pathology are rarely made in career counseling and organizational development settings, here too counselors maximize their effectiveness through the use of assessment and treatment planning. Theories of career and organizational development counseling are presented, as well as a case study.

Documentation, Report Writing, and Record Keeping in Counseling are reviewed in Chapter 11. This chapter discusses the importance of writing and record keeping in counseling and provides models for progress notes, interim reports, assessment reports, professional disclosure statements, safe-keeping contracts, case conferences and other reports prepared by counselors.

Chapter 12, a completely new chapter in this edition of the book, discusses the Importance of Ethical and Professional Development for Counselors. Whether mental health professionals are engaged in diagnosis, treatment, or any of the other roles of the counselor, they must always have the ethical standards of the profession in mind and follow those standards in their work. The second part of this chapter focuses on you, the reader. It presents information on counselors' professional development and provides a format for you to plan out your own professional development.

Future Trends and Predictions in Counseling are presented in Chapter 13. This chapter reviews the predictions made in the first and second editions of this book and discusses their current status. In addition, predictions are made about the future of the counseling profession, based primarily on information and issues discussed throughout this book.

Acknowledgments

I would like to express my appreciation to some of the people who contributed to this book.

Many thanks to:

- My husband, Dr. Robert Zeskind, for all his love and support.
- My friend, Bettie MacLennan Young, for her friendship, good advice, and understanding.
- Dr. Shannon Peters of George Washington University. Dr. Peters provided considerable assistance with the research for this book and coauthored Chapter 11.
- Dr. Brian Peters, organizational consultant, who coauthored Chapter 11.
- Michele Lewis, NCC, consultant, teacher, career counselor, and researcher, who used her knowledge of both editing and counseling in reviewing this manuscript.
- Dr. Bonnie Moore and Dr. Stephanie Hardenburg, who contributed to the second edition of this book and whose ideas are still reflected in this edition.
- My clients, who helped me to really understand diagnosis and treatment planning, many of whom are reflected in composite versions in the cases presented in this book.
- The participants in my courses and workshops on diagnosis and treatment planning who contributed greatly to my knowledge of how to teach diagnosis and treatment planning.

About the Author

Dr. Linda Seligman received the Ph.D. degree in Counseling Psychology from Columbia University. She is a faculty member at Walden University and a faculty associate at Johns Hopkins University. In addition, she is a professor emeritus at George Mason University, where she was codirector of the doctoral program in education and head of the graduate program in Counseling.

Dr. Seligman is a licensed psychologist and licensed professional counselor. She has experience in a variety of clinical settings, including psychiatric hospitals, community mental health centers, substance abuse treatment programs, foster care, corrections, and private practice. She is currently the Director of the Center for Counseling and Consultation, a private practice with offices in Fairfax, Virginia, and Bethesda, Maryland.

Dr. Seligman's research interests include diagnosis and treatment planning, counseling people with chronic and life-threatening illnesses, and the mind-body-spirit connection. She has completed 10 books, including *Selecting Effective Treatments*; *Technical and Conceptual Skills for Mental Health Professionals*: *Systems, Strategies, and Skills of Counseling and Psychotherapy*; *Promoting a Fighting Spirit*; and *Developmental Career Counseling and Assessment*. She also has authored over 50 professional articles and book chapters. In addition, she has lectured throughout the world on diagnosis and treatment planning.

Dr. Seligman has been the editor of *The Journal of Mental Health Counseling* and has served as president of the Virginia Association of Mental Health Counselors. She was selected as a Distinguished Professor by George Mason University and as a Researcher of the Year by the American Mental Health Counselors Association.

Contents

10. Counseling For Career and Organizational Development   291

Shannon Peters, Brian J. Peters, and Linda Seligman

The Evolving Role of the Counselor

The counseling profession is now approximately 100 years old and, in 2003, the American Counseling Association celebrated its 50th anniversary. The growth and change in the counseling profession reflect a dynamic field full of energy and innovation. Rapid changes over the past 25 years have led to expansion and flexibility in the counseling profession as well as increasing responsiveness to the needs of our multicultural society.

During the first 75 years of the profession, the term "counselor" usually meant only school or career counselor. However, beginning in the early 1980s, the profession was transformed by the emergence and rapid growth of mental health counseling, family counseling, and multicultural counseling. By the early 1990s, graduate programs for these new counseling areas outnumbered programs to train school counselors (Cowger, Hinkle, DeRidder, & Erk, 1991).

Many changes and trends have contributed to the growth of these areas. Among them are social, economic, and cultural stressors; growing awareness of the prevalence and impact of dysfunctional families; and expansion of and appreciation for diversity. Other developments that contributed to this growth include the high incidence of chronic and life-threatening illnesses; increased media attention to such pervasive problems as substance abuse, physical and sexual abuse, and mental illness; a growing awareness of violence in our society, including hate crimes, school shootings, terrorist attacks, and wars; and a greater emphasis on family unity and emotional health. The Internet, with its instantaneous transmission of vast amounts of information, promoted widespread awareness of these changes. All of this has led to a growing acceptance of counseling and the many ways it can help people deal with life's challenges. A broad range of opportunities for counselors emerged, not only in mental health settings but also in business and industry, private practice, community organizations, and elsewhere. Counselor education programs responded to an increased demand for mental health professionals by training more counselors.

DEFINITIONS OF COUNSELING

Many writers have struggled to define counseling and to clarify what distinguishes it from the other mental health professions such as social work, psychology, and psychiatric nursing. Numerous efforts also have been made to explain how mental health counseling differs from other specializations within counseling and from counseling in general. While an increased clarity has been achieved in distinguishing the professions, some identity confusion continues. According to Pistole and Roberts (2002, p. 8), "Persons newly admitted to training in the 21st century are faced with forming a professional identity within a complex and bewildering array of overlapping and related, but separate, human service delivery paths. In such a context, development of a professional identity, especially initially may be a confusing task ... ." Nevertheless, they emphasize that a sense of professional identity promotes feelings of "belongingness and uniqueness" (p. 1).

Ohio State Law (section 4757.01) provides a concise legal definition of counseling: " 'Practice of professional counseling' means rendering or offering to render a counseling service involving the application of clinical counseling principles, methods, or procedures to assist individuals in achieving more effective personal, social, educational, or career development and adjustment, including the diagnosis and treatment of mental and emotional disorders."

Older definitions, formulated to shape mental health counseling in its early years, continue to provide clarification of the profession. Ivey (1989, pp. 28–29), for example, advanced a definition of mental health counseling, broad enough to encompass the work of all counselors: "Mental health counseling is a profession which conducts its developmental practice with both the severely distressed and those facing normal developmental tasks. This developmental practice exists within a multicultural awareness and seeks to address clients and the systems in which they live." According to Ivey, counseling interventions help individuals and systems (families, groups, and organizations) to fulfil their potential, effect positive change, and grow, regardless of the severity of their concerns. He believes that "[m]ental health counseling recognizes that individual change may not be possible unless family, school, community, and sociocultural systems are also in place. Mental health counseling, then, does not focus narrowly on individual change, but on a careful assessment of both individual and environment and then acts on or treats both personal and systemic variables."

Fong's (1990, p. 108) definition of mental health counseling also is broad. She views mental health counseling as encompassing a " ... continuum of services that is developmental, environmental, and ecological, as well as remedial." It emphasizes interventions that "focus on competencies, strengths, coping, resources, negotiating life transitions, and managing stressors."

Spruill and Fong (1990, p. 21) provided further understanding of mental health counseling in the following definition: "Mental health counseling, a core mental health care profession, is the aggregate of the specific educational, scientific, and professional contributions of the disciplines of education, psychology, and counseling, focused on promotion and maintenance of mental health, the prevention and treatment of mental illness, the identification and modification of etiologic, diagnostic, and systems correlates of mental health, mental illness, and related dysfunction, and the improvement of the mental health service delivery system."

Mental health counseling, then, is characterized by:

1. taking a holistic, systemic, and developmental view of people, their families, their environments, and their interrelationships;
2. using approaches that are preventive, remedial, rehabilitative, and enhancing;
3. advocating an understanding of pathology and dysfunction, but maintaining an emphasis on health, wellness, and growth;
4. enabling people to identify and build on their strengths so that they can help themselves;
5. emphasizing the need for awareness of and sensitivity to individual, gender, cultural, and other differences and reflecting that understanding in multicultural counseling competencies;
6. taking place in a wide range of settings with a diverse clientele;
7. being multifaceted and interdisciplinary, and encompassing a broad range of theories and interventions that can be adapted to meet the needs of a particular person or group.

Despite the apparent consistency in these definitions, professional identity continues to be an important issue; counselors still strive to establish a clear, distinctive, and positive image of themselves in the minds of the general public. The information in this book, including definitions of the counseling profession, a review of its history and organization, important counseling competencies, and some of the counselors' important roles and tools, will help readers formulate a meaningful definition of their profession.

EARLY HISTORY OF THE COUNSELING PROFESSION

In the decades before the beginning of the counseling profession, Freud and his colleagues focused the attention of Europe and the United States on the development of the psyche. Although considerable stigma was still attached to mental illness, psychoanalysis, with its promise of understanding and alleviating some forms of emotional difficulties, shifted perceptions and sparked interest in the mind. The climate was right for the development of new approaches that would promote adjustment and help people with milder forms of emotional upset and uncertainty.

At its inception in the early 1900s, the field of counseling was a relatively well-defined and circumscribed one. The primary task of the counselor was helping people make occupational choices by seeking a good match between person and job. The guiding theory was the trait-and-factor approach advanced by Frank Parsons in his 1909 book *Choosing a Vocation*. Vocational or career counseling, then, was the counselor's primary role for more than 30 years. This was reflected by the first national professional organization for counselors, the National Vocational Guidance Association (NVGA), founded in 1913.

COUNSELING IN THE 1940s, 1950s, AND 1960s

The role of the counselor changed and expanded through the 1940s and 1950s. World War II and the Korean War led to a need for counselors to facilitate the readjustment and rehabilitation of veterans. In 1944, the Veterans Administration established a nationwide network of guidance services. In that same year, the United States Employment Service was initiated, eventually establishing well over 1,000 offices throughout the United States. Counselors soon realized they could best meet people's needs by considering their emotional development as well as their physical concerns and occupational aspirations. They became increasingly interested in helping healthy people deal with transitions and developmental concerns.

Carl Rogers contributed to the shift in the counselors' role with the 1942 publication of *Counseling and Psychotherapy* and his theory, then called nondirective or client-centered counseling. Rogers encouraged counselors to define goals based on people's needs, to attend to clients' emotions and self-esteem, to use a broad and flexible array of interventions, and to promote a positive counseling alliance with their clients.

In 1951, the Personnel and Guidance Association (PGA) was founded, the organization that would evolve into today's American Counseling Association (ACA). At its inception, the PGA had four divisions reflecting the primary roles of counselors at that time: the American College Personnel Association; the National Association of Guidance Supervisors and College Trainers, forerunner of the modern Association for Counselor Education and Supervision (ACES); the National Vocational Guidance Association; and the Student Personnel Association for Teacher Education. The American School Counselors Association (ASCA) soon became a fifth division and in 1957 the American Rehabilitation Counseling

Association became division six. In the 1960s, the Association for Measurement and Evaluation in Guidance and the National Employment Counselors Association became additional divisions.

Professional associations for other helping professions were initiated during these years, reflecting the growth in those professions as well as in the counseling field. The American Association of Marriage and Family Therapists was established in 1945 and, in 1955, the National Association of Social Workers was founded (Nugent, 1990).

During the 1950s and 1960s, Erik H. Erikson (*Childhood and Society*), Rollo May (*Man's Search for Himself*), Fritz Perls (*Gestalt Therapy*), Leona Tyler (*The Work of the Counselor*), Robert J. Havighurst (*Human Development and Education*), and Albert Bandura (*Principles of Behavior Modification*) all published influential texts that focused attention on people's developmental needs. Counselors began to address prevention and the personal growth of their clients as well as remediation of difficulties. Humanistic psychology gained interest and was called the third force in psychology, along with behaviorism and psychoanalysis.

The 1960s were a transitional period. Civil rights issues, campus unrest, increasing drug abuse, and antiwar demonstrations contributed to a growing national feeling of discontent, especially among the poor and ethnic minorities who had not been well served by traditional helping agencies. Many programs developed during the 1960s responded to this dissatisfaction. Among them were the Peace Corps, VISTA, the War on Poverty, and Operation Headstart. In addition, strong special interest groups formed to promote racial equality and women's rights.

Those movements had a strong effect on the role of the counselor. They brought increasing recognition to the importance of the family, community, and social system in a person's emotional development. People were less often thought of as abnormal or "sick" and more often as unable to cope successfully with a stressful or destructive environment.

However, mental health professionals were reaching only a small fraction of people needing help. The medical model, emphasizing one-to-one contact with troubled people who actively sought help, increasingly seemed outmoded and ineffective. Progress required changes in communities as well as in individuals.

In 1963, the Community Mental Health Centers Act was passed, necessitating redefinition of the field of counseling. That act mandated establishment of a nationwide network of approximately 2,000 community mental health centers (CMHCs), multifaceted and comprehensive agencies offering a broad range of readily accessible services. Preventive approaches were emphasized as mental health workers became change agents in the community.

The importance of CMHCs was accelerated by a move toward deinstitutionalization, in order to curtail the length of inpatient treatment for people with serious mental illness, and a shift to outpatient care of the chronically mentally ill.

This effort was facilitated by more effective psychotropic medication to treat Schizophrenia and other mental disorders. Although deinstitutionalization was cost-effective in the short run and helped some people regain independence, it complicated the treatment process. Some people did not receive needed treatment because of difficulty in accessing services.

At the outset, CMHCs were staffed largely by the well-established helping professionals, the psychiatrists and doctoral-level psychologists. In order to fulfill the mission of the CMHCs, however, community psychology, a new area of specialization, soon evolved. Community psychology emphasizes the role of environmental forces in both causing and alleviating people's problems. The growth in CMHCs as well as their community focus led to the hiring of masters-level helping professionals (counselors, psychologists, and social workers) in addition to people without advanced degrees to meet staffing needs and provide community representation.

Counselor education programs, responding to growth in employment of both school and mental health counselors, began to expand and diversify. In the early 1960s, the National Institutes for Mental Health funded pilot training programs for mental health counselors. National Defense Education Act Institutes, initiated in 1958 primarily for school counselors, also lent credibility and refinement of skills to the profession. These Institutes stemmed from the government's perception that trained counselors who could identify talented youth to help the United States compete with the Soviet Union were urgently needed.

Counseling became well established in colleges and universities, as it was in secondary schools and mental health centers. By the early 1960s, most colleges and universities offered counseling to their students. Legislation at that time also helped expand the numbers and responsibilities of counselors in elementary schools.

COUNSELING IN THE 1970s

Between 1964 and 1976, the number of counselor education programs increased by about 35% (Shertzer & Stone, 1980). Important ideas and writings by C. Gilbert Wrenn (*The Counselor in a Changing World*), Albert Ellis (*Reason and Emotion in Psychotherapy*), John Krumboltz (behavioral counseling), Robert Carkhuff and C. B. Truax (facilitative conditions), and Norman Kagan (Interpersonal Process Recall) further expanded the counselors' repertoire of skills and promoted diversification and growth in the profession.

The 1970s was a time of reorientation for the profession. Counseling was maturing, and the influx of counselors into staff positions at mental health facilities continued. However, the declining birthrate, coupled with nationwide budgetary constraints, led to a decline in the employment of school counselors. In 1976, the ratio of trained school counselors to available positions was 2.4 : 1, although counselor–student ratios had increased by 50% (Shertzer & Stone, 1980). At the same time, however, many counselor education programs, some only recently initiated, were being forced to increase enrollments due to universities' financial concerns.

Clearly, then, the way to meet the needs of people who wanted to counsel and of programs that needed to grow was in a redefinition of the counselors' role and the expansion of the field of mental health counseling. This trend has been evident on many fronts over the past three decades.

The events of the 1970s also shaped the role of the counselor. The men and women returning from the Vietnam war brought to the counselors' offices problems of adjustment, family conflict, and Posttraumatic Stress Disorder (PTSD). Drug abuse became a growing problem, spreading into the middle classes and necessitating additional treatment programs. Correspondingly, interest grew in multicultural counseling and in group counseling, particularly effective in treating substance use, PTSD, and other disorders that proliferated during the 1970s.

In addition, the Human Potential Movement, spearheaded by a group of therapists including Fritz Perls, Virginia Satir, and others, expanded the repertoire of counselors' skills and led to marathon therapy sessions, personal growth groups, and other innovative approaches. Important counseling theorists, including Ivey and Carkhuff, focused on the identification and teaching of effective counseling and communication skills.

These developments were reflected in the addition of more divisions to ACA during the 1970s and 1980s. These included the Association for Non-White Concerns in Personnel and Guidance (forerunner of the Association for Multicultural Counseling and Development), the Association for Specialists in Group Work, the Association for Religious and Value Issues in Counseling (forerunner of the Association for Spiritual, Ethical, and Religious Values in Counseling), and the American Mental Health Counselors Association.

COUNSELING IN THE 1980s

Important changes in the field of counseling during the 1980s included a growing emphasis on brief, active, and structured approaches to counseling. Aaron Beck promoted cognitive therapy and Jay Haley, Cloé Madanes, Steve deShazer, and others developed strategic and brief models of counseling. As counselors moved into mental health settings, their need to develop expertise in diagnosis and treatment planning grew. I was the first to offer nationwide training for counselors on these topics through the ACA. The first edition of this book, *Diagnosis and Treatment*

Planning in Counseling, published in 1986, was the first volume on that subject directed specifically toward counselors and one of the first books published that focused on the work of the mental health counselor.

In 1980, 552 counselor education programs were identified in the United States and its territories (Wantz, Scherman, & Hollis, 1982). Between 1978 and 1980, nearly all of the programs expanded and added an average of 2.76 new courses, typically in areas such as (in order of frequency) family counseling, consultation, geriatric counseling, career and life planning, and women's studies. Specializations in mental health counseling were offered under a variety of names: agency, social agency, community agency, or clinical counseling; human development; marriage and family counseling; corrections counseling; pastoral counseling; personal counseling; rehabilitation counseling; and, of course, mental health counseling. Although most of the programs were housed in schools or colleges of education, mental health counselors were being graduated in numbers equal to or greater than school counselors (Wantz et al., 1982). By 1986, 90% of the graduate training programs in counseling offered a specialization in community agency counseling (Spruill & Fong, 1990). Other changes in counselor preparation included a stronger emphasis on developmental counseling and client diversity, an increase in practicum and internship requirements, and a focus on integrating and applying existing counseling modalities rather than searching for new approaches.

These changes were reflected in the counselors' primary professional organization called the American Association for Counseling and Development in the 1980s and, as of 1992, the American Counseling Association. That organization had grown rapidly since its inception and had over 42,000 members in 1984, as well as state and local divisions throughout the United States. In 1984, the *Occupational Outlook Handbook* included listings for both general counselors and mental health counselors, providing further national recognition of the establishment of the counseling profession (Glosoff, 1992). A few years later, in 1988, the Civilian Health and Medical Program of the Uniformed Services (CHAMPUS) included mental health counselors as approved service providers.

Changes in the counseling profession also were mirrored in the establishment of the American Mental Health Counselors Association (AMHCA), founded in 1976 by Nancy Spisso and James Messina as an independent professional organization for community and mental health counselors and allied professionals. AMHCA clearly met a need, and its membership grew rapidly. In 1978, it became the 13th division of ACA. Throughout the 1980s and into the 1990s, the number of mental health counselors grew, as did membership in AMHCA. By the 1990s, AMHCA had over 12,000 members and vied with ASCA for the distinction of being the largest division of ACA.

During the 1980s, the specialty of mental health counseling developed subspecialties. Interest grew in such areas as family counseling, counseling older adults, and treatment of substance use disorders. Several new divisions, including the Association for Adult Development and Aging, were added to the ACA. In 1990, the International Association of Marriage and Family Counselors (IAMFC), developed by Robert Smith, Jon Carlson, Don Dinkmeyer, and others, became one of the fastest growing divisions of ACA.

Graduate students in counseling got their own organization in 1985 with the establishment of Chi Sigma Iota, an academic and professional honor society in counseling. By the 1990s, this international society had over 90 chapters and 3,000 members, including students, faculty, and practitioners in counseling. According to Article I of its bylaws, the purposes of Chi Sigma Iota are "To promote scholarship, research, professionalism, and excellence in counseling, and to recognize high attainment in the pursuit of academic and clinical excellence in the field of counseling."

Several legislative and regulatory changes during the 1980s led to clarification and expansion of the counselors' roles. State licensure for counselors, initiated in Virginia in the late 1970s, expanded throughout the country. In addition, the National Academy of Certified Clinical Mental Health Counselors (NACCMHC) was formed; certification of mental health counselors, which began in 1979, expanded through the 1980s and 1990s. (More will be said on credentialing for counselors later in this chapter.) By the late 1980s, many states mandated counselor availability in elementary schools. This led not only to an increased demand for counselors trained in working with children but also promoted early identification of troubled children. This, in turn, has increased attention to the problems of abuse and dysfunction in families and promoted greater collaboration between schools and mental health agencies.

COUNSELING IN THE 1990s

The ACA remained strong and its membership continued to grow, although some years saw a decline in membership. Some divisions were disillusioned with the parent organization and, in 1992, the American College Personnel Association disaffiliated from ACA and became a separate organization. The AMHCA and the ASCA would also loosen their ties with ACA. Nevertheless, by the mid-1990s, ACA had well over 50,000 members.

By the early 1990s, the number of programs to train school counselors and the number of programs to train community agency counselors was approximately equal (Cowger et al., 1991). Specialties such as marriage and family counseling, adult development and aging, substance abuse counseling, multicultural counseling, and child counseling were becoming popular, as the field of mental health counseling became further delineated. The 30-credit master's degree of the 1970s was rare, and most programs required at least 45 credits, with a requirement of 60 credits for a master's degree in counseling becoming increasingly common.

The Orlando Model Project

Assessment of qualifications, credentialing, and accountability became important areas of inquiry for counselors and counselor educators. To address these areas, the AMHCA and the ACES collaborated in developing the Orlando Project to promote the reputation, quality, and development of mental health counseling. The Orlando Project established minimum preparation standards for mental health counselors of 60 graduate credits of coursework, 1,000 hours of internship, 2 full years or residency or postgraduate supervised experience, and 20 hours a year of continuing education (Messina, 1995).

Impact of Managed Care

Perhaps the biggest impact on the role of counselors in the 1990s came from changes in health insurance plans and the way that health care was provided. A nationwide movement to provide all people access to treatment for physical and emotional problems gained considerable attention during the Clinton administration. The value of a preventive approach to health maintenance also was recognized. At the same time, the escalation of health care costs led health insurance companies to seek more economical methods of providing health care. Causes of the increase in health care costs included the growing number of people over 65, rising health care expectations, costly malpractice suits, improved and expensive medical technology, and the high cost of health care system administration. New approaches to approving and providing services resulted from these potentially conflicting thrusts.

The most obvious change was the rapid growth in managed care organizations (MCOs) as well as the consolidation of MCOs into a small number of large organizations such as Magellan, Value Options, Managed Health Network, and United Behavioral Health. Today, MCOs oversee the utilization of both mental health and medical services for the vast majority of people with health insurance.

According to Lawless, Ginter, and Kelly (1999, p. 50), "Managed care is a general term used to describe the constellation of businesses and organizations that arrange for the financing and delivery of mental health services." MCOs typically contract with providers, referred to as participating or preferred providers, to offer services for a fixed fee to members of the health insurance program associated with the MCO. Ideally, MCOs should insure that delivery of services is cost-effective, responsive to the needs of the treatment providers, and compatible with clients' needs and interests (Smith, 1999). They should have procedures in place to promote high-quality services, to make sure that participating providers have appropriate credentials and experience, and to make services easily and widely available to members.

MCOs have created benefits as well as difficulties for subscribers. Many MCOs require that each member has a primary physician who determines the member's need for services and, if indicated, makes a referral for those services. This can serve as a roadblock or can help direct a person to the appropriate referral source. Subscribers who choose providers participating with their insurance companies also benefit financially; generally their copayment, the part of the cost paid by the person, is reduced or eliminated. In addition, MCOs generally screen providers to insure that they have appropriate degrees and licensure. However, the need to select an approved provider may require that subscribers select a counselor from a limited pool of providers who may not have expertise in their area of concern and may not have convenient hours and locations.

Similarly, MCOs present both benefits and drawbacks for providers. Mental health counselors typically give MCOs mixed and often negative reviews. In a survey of mental health counselors conducted by Danzinger and Welfel (2001), over 90% of the respondents said that managed care has affected their practice of counseling. Important areas of concern emerging from this study included:

- Conflict of interest and divided loyalties between their clients and the MCOs
- Restricted treatment options and number of sessions
- Limited choices of treatment providers available to clients
- Possible violations of client privacy because of documentation required by MCOs
- Pressure to exaggerate or modify a diagnosis in order to obtain payment.

Many treatment providers also express considerable concern about the paperwork required by MCOs, difficulty in dealing with their bureaucratic structures, and delays and denials of payments. Many third-party payers require preauthorization of treatment. Approvals for mental health services are rarely open-ended; generally they authorize a specific number of sessions, typically ranging from 3 to 10. If additional sessions are needed as counseling proceeds, providers must usually submit a request to the MCO for a utilization review. In addition, participating providers generally receive a lower fee per session than they would in a fee-for-service model.

On the other hand, referrals from MCOs can contribute greatly to filling counselors' caseloads. The need for counselors has increased, as has their opportunity to treat people with a broad range of mental disorders. Documentation required by the MCOs may initially be time-consuming. However, familiarity with the policies and procedures of MCOs also can streamline providers' record-keeping, marketing, and administrative procedures. In addition, MCOs have helped to promote the use of diagnosis and treatment planning.

Because most third-party payers are trying to contain the escalating cost of health care, they typically encourage treatment that is short and efficient. By the mid-1990s, brief solution-focused therapy, with mental health service providers taking an active and directive role, permeated the field. Short-term counseling can have a powerful and beneficial impact when used appropriately. Hill (1990), for example, reported that as few as six visits to a counselor were associated with a reduction in clients' medical bills by as much as 75% over 5 years.

Despite its shortcomings, managed care has encouraged mental health professionals to use more effective and efficient modes of intervention. Today's counselors are skilled in diagnosis, goal setting, treatment planning, and assessment, in part because of the influence of managed care.

Some form of managed care will almost certainly be in place for the foreseeable future. Efforts are being made by all the helping professions to improve their interactions with managed care. That effort is promising, and MCOs may well improve their dealings with both subscribers and treatment providers. Although some counselors have stopped participating with MCOs and only accept clients on a fee-for-service basis, most are trying to find successful ways to practice within a managed care environment.

To deal with managed care successfully, counselors need to demonstrate their competence. They need to develop knowledge and expertise in such areas as brief therapy and cognitive-behavioral counseling, treatment of drug and alcohol problems, relapse prevention, treatment effectiveness, dual diagnoses, crisis intervention, use of community resources, and pain and stress management. Facility with diagnosis and treatment planning, as well as knowledge of assessment to demonstrate progress and accountability, are essential. Flexibility and breadth in skills, the ability to match technique to disorder, and involvement in a multidisciplinary group practice also are viewed as desirable in the managed care arena. Managed care can prompt counselors to find better and more efficient ways to help people, as long as counselors remain proactive in their relationships with managed care.

THE MENTAL HEALTH COUNSELOR OF THE 21st CENTURY

The National Standards for the Clinical Practice of Mental Health Counseling (1999, pp. 1–2), developed by the AMHCA, presents the following definition: "Clinical mental health counseling is the provision of professional counseling services involving the application of principles of psychotherapy, human development, learning theory, group dynamics, and the etiology of mental illness and dysfunctional behavior to individuals, couples, families and groups, for the purposes of promoting optimal mental health, dealing with normal problems of living and treating psychopathology." That document describes the practice of clinical mental health counseling as including, but not being limited to, diagnosis and treatment of mental disorders, psychoeducation designed to prevent emotional problems, consultation, and research into more effective "psychotherapeutic treatment modalities." This broad definition captures the essence of mental health counseling.

Changes in Theory and Practice

Many forces have shaped the counseling profession of the 21st century. D'Andrea (2000) identified three of the most important:

1. *Postmodernism* emphasizes subjective experience and social context and takes the position that objective or essential truths do not exist (Held, 2001). Knowledge is seen as changing and relative. People are encouraged to question their assumptions and understand and accept multiple perspectives as legitimate. The postmodern counselor seeks to understand each person's unique perspective and life experiences.
2. *Constructivism* stresses the human drive to construct meaning and significance out of our experience (D'Andrea, 2000). Compatible with postmodernism, constructivist counseling encourages people to tell their stories and then client and counselor cocreate new and more helpful meanings and solutions.
3. *Multiculturalism* refers to differences associated with age, gender, ability, ethnicity, race, culture, religious and spiritual beliefs, sexual orientation, and socioeconomic status. Counselors with multicultural competence understand and respect diversity. They develop interventions that reflect knowledge of and sensitivity to diversity and that take account of environment. The development of feminist therapy and the growing emphasis on spirituality, both discussed later in this book, reflect the influence of multiculturalism.

These three forces are relatively compatible, although multiculturalism encourages counselors to advocate for social justice while constructivism and postmodernism emphasize intrapsychic experiences. Other trends in counseling in this century, however, seem in conflict with the three forces identified above. These trends include:

- A growing emphasis on the role of biology, genetics, and neurophysiology in emotional difficulties, accompanied by recognition of the positive and often synergistic impact of combining counseling and psychotropic medication.
- Increasing reliance on empirically supported counseling approaches, sometimes leading to the use of well-researched treatment manuals to guide the counseling process.

- Growing importance of the role of technology in the counseling process. New tools and skills offer counselors and clients a variety of ways to communicate.
- Broadening the role of the counselor to include advocacy, activism promoting social action and social justice, and outreach to underserved groups.
- Use of both qualitative and quantitative research to determine treatment effectiveness, develop new interventions and inventories, and demonstrate accountability.

Other trends characterizing today's counselor are:

- The development of positive psychology and other approaches that emphasize people's strengths and nurture resilience, empowerment, and self-efficacy.
- Increases in the breadth and severity of disorders that counselors are addressing in their work. While only a small percentage of the work of counselors focuses on people with severe mental disorders such as Schizophrenia and Dementia, many are dealing with such serious concerns as school violence, PTSD, Major Depressive Disorder, and personality disorders.
- The increasing incorporation of what have been called power therapies and energy therapies such as eye movement desensitization and reprocessing, thought field therapy, traumatic incident reduction, and other approaches into the counseling process.

Legislation Affecting the Counselor of the 21st Century

Several pieces of legislation in the early years of the 21st century are likely to have a significant impact on all mental health professions. Even though the nature of this impact is not yet clear, resulting change is inevitable.

On April 14, 2003, the Health Insurance Portability and Accountability Act (HIPAA) went into effect. This act governs how health care providers handle the use or disclosure of protected health information, including individually identifiable information regarding people's mental or physical health, their care, and their payment for their services. All providers who transmit patient or client information electronically are subject to this act, including any counselors who send information via the Internet to MCOs, insurance companies, billing services, or other professionals. This law is intended to protect people's confidentiality by mandating that treatment providers give them written information regarding policies and procedures for disclosing their information. Under most circumstances, providers are required to obtain clients' written consent before sharing person-identifiable information.

This should lead to more careful handling of client information as well as standardization of protocols for sharing information.

Laws such as the Mental Health Parity Act require that health insurance plans encompassing mental health benefits provide the same lifetime and annual dollar limits for mental health services as for medical and surgical care. These laws are intended to ensure that third-party payers provide adequate coverage for treatment of mental disorders.

A final piece of legislation, not yet passed as this book is being written, seems likely to gain approval. Although most MCOs provide payment for the services of licensed counselors, Medicare has not included mental health counselors among its roster of approved providers. Legislation is under consideration to rectify this omission. This should expand counselors' services to many people who are disabled or over 65.

Profile of the Counselor of the 21st Century

The mental health field today is a broad and diverse one that calls for counselors who are flexible and knowledgeable and who can draw on a wide range of skills and approaches to meet the multifaceted needs of their clients. It calls for people who can make good use of community resources, managed care, consulting, program development, and collaboration with other mental health service providers. It calls for counselors who can assess and deal sensitively with developmental, multicultural, and family contexts; who are skilled in diagnosis and treatment planning; who have effective and innovative preventive and remedial approaches; and who can provide good role models and supervision to students and other counselors.

Effective counselors have a high tolerance for ambiguity and change and a low need for power and immediate gratification; their rewards often come from developing the strengths of the community and the individual, mobilizing people's resources, and increasing opportunities for growth, rather than from displaying their own ability to heal others. Counselors need to be self-motivated and proactive. They need to relate successfully to people who seem different from themselves and learn to prize and foster the individuality of those people. Counselors must deal with reluctant clients by demonstrating quickly and effectively that they have something to offer and are capable of meeting client needs. They have to be politically aware and assertive and assume the role of client advocate, often focusing on issues and groups rather than on individuals. They need to be familiar with legal and ethical standards that may have an impact on their work and on their clients and must practice in accord with those guidelines.

Counselors must establish a true partnership with their colleagues, their clients, and their communities. In order to accomplish this, counselors will need a broad range of skills, active participation in their professional associations and their profession, state and national credentials, knowledge of advances in technology and in the profession, and commitment to exemplifying ethical behavior and a high level of skills. Rather than advocating a single model of change or intervention, mental health counselors are increasingly individualizing treatment in integrative and creative ways. Counselors' personality and style as well as their ability to form a positive therapeutic alliance are now being recognized as key elements in the success of treatment.

CREDENTIALING FOR COUNSELORS

As the field of counseling grew, so did the need for credentials that would establish and maintain standards for the profession as well as advance its reputation. Credentialing of counselors and counselor education programs has become increasingly important.

Credentials for counselors include two types: licensure or certification issued by the state in which the counselor practices and certification granted by a national professional organization. Both credentials indicate that counselors have met specified levels of training, experience, and knowledge. These credentials are important to counselors as well as to the general public. They safeguard the consumer from unqualified practitioners, protect counselors' right to practice, increase the likelihood of third-party payments and privileged communication, and generally promote the reputation and importance of the profession (Alberding, Lauver, & Patnoe, 1993).

National Certification for Counselors

Emphasis on well-defined standards, reflected in credentials, has been one of the greatest contributions of AMHCA leaders to the counseling field. In 1979, AMHCA established the NACCMHC with James Messina as its first chair. NACCMHC determined criteria for certification as a mental health counselor and awarded that credential to applicants who passed a rigorous screening process, including a written examination and submission of work samples.

NACCMHC initiated an emphasis on national certification for counselors that has continued up to the present. Recognizing that not only mental health counselors needed certification, ACA established an independent credentialing body, the National Board of Certified Counselors (NBCC), in 1982 to promote quality counseling. The role of NBCC is to "establish and monitor a national certification system, to identify those counselors who have voluntarily sought and obtained certification, and to maintain a register of those counselors." The two national bodies to certify counselors, NACCMHC and NBCC, coexisted for over 10 years, creating considerable confusion in the minds of many counselors as to their differences as well as their respective benefits. Finally, in 1993, NBCC merged with the Academy of Clinical Mental Health Counselors and now oversees the certification process. Over 31,000 counselors have been certified by NBCC, which offers the following credentials:

- National Certified Counselor (NCC), a generic credential for all types of counselors. Certification requirements include at least 48 semester hours of graduate coursework in counseling, at least 3,000 hours of subsequent relevant work experience, at least 100 hours of face-to-face counseling supervision over a minimum of 2 years, and satisfactory performance on an examination.
- Three specialty certifications: The National Certified School Counselor (NCSC), The Certified Mental Health Counselor (CCMHC), and The Master Addictions Counselor (MAC).

NBCC offers two examinations of particular importance to counselors. The National Counselor Examination (NCE), consisting of 200 multiple-choice questions, is administered to people seeking the generic credential of NCC. This examination covers the following eight content areas, paralleling courses required for that certification: Human Growth and Development; Social and Cultural Foundations; Helping Relationships; Group Work; Career and Lifestyle Development; Appraisal; Research and Evaluation; and Professional Orientation and Ethics. Question content is based largely on five work behaviors: Fundamentals of Counseling, Assessment and Career Counseling, Group Counseling, Programmatic and Clinical Intervention, and Professional Practice Issues.

NBCC also offers the National Clinical Mental Health Counseling Examination (NCMHCE), used exclusively by state credentialing boards. This examination consists of 10 clinical mental health counseling cases, with each case followed by multiple-choice questions focused on information-gathering or decision-making. According to NBCC, these questions are designed to "assess clinical problem-solving ability, including identifying, analyzing, diagnosing, and treating clinical issues." This examination taps a broad range of clinical skills including conducting a mental status examination, taking a client history, formulating a diagnosis, developing a treatment plan, making a referral, and demonstrating knowledge of ethical and legal issues. All of these competencies are presented in this book.

Certification by professional associations is an important credential for counselors, although it is less restrictive and less powerful than state licensure. Sometimes certification standards are more relevant because they have been developed by counselors rather than legislators. Certification establishes and maintains standards and identifies people who have met those standards. Certifying bodies advocate for the profession and promote its visibility and accountability. Registries of people who are certified facilitate referrals as well as networking. Certification also is valued by many employers and is a way to demonstrate competence and support the profession. NBCC, like most certifying bodies, also encourages professional development; maintenance of certification requires at least 10 continuing education units (CEUs) or 100 hours of professional development (e.g., coursework, workshops) every 5 years.

Other Certifications for Counselors

Several other certifications are available to members of the counseling profession. The Center for Credentialing & Education (CCE), a corporate affiliate of NBCC, offers two credentials: the Approved Clinical Supervisor credential and the Global Career Development Facilitator certification. In addition, the IAMFC, a division of ACA, offers certification for marriage and family therapists.

State Licensure and Certification for Counselors

When counselors moved beyond schools and colleges to join the staffs of mental health agencies and establish private practices, state licensure was needed to give counselors credibility and autonomy, to help the public identify qualified practitioners, and to enhance professional identity so counselors could achieve the status of the other credentialed mental health practitioners (social workers and psychologists). In 1972, in *Weldon v. Board of Psychological Examiners*, the Virginia Supreme Court found that "the profession of personnel and guidance counseling is a separate profession from psychology and should be so recognized" (Seiler & Messina, 1979, p. 4). This paved the way for Virginia to become, in 1976, the first state to license counselors. As of 2003, 46 states plus the District of Columbia and Puerto Rico have passed credentialing laws for counselors.

State credentials are necessary for independent practice. In addition, state licensure is increasingly required for employment beyond entry level. Even when that credential is not required, licensed counselors have a competitive edge in the employment market. As of 1998, more than 96,000 professional counselors were licensed or certified for independent practice in the United States (Mental Health, United States, 1998).

Although licensure requirements vary from state to state, most states require a master's or doctoral degree in counseling (or a related profession) with 45–60 semester hours of graduate coursework, at least 3,000 hours of clinical experience, at least 100 hours of face-to-face supervision, and an examination, usually one of the NBCC examinations discussed previously. Many states require coursework in the eight core areas assessed on the NCE examination described earlier.

State legislation also establishes the scope of the counselors' practice. Most states grant, or permit by implication, the right of counselors to diagnose and treat mental disorders (Throckmorton, 1992). In states that regulate the profession of counseling, no unlicensed people can legally practice counseling, call themselves counselors, or perform the work of counselors, even if they are certified, except while under approved supervision or employed by schools or mental health agencies.

Licensing of counselors has facilitated counselors' efforts to receive third-party payments and to become participating providers in MCOs. In addition, in many states, they benefit from so-called Freedom of Choice legislation. This requires MCOs providing third-party payments for any mental health treatment providers to make third-party payments for the services of all licensed mental health professionals.

Another benefit of licensure for counselors, portability, is still on the horizon. Presently, because of the variation in state licensure requirements, counselors licensed in one state cannot be sure of licensure reciprocity if they move to another state. The American Psychological Association has two vehicles to facilitate nationwide reciprocity, the National Register of Health Service Providers in Psychology and a Certificate of Professional Qualifications issued by the Association of State and Provincial Psychology Boards. The ACA is considering establishment of a credentialing bank, as well as a professional qualifications certification, to facilitate licensure portability.

Accreditation of Counselor Education Programs

Like licensure and certification, the credentialing procedure for counselor education programs also experienced considerable modification over the last 25 years. Previously, most counselor education programs were reviewed for approval by the National Council for the Accreditation of Teacher Education (NCATE). When counselor preparation focused primarily on school counselors, the well-established NCATE was an appropriate evaluator for such programs. However, with the growth of mental health counseling, the field needed a credentialing body that was familiar with and had criteria for evaluating the increasing range of counseling specialties.

In 1981, ACA led the development of the Council for Accreditation of Counseling and Related Educational Programs (CACREP) to establish more uniform and rigorous standards for counselor preparation and further enhance the reputation of the profession. As of 2003, CACREP had accredited approximately 175 institutions (close to one half of the institutions offering graduate degrees in counseling), with the following numbers of accreditations in each of the nine program areas: Career Counseling, 6; College Counseling, 35; Community Counseling, 130; Gerontological Counseling, 2; Marital, Couple, and Family Counseling/Therapy, 26; Mental Health Counseling, 29; School Counseling, 148; Student Affairs, 12; and Counselor Education and Supervision (doctoral-level only), 44.

To receive CACREP approval, entry-level degree programs must require a minimum of 72 quarter/48 semester hours of graduate studies. Mental Health Counseling and Marital, Couple, and Family Counseling programs must require at least 90 quarter/60 semester hours of graduate study. Approved doctoral programs must have a minimum of 144 quarter/96 semester hours, including entry-level preparation. CACREP-accredited programs must have at least three core faculty members, require supervised experience (practicum and internship), have a comprehensive mission statement, and require coursework in the following eight core areas: Professional Identity and Ethics, Social and Cultural Diversity, Human Growth and Development, Career Development, Helping Relationships, Group Work, Assessment (or Appraisal), and Research and Program Evaluation.

THE EDUCATION OF THE MENTAL HEALTH COUNSELOR

During the early years of the 21st century, approximately 380 institutions offered counselor education programs. While the master's degree is the minimum standard for the profession, many programs also offered doctoral degrees in counseling.

The Master's Degree in Counseling

Admission requirements, of course, vary from one program to the next, but programs typically require an undergraduate grade point average of 3.0 or higher and letters of recommendation. About half of the programs require courses in psychology as a prerequisite for admission. Many programs have additional requirements, including prior relevant employment or volunteer experience, an admissions test, a writing sample, and an individual or group interview.

Programs to train mental health counselors generally entail the equivalent of 2 years of full-time academic study and 45–60 semester hours of coursework. Distance education, self-instructional training, and other alternative models of teaching have begun to be incorporated into counselor education programs. In keeping with CACREP requirements, programs typically require a supervised practicum of at least 100 clock hours as well as 600 clock hours of internship. Programs may award the M.A., M.S., or M.Ed. degree.

Students aiming toward a career in mental health counseling can choose from a range of concentrations. These include general mental health counseling, community counseling, community agency counseling, marriage and family counseling, pastoral counseling, rehabilitation counseling, adult development and aging, multicultural counseling, addictions counseling, career development, gerontological counseling, and child counseling.

The Doctoral Degree in Counseling

Many more people receive the master's degree in counseling than receive the doctorate in counseling. Doctoral students in counseling commonly are embarking on a second or modified career and typically are well into their thirties when they receive their degree. Most have master's degrees in counseling or related areas and are employed in the human services field.

Many students who hope to teach at the university level where a doctoral degree is usually required pursue their doctorate in counselor education. However, others seek the doctorate in counseling to advance in their careers, develop research skills, improve their clinical skills, develop a new area of specialization, or simply to satisfy their eagerness to continue learning.

PROFESSIONAL ASSOCIATIONS FOR COUNSELORS

Membership and active participation in professional associations are important for counselors for many reasons:

- Conferences, newsletters, journals, books, home-study programs, continuing education programs, and listservs produced by professional associations help counselors to develop sound and up-to-date knowledge and skills in their field.
- Conferences and publications offer counselors a forum for disseminating their own research and ideas.
- Membership in a professional association facilitates networking, employment, and identification of colleagues with similar interests or important areas of expertise.
- Professional associations have made great strides over the years in promoting the field of mental health counseling, in obtaining state licensure for counselors, and in obtaining parity for counselors in managed care, privileged communication, and other areas. By supporting professional associations through service and dues, counselors contribute to the advancement of their profession.

The American Counseling Association

The primary professional association for counselors is the ACA. This organization has approximately 55,000 members and recently celebrated its 50th anniversary. The mission of ACA is "to enhance the quality of life in society by promoting the development of professional counselors, advancing the counseling profession, and using the profession and practice of counseling to promote respect for human dignity and diversity" (ACA, 2003). Important values of the association include caring for self and others, facilitating positive change, acquiring and using knowledge, promoting leadership, and encouraging networking. The fundamental purposes of ACA include human development, human rights, interprofessional and international collaboration, organization and management, professional development, professionalization, public awareness and support, public policy and legislation, and research and knowledge. ACA helps graduate students become integrated into their profession by offering a listserv specifically for graduate students, a career center to facilitate employment, and special programs for students and first-time attendees at the national conference.

Headquartered in Alexandria, Virginia, ACA presently includes 56 state and regional branches in the United States, Europe, and Latin America. It also includes the following 17 chartered divisions, reflecting special interests within the counseling field:

- Association for Assessment in Counseling and Education
- Association for Adult Development and Aging
- American College Counseling Association
- Association for Counselors and Educators in Government
- Association for Counselor Education and Supervision
- Association for Gay, Lesbian, and Bisexual Issues in Counseling
- Association for Multicultural Counseling and Development
- American Mental Health Counselors Association
- American Rehabilitation Counseling Association
- American School Counselor Association
- Association for Spiritual, Ethical, and Religious Values in Counseling
- Association for Specialists in Group Work
- Counseling Association for Humanistic Education and Development
- Counselors for Social Justice
- International Association of Addictions and Offender Counselors
- International Association of Marriage and Family Counselors
- National Career Development Association
- National Employment Counseling Association.

In addition to the national branches and divisions, each state has organizations paralleling some or all of these divisions, as well as local groups for counselors in particular geographic areas. These organizations are helpful in promoting networking and involvement in the profession.

The American Mental Health Counselors Association

Although AMHCA continues to be a part of ACA, it has loosened its ties to that organization and is considered an independent division. AMHCA currently has its own dues, membership, journal, newsletter, code of ethics, and annual conference. In this way, the leaders of AMHCA believed they could better serve the needs of mental health counselors.

As stated in the AMHCA web site (www.amhca.org), the organization's mission is "to enhance the profession of mental health counseling through licensing, advocacy, education, and professional development." According to its Vision Statement, "The American Mental Health Counselors Association will be the national organization representing licensed mental health counselors, and state chapters, with consistent standards of education, training, licensing, practice, advocacy and ethics."

COMPETENCIES OF THE MENTAL HEALTH COUNSELOR

In the 1990s, counselors became increasingly aware of the importance of demonstrating their competence and accountability to other mental health service providers, consumers, and managed care organizations. This accelerated interest in the development of standards of practice. According to AMHCA's Standards for Clinical Mental Health Counseling (1999), mental health counselors should have a minimum of 60 graduate semester hours of coursework, including a 48-hours core curriculum and 12 hours in mental health counseling, as well as a clinical counseling practicum and internship. They should have at least 3,000 hours of supervised postgraduate clinical experience over at least 2 years and a minimum of 200 hours of supervision. Clinical experience is identified as the direct delivery of counseling to clients who have been diagnosed as having a mental disorder as defined by the latest edition of the *Diagnostic and Statistical Manual of Mental Disorders* (discussed in Chapter 3 of this book) or the *International Classification of Diseases, Clinical Modification.* Mental health counselors should comply with the state regulations governing their practice as well as with the code of ethics for mental health counselors.

A synthesis of CACREP requirements for mental health counselors, the AMHCA Standards for Clinical Mental Health Counselors, and a survey of mental health counselors on their perceptions of important competencies, skills, attitudes/styles, and training (Sexton, 1995) suggests that mental health counselors should have the following skills and knowledge, grouped into 10 core areas.

Core Area 1: Professional Orientation, Identity, and Ethics

1. Knowledge of the history and philosophy of the counseling profession.
2. Understanding of the professional roles and functions of the counselor.
3. Knowledge of other mental health professionals and ways to collaborate with them.
4. Computer literacy, as well as technological competence.

5. Awareness of professional organizations for counselors and their benefits and activities.
6. Knowledge of credentials relevant to the profession, including licensure, certification, and accreditation, and their guidelines and standards.
7. Ability to use technology and its applications to facilitate the counseling process.
8. Knowledge of the ethical standards of the profession as well as relevant legal guidelines.

Core Area 2: Social and Cultural Foundations

1. Familiarity with theories of multicultural counseling and identity development and ability to take account of the impact of cultural and environmental background on development.
2. Understanding of multicultural trends and developments.
3. Knowledge of characteristics and concerns of diverse groups.
4. Multicultural counseling competence, along with the ability to use that competence effectively with individuals, couples, families, groups, communities, and organizations.
5. Cultural self-awareness.
6. Awareness of and sensitivity to issues of bias, discrimination, and other oppressive behaviors along with skills that can counter these negative forces.
7. Awareness of and appreciation for individual, lifestyle, and cultural diversity.
8. Ability to build coalitions and collaborate with others to help people develop and use support systems.
9. Understanding of the principles of social change, community intervention, and organizational development, as well as the ability to assess the need for social change.
10. Ability to identify and work effectively with both community strengths and growth-inhibiting aspects of the community.
11. Understanding of the importance of counselor advocacy for both the profession and society, as well as knowledge of approaches to advocacy that will improve social justice and equity, reduce barriers, and facilitate the strengthening of socially devalued groups.
12. Ability to involve the community or organization in efforts to effect positive change, drawing on existing leadership.
13. Knowledge of causes and dynamics of important social problems (e.g., addictions, physical and sexual abuse, suicide, divorce, violence) as well as ways to treat or prevent them.

14. Ability to view people holistically and in context.
15. Understanding of and ability to use outreach and prevention strategies.

Core Area 3: Human Growth and Development

1. Understanding of the theories and principles of normal individual and family development across the life span and the typical concerns of various age groups.
2. Ability to discriminate between healthy and disturbed development.
3. Understanding of theories of learning and cognitive development.
4. Familiarity with theories of personality development as well as knowledge of common personality types and patterns.
5. Understanding of sexual development and behavior.
6. Ability to help others to understand their own development as well as strategies for promoting optimum development over the life span.
7. Awareness of human behavior, including the impact of developmental crises, disability, situational and other factors and changes that can affect development.

Core Area 4: Lifestyle and Career Development

1. Understanding of the changing patterns and meaning of work in society, including the interrelationships of work and family.
2. Appreciation of the lifelong process of career development, the broad scope of career counseling, and the impact of diversity, gender, and other factors on career development.
3. Familiarity with theories of career development and decision-making.
4. Ability to skillfully use a broad range of career counseling interventions and resources and adapt them to specific populations.
5. Familiarity with a broad range of inventories relevant to career counseling and decision-making as well as skill in using them to assess interests, abilities, and values and to integrate them into the counseling process.
6. Familiarity with sources of career, occupational, avocational, educational, and labor market information and resources as well as knowledge of how to help people acquire and use that information.
7. Ability to use technology to facilitate career counseling and development.
8. Ability to help people with effective job seeking, educational planning, and placement.
9. Facility for designing career development programs and engaging in organization, implementation, administration, follow-up, and evaluation of interventions at both individual and school or agency level.

Core Area 5: Counseling Theory and Helping Relationships ————————

1. Skill in developing a positive and collaborative therapeutic alliance that maintains appropriate professional boundaries.
2. Knowledge of the developmental stages of the helping relationship, as well as ability to deal effectively with common reactions to that process, including transference and countertransference, resistance, identification, and multiculturally related responses.
3. Knowledge of and ability to establish therapeutic conditions likely to facilitate positive development and change.
4. Understanding of essential interviewing and counseling skills, as well as ability to successfully establish counseling goals, design appropriate interventions, implement a treatment plan, evaluate outcome, and terminate the counseling process.
5. Knowledge of a broad range of established and effective counseling theories and treatment approaches, their historical development, and appropriate use.
6. Ability to take a systems perspective to working with individuals and families.
7. Knowledge of a framework for understanding and practicing consultation and understanding of the development of the field of consultation as well as of the consulting relationship.

Core Area 6: Group Counseling ————————————————————

1. Understanding of principles of group process and dynamics, including developmental stage, and member roles and behaviors.
2. Knowledge of the strengths and limitations of group counseling and the ability to determine when and how it is likely to be helpful.
3. Familiarity with theories and research on group counseling.
4. Competence in group counseling methods including orientation, selection, promoting growth, overcoming obstacles, and achieving goals.
5. Ability to work effectively with groups of various sizes, in diverse settings, and with a wide range of client groups including both homogeneous and heterogeneous groups.
6. Understanding of the goals and procedures of various types of groups (e.g., personal growth, therapy, support, psychoeducational, task groups).
7. Knowledge of styles and approaches of group leadership, characteristics of effective group leaders, and preparation standards for leaders.

Core Area 7: Assessment and Appraisal

1. A historical perspective on the nature and importance of assessment.
2. Knowledge of the indications and contraindications, benefits and limitations of an assessment or appraisal procedure.
3. Ability to effectively plan and discuss assessment with clients as well as to integrate assessment into the counseling process.
4. Familiarity with the appropriate use, administration, interpretation, strengths, and limitations of instruments that are widely used in assessing development, intelligence, abilities, interests, values, personality, and other relevant dimensions.
5. Understanding of relevant statistical concepts such as norms, sample groups, reliability, validity, scales of measurement, types of distributions, correlation, and error of measurement.
6. Ability to conduct intake interviews, behavioral observations, and mental status examinations.
7. Ability to take account of characteristics such as age, ethnicity, language, disability, gender, and other factors when planning and conducting assessments.
8. Knowledge of when and how to refer clients for physical, neurological, and other assessment procedures not generally performed by counselors.

Core Area 8: Research and Program Evaluation

1. Awareness of the importance of research as well as its benefits and challenges.
2. Knowledge and understanding of important research in the field of counseling.
3. Knowledge of how to plan and conduct research to assess and improve the counseling process.
4. Familiarity with important research methods, including qualitative, quantitative, single-case, action research, and outcome-based research.
5. Appreciation for the importance of evaluating the impact and effectiveness of one's own efforts and the need for accountability.
6. Knowledge of how to conduct needs assessments, program evaluations, and research on one's own practice.
7. Ability to effectively use statistical methods, the Internet, and other forms of technology to conduct research.

Core Area 9: Diagnosis and Psychopathology ——————————————————

1. Understanding of and ability to recognize the differences between normal and pathological personality dynamics and functioning.
2. Sound knowledge of the current edition of the *Diagnostic and Statistical Manual of Mental Disorders (DSM)*.
3. Ability to use the *DSM* to make an accurate multiaxial assessment.
4. Ability to conduct psychosocial histories, intake interviews, and mental status examinations to facilitate diagnosis and treatment planning.
5. Knowledge of how to determine when clients present a danger to themselves or others, as well as steps to take to prevent harm.
6. Ability to use both general and specific personality inventories to clarify diagnoses.
7. Ability to develop comprehensive and sound case conceptualizations.
8. Basic understanding of neurophysiology.
9. Knowledge of when and how to make a successful referral.

Core Area 10: Psychotherapy ——————————————————————

1. Ability to develop comprehensive and effective treatment plans.
2. Skill in using a broad range of theories and techniques of individual, family, and group counseling and psychotherapy to ameliorate emotional difficulties and improve functioning.
3. Ability to make effective use of brief and solution-focused therapy.
4. Skill in crisis intervention and management.
5. Knowledge of theories and techniques of relaxation, exercise, nutrition, stress management, holistic health, and their appropriate uses.
6. Understanding of the application of behavioral and other counseling approaches to such problems as smoking, eating disorders, and substance use disorders.
7. Knowledge of the circumstances under which individual, couples/family, or group counseling or a combination of these is likely to provide the most effective treatment.
8. Ability to plan and implement psychoeducational and prevention programs.
9. Knowledge of the benefits and side effects of psychotropic medication, as well as when and how to refer clients for a medication or medical evaluation.

In addition to these 10 groups of competencies, the professional literature, as well as Sexton's (1995) survey, suggest three other areas in which counselors must be competent. These include emotional health and self-awareness, communication skills, and supervisory skills. Although NBCC does not test the emotional health of future counselors, graduate programs in counseling look for people who have not only the intelligence to become effective counselors, but also the stability, the personal characteristics, the self-awareness, and the communication skills to interact well with others. Therefore, I suggest the following additional competencies:

Additional Competence Area 1: Emotional Health and Self-awareness

1. Interest in and active pursuit of personal growth and lifelong learning.
2. Establishment of an emotionally stable and rewarding lifestyle.
3. Close and trusting relationships with at least a few people.
4. Positive but realistic self-esteem and a good capacity for self-efficacy.
5. Ability to provide a relatively objective picture of themselves, including both strengths and weaknesses, as well as willingness to take steps to remediate weaknesses.
6. Insight into the nature and impact of their family background as well as ability to prevent that background from intruding on their activities and relationships.
7. Strong belief that individuals, families, groups, organizations, and communities can change and improve.
8. Attitudes that are open-minded and optimistic.
9. Understanding of own multicultural background and issues and a valuing of diversity.
10. Flexibility and ability to cope with ambiguity, uncertainty, and change.
11. Ability to function well both independently and in the roles of leader and team member.
12. Commitment of ethical behavior.
13. Objectivity, empathy, and insight.
14. Reliability, trustworthiness, caring, genuineness, and persuasiveness, as well as the ability to instill hope and to affirm others.
15. Sense of humor, friendliness, patience.

Additional Competence Area 2: Communication Skills

1. Possession of good verbal and interpersonal skills and the ability to model those skills.
2. Ability to write clearly and correctly and prepare well-written progress notes, reports, letters, and other communications.
3. Ability to listen well and respond appropriately to both overt and covert, verbal and nonverbal messages.

4. Ability to communicate empathy, positive regard, genuineness, and acceptance as well as to use constructive confrontation and other essential listening behaviors needed in counseling.
5. Ability to describe to people the nature of the counseling process and help them understand both its value and its limitations.
6. Ability to effectively conduct an interview or discussion with people from various educational, cultural, socioeconomic, and other backgrounds.

Additional Competence Area 3: Training, Supervisory, and Other Management Skills

1. Ability to supervise, train, and work effectively with professional, paraprofessional, and indigenous workers.
2. Strong administrative and program development skills.
3. Understanding of models of supervision, as well as the differences among counseling, consultation, and supervision.
4. Comfort in a teaching role, as well as ability to integrate teaching and counseling skills.
5. Ability to conduct in-service and other types of training programs.

The state licensure boards and ACA, AMHCA, CACREP, and NBCC are working to advance the competence of all counselors. This book seeks to help its readers develop and improve both general counseling skills and those that are especially relevant to the mental health counselor. The growing breadth of the role of the mental health counselor and the diverse range of employment opportunities open to counselors suggest that the most effective and employable counselors will be those who have acquired these skills.

I encourage you to review the 13 skill areas presented in this chapter, identifying those in which you already have considerable competence as well as those in which you need improvement. As you continue reading this book, pay particular attention to those areas in which you would like to improve your skills, but be sure to congratulate yourself for the progress you have already made en route to becoming a skilled and knowledgeable counselor.

Opportunities for the
Mental Health Counselor

Today's mental health counselor has a wide range of roles and employment opportunities. For example, counselors can be psychotherapists, teachers and trainers, case managers, coaches, consultants, grant writers, coordinators and program developers, marriage and family counselors, evaluation specialists, writers, researchers, and supervisors. Additional roles for counselors continue to evolve.

As of 1994, Hollis and Wantz found that, upon receiving the master's degree in mental health counseling, about half of recent graduates found employment in public agencies, 25% entered private agency practices, 12% continued their education, 8% worked in managed care settings, and the remaining 7% made other choices. Counselors with experience as well as credentials beyond the master's degree were more likely to be in private practice, although they are also found in a broad range of employment settings including university teaching. That pattern seems to have remained relatively stable, although the spread of licensure throughout the country has led more counselors into private practice, typically after several years of employment in a public agency.

The primary roles of nearly all mental health counselors include case management and treatment of clients, conducting intake interviews, and diagnosis and treatment planning. Testing and assessment, to provide additional information on people's abilities, interests, values, personalities, and symptoms, are other essential roles of the counselor. Nearly all counselors spend at least part of their time with adult clients and conduct individual, group, and family therapy, although the proportion of time each counselor devotes to these activities varies widely. In addition, many counselors specialize in treating families or in working with children and adolescents. Most counselors are also involved in consultation and education, community services and outreach, supervision (either providing or receiving), and evaluation of services; nearly all document their work via case notes, written reports, and closing summaries.

Counselors' roles may be described in terms of the client population and issues they address, the settings in which they work, and the responsibilities they have. This chapter looks at mental health counselors from all three perspectives.

CLIENT ISSUES OF SPECIAL INTEREST TO MENTAL HEALTH COUNSELORS

Mental health counselors are encountering increased diversity and severity of client problems in their counseling. As a result of this, counselors have many new challenges and areas of focus in their work, as well as new ways to define their areas of specialization.

Age- and Stage-related Issues

Counselors have long recognized that, although people in the same age group and stage of life have many individual differences, they also are likely to have some common issues and concerns. Anticipating these, and developing both preventive and remedial interventions to address them, can facilitate healthy negotiation of each stage of life. While some counselors may not focus their work on a particular age group, many do specialize in treatment of an age-defined group such as children and adolescents, adults between 21 and 65, or people over 65.

Issues of Children and Adolescents

According to the U.S. Bureau of Health, the demand for mental health services for children is expected to increase by 100% by the year 2020 while the number of professionals in the field (e.g., counselors, school psychologists, social workers, child psychologists) will probably increase by only 30%. Estimates suggest that 21% of children and adolescents in the United States have a mental disorder but only about one third of these receive treatment. Counseling youth is a high-need area and legislation is under consideration to provide incentives to attract people to professions focused on children's mental health (Powell, 2002).

New areas of problems and inquiry related to the mental health of youth have attracted attention in recent years. For example, some theorists believe that increases in early attachment problems, resulting from the decrease in intact families and corresponding increase in family dysfunction and pressures, is a major cause of subsequent problems in intimacy and autonomy (Bartholomew & Horowitz, 1991; Bowlby, 1988).

Probably related to the growth in attachment problems is an increase in school violence. The two troubled students who killed students and teachers at Columbine High School left an indelible impression of extreme school violence. While such incidents are relatively rare, as Daniels (2002, p. 218) stated, " ... the incidence of school-related targeted violence is a major social issue in the United States .... A climate of fear pervades many schools." Counselors working with youth now need to engage in threat assessment, early identification of children who present a danger to themselves and others, conflict resolution, and critical incident stress debriefing following episodes of violence and upheaval.

Bullying and harassment also are significant issues in large numbers of schools. Over 75% of adolescents report having been bullied, with most stating it had a negative impact on them, including loss of friends, isolation, and discouragement (Espelage, Bosworth, & Simon, 2000). Bullying takes many forms, including name-calling, teasing, verbal threats, theft, and physical violence. Regardless of the form, bullying is about a power imbalance and is harmful to both the bully and the victim (often a special needs student or a young person who has difficulty with assertiveness and self-protection). Many schools are establishing bullying protection programs, only one illustration of the growing importance of prevention programs and the role of the counselor in developing such programs in the school system.

Identification and prevention of self-harm via cutting oneself and other forms of self-mutilation is another growing challenge for the counselor. Girls in early adolescence seem particularly prone to use self-harm as a way to deal with stress and unhappiness.

The nature and severity of problems presented by young people have changed over the years, with issues becoming more complex and serious. Counselors working with children now have a broad and multifaceted role; they must become knowledgeable about play therapy, child and adolescent development, effective parenting, stress management, crisis intervention, and diagnosis and treatment of the prevalent disorders of children and adolescence described in Chapter 3.

Issues of Adults

Like children and adolescents, adults present a vast array of problems and disorders. Most counselors who treat adults narrow the scope of their work, delineating some issues as within the scope of their practice while viewing others as outside their areas of expertise. The most common presenting concerns of an adult clientele include adjustment to crises and life changes, depression, anxiety and stress, relationship concerns, and career-related concerns. Other issues frequently presented include substance use problems, health-related concerns, and emotional, sexual, and physical abuse. Loss of contact with reality and cognitive impairment are symptoms less often seen for treatment and, when they are, it is usually in an agency specializing in such concerns.

Some of the problems of the later years can be prevented or ameliorated through counseling during midlife. The counseling literature has been paying more attention to the years between 40 and 60 (Sundel & Bernstein, 1995). For most, these are years of increased freedom and self-confidence as well as of introspection and pursuit of goals as yet unrealized. Counseling can help people in midlife to make the most of this period of their lives and develop plans and skills that will help them as they grow older.

Issues of People over 65

Counselors are paying more attention to the needs of older people and their caregivers. According to Myers (1990, p. 245), "Mental health counseling with older persons is a … specialty, stimulated by changing demographics and dramatic increases in the numbers of older persons …." As of 2000, the U.S. population included approximately 35 million people age 65 and older. Twenty percent of these need support services to help them remain in their communities, although 80% of people in this age group are able to live independently and are in good health. The percentage needing care is likely to grow since people 85 and older represent the fastest growing segment of the population. Usually adult children provide this care, most often daughters between the ages of 40 and 70, who typically must balance many responsibilities and may benefit from their own counseling (Schwiebert & Myers, 1994).

Common issues of older people include planning for and coping with retirement; losing their roles; seeking intimacy and identity; coping with change and loss; establishing new goals; declining independence; experiencing grief, depression, and loneliness; chronic medical problems; adjusting to the finiteness of life; and ultimately dealing with dying. They must contend with the sometimes negative and devaluing perceptions of society and even with bias from their counselors, who may not appreciate their great abilities and continued need for challenge and growth (Myers, 1990). In fact, some research suggests that older people are more receptive to changing their beliefs and attitudes than are people in midlife (Danzinger & Welfel, 2001).

Counselors working with older people typically use approaches that enhance their dignity, worth, and independence; take account of their culture, environment, historical context, and physical capacities; improve socialization and relationships; reduce anxiety and depression; and address difficulties in a problem-focused way (Gross & Capuzzi, 2001). Counselors have some specialized techniques for working effectively with this population, including remotivation therapy, reminiscing groups, milieu therapy, and life review. They also need to become familiar with physical and emotional disorders that are especially common in this group.

Multicultural Counseling

By 2010, the term minorities will be a misnomer, when so-called racial and ethnic minorities will comprise 50% of the population. By 2050, estimates suggest that only 52.8% of the U.S. population will be Caucasian (Kocarek, Talbot, Batka, & Anderson, 2001). Two trends are primarily responsible for this growth: immigration patterns and relatively high birth rates among many visible racial and ethnic groups. Pedersen (1990, p. 93) wrote, "Just as humanism became a third force to supplement the psychodynamic and behavioral perspectives, multiculturalism is becoming a 'fourth force' in its influence on … mental health counseling."

The counseling profession's understanding of multiculturalism has changed greatly over the past 50 years, from the color blindness of the 1950s and 1960s, through the 1970s' effort to tailor treatment to each specific ethnic group, to a recognition in the 1980s of the need for general principles and competencies, and finally in the 1990s and 21st century to a broad definition of multiculturalism. Now, multiculturalism refers not only to race and ethnicity but also to the whole spectrum of diversity. Arredondo et al. (1996) identify the following three dimensions for describing and understanding human diversity:

- Dimension A includes age, culture, ethnicity, gender, language, physical ability, race, sexual orientation, and social class.
- Dimension B includes educational background, geographic location, income, marital status, religious and spiritual beliefs, work experience, citizenship status, military experience, and leisure activities and interests.
- Dimension C includes the person's historical context and events.

Multicultural counseling competence is reflected in beliefs and attitudes, knowledge, and skills (Kwan, 2001; Sue, Arredondo, & McDavis, 1992). Multiculturally competent counselors:

1. Seek awareness of their own assumptions about people; understanding of their own multicultural aspects; and knowledge of the impact that oppression and bias have on people.
2. Attempt to understand their clients holistically, looking at all the aspects of diversity previously listed.
3. Actively pursue strategies and skills that enable them to work effectively with their culturally different clients as well as to reduce or eliminate discrimination on all levels (although multicultural counseling entails attending not only to the special needs of underserved groups and people of color but also to groups that are generally successful and not so visible).

Multicultural counseling entails addressing issues directly related to cultural background such as acculturation, identity development, religious and spiritual problems, and generational conflicts. In addition, all other issues should be viewed and understood from a multicultural perspective. For example, a young woman, born in South America, recently gave birth to her first child and sought counseling for help in becoming a good mother. Her concern is more clearly understood in light of her having been separated from her own mother for nearly 10 years before joining her in the United States.

Religious and Spiritual Issues

As recently as 25 years ago, many counselors shied away from discussion of religious and spiritual issues, viewing these topics as inappropriate to address in a secular setting. Our perspective on these topics has shifted dramatically. Now most counselors recognize that religious and spiritual beliefs (as well as their absence) typically affect all aspects of people lives. Examples include the man diagnosed with cancer who felt anger toward God for "giving me this disease" and the woman married to a physically abusive man who refused to leave her marriage because of her religious beliefs. Although mental health professionals trained in pastoral counseling are particularly likely to help people with religious and spiritual issues, and even to pray with them and discuss theology, mental health counselors in secular settings also should encourage clients to discuss their religious and spiritual beliefs, their impact on their concerns, and any comfort they may be able to gain from those beliefs.

Gender Issues

Just as culture shapes personality and behavior, so does gender. Attention has been paid to the special needs of women in counseling since the 1970s, with a particular emphasis on women's strong interpersonal values, problems in self-esteem, and restricted opportunities. The 1990s witnessed a growing interest in feminist therapy and in the common problems of women in middle age and older, including midlife transitions, gynecological cancers, menopause, caring for elderly parents, and widowhood.

Increased sensitivity to women's difficulties sometimes led to a view of men as their oppressors. This attitude fortunately has been changing since the 1990s with the recognition that men, too, have been shaped and often limited by gender stereotypes. Men now are receiving special attention in counseling, where they are typically encouraged to develop, celebrate, and affirm their strengths and abilities and to develop closer relationships with other men, especially their fathers (Kelly & Hall, 1992). These efforts are dispelling the myth of the inexpressive male and are helping people see that men and women both value relationships but generally prefer different ways of achieving closeness (Twohey & Ewing, 1995). Men typically develop closeness by engaging in side-by-side interactions, while women usually seek conversation, shared activities, and self-disclosure as paths to intimacy.

Issues of Sexual Orientation

Gender issues may be compounded by issues of sexual orientation, another multicultural variable. The American Counseling Association (ACA) and other organizations have paid increasing attention to issues faced by people who are gay, lesbian, bisexual, or transgendered. These people face homophobia (fear or hatred of those who define themselves as gay or lesbian), heterosexism (the assumption that heterosexuality is the normal and superior orientation), highly controversial efforts to change their sexual orientation (sexual reorientation therapy), and other societal messages that they are flawed and need to be changed. In addition, knowledge of these negative societal reactions can lead to or exacerbate inner conflicts and issues (Carroll, Gilroy, & Ryan, 2002). Concerns that are particularly prevalent in this population include acknowledging their sexual orientation to themselves and others, developing an integrated and valued sense of themselves, achieving intimacy and commitment in relationships, finding their place in society, parenting, religious and spiritual issues, guilt, loneliness and depression, and HIV and AIDS.

Family Issues

The rapid growth of family counseling as a specialization within mental health counseling reflects its importance in treating nearly all problems. Many client concerns, such as harmful use of substances, physical and sexual abuse, children's misbehavior, and even depression and anxiety, can be best understood, and often treated, in their family context. Helping people with family issues also necessitates understanding of nontraditional families. Single-parent and blended families comprise nearly half of all families. These families have special characteristics, as do families with adopted children, gay and lesbian family members, and people with serious mental or physical disabilities. Chapter 8 of this book provides additional information on theories and techniques of family counseling, as well as ways to understand family dynamics.

Conflict Resolution and Mediation

Conflict resolution and mediation are special skills that are very useful in helping people address family dissension and marital dissolution. These tools are also used in a variety of other settings, including schools, the military, and business and industry. Using such skills as role reversal and negotiation and encouraging empathy and active listening, counselors help people clarify their concerns and conflicts and reach mutually agreeable solutions based on cooperation rather than competition (McFarland, 1992).

Trauma and Crisis

The aftermath of the Vietnam War provided counselors with much greater understanding of trauma. Its impact is usually profound and often delayed, complicating diagnosis and treatment. Symptoms of Posttraumatic Stress Disorder (PTSD) often occur in people who have been abused, people who have experienced accidents or natural disasters, and people who have faced other traumatic or life-threatening experiences. Trauma-related symptoms also are prevalent in people such as police and firefighters who deal with the consequences and aftermath of such experiences. Large-scale traumatic events such as wars, floods, airplane crashes, and terrorist attacks expose many people to the potential of developing PTSD.

Counselors and others are being trained in critical incident stress debriefing and other approaches to prevent the development of PTSD symptoms in people who have been exposed to trauma or violence. Morrissey (1994) reported that there are hundreds of trained critical incident response teams in the United States. They provide rapid intervention (within no more than 48 hours), usually including the following seven phases: introductions and guidelines; description of the facts of the experience; description of thoughts about the experience; discussion of emotional reactions to the incident; identification and normalization of specific symptoms; teaching and mobilization of coping techniques such as stress reduction, thought stopping, image replacement, and relaxation; and facilitation of reentry, with continuing help.

Sexual and Physical Abuse

Among the most challenging and troubling problems counselors address and that often have a traumatic impact are sexual and physical abuse. Although these problems have probably always been present, public awareness of their prevalence is relatively recent. According to Jones, Robinson, Minatrea, and Hayes (1998, p. 332), "...32% of females and 13% of males reported a history of child sexual abuse involving physical contact." Rates of childhood sexual abuse among women in therapy range from 36 to 70%. Of course, abuse is not confined to the young. Many adults are verbally and physically abused by their partners. In addition, 3–4% of people over age 65 experience abuse and maltreatment, including neglect, violence, psychological abuse, financial exploitation, and violation of rights (Welfel, Danzinger, & Santoro, 2000).

The increased awareness and attention to sexual and physical abuse have led counselors to address several related problem areas. Mental disorders such as

Dissociative Identity Disorder, Borderline Personality Disorder, and PTSD are especially prevalent among people who have been physically or sexually abused and often require long-term intensive treatment. Memories of early abuse may have been partially or completely repressed, surfacing years later in confusing and upsetting ways. Helping people deal with and make sense of these memories is an important and difficult aspect of counseling, complicated by questions that have been raised about the veracity of these memories, the so-called false memory syndrome. Even counselors who focus on current and developmental concerns such as career or relationship issues must be attuned to the possibility that a long-standing issue such as abuse contributes to the present concern and must be addressed. Many counselors treating trauma, including abuse, have enhanced their effectiveness by using hypnotherapy, critical incident stress debriefing, and eye movement desensitization and reprocessing.

People who commit sexual or physical abuse constitute another important focus for counselors. This dysfunctional behavior pattern is more likely to develop in people who have experienced abuse. Counselors should be alert to the possibility of abuse in their clients.

Counseling people who have experienced or committed abuse can be challenging and can raise many issues and emotions in counselors. Questions such as when and how to report abuse as well as how best to protect their clients are difficult ones. In addition, counselors may experience rage, overinvolvement with their clients, and shock, as well as cynicism, loss of empathy, guilt for their own happy lives, and even vicarious traumatization or arousal (Jones et al., 1998). They may find it hard to maintain appropriate boundaries. Such responses are normal and understandable, but often call for consultation with a trusted colleague or supervisor.

Suicidal Ideation and Self-harm

Other highly charged issues for counselors include client suicidal ideation and self-harming behavior. As with abuse, counselors must be alert to the presence of suicidal thoughts in their clients and the need to keep clients safe. This may sometimes include breaking confidentiality to get clients the help they need. Chapter 4 includes more information on identifying and addressing suicidal thoughts.

Self-mutilation or self-harm, an increasingly prevalent symptom, especially in adolescent females, may appear to be a precursor to suicide but usually serves a different function. Self-mutilation can take a variety of forms, including scratching, cutting the skin, and burning or hitting oneself. This usually repetitive behavior serves the purpose of giving the perpetrator a sense of self-control and relieving stress and tension. Often done in a dissociative state, the self-harm may not cause pain. Counselors often have strong reactions to self-mutilation; common counselor responses include fear, confusion, frustration, and revulsion (Zila & Kiselica, 2001).

However, knowing that many effective treatments for self-mutilation have been developed can be reassuring to counselors. Some of these include replacing actions with words, vigorous exercise, drawing and writing, and self-soothing via warm baths, rocking, music, calling a friend, meditation, self-talk and other strategies (Ferentz, 2002).

Harmful Use of Substances

Harmful use of substances is another prevalent problem. At some point in their lives, nearly 20% of all people in the United States will have a Substance-Related Disorder (Maxmen & Ward, 1995). Most of these people have a coexisting mental disorder such as depression, Antisocial Personality Disorder, or an Impulse-Control Disorder. These dually diagnosed people constitute another growing segment of the counselor's work. Their diagnosis and treatment are difficult due to the interaction of the disorders, and relapse prevention is a great concern.

Counselors encounter problems of substance use, as they do problems of physical and sexual abuse, in nearly all settings, from elementary schools to nursing homes. They often find that substance-related problems underlie people's presenting concerns, particularly in employee assistance counseling. Experience with these disorders has led counselors to broaden their repertoire of interventions; they now have to become knowledgeable about the physical and psychological impact of chemical abuse, detoxification, inpatient and outpatient treatment, 12-step programs (e.g., Alcoholics Anonymous, Narcotics Anonymous), interventions to overcome resistance, and relapse prevention strategies.

Sexual and Other Addictions

The concept of addictions has become important for counselors. In an addiction, also known as an Impulse-Control Disorder, people are strongly drawn to engage frequently in a self-destructive or otherwise harmful behavior. Although they may recognize the undesirable nature of the behavior, mounting tension, craving, and weak coping skills lead them to engage in the behavior nonetheless. Of course, counselors are familiar with addiction to substances, but the literature also describes addictions to violence, food, gambling, the Internet, and sex.

The dramatic rise in computer and Internet use in recent years seems to have fueled two addictions. These have been labeled Internet Behavior Dependence and Cybersex Addiction. Hall and Parsons (2001) believe that 6% of the population can be diagnosed with Internet Behavior Dependence, primarily well-educated students and homemakers. These people neglect other aspects of their lives in favor of the Internet and have difficulty fulfilling major obligations. They tend to be irritable and anxious when not at the computer and experience diminished pleasure, along with depression and low self-esteem.

People who engage in Cybersex as well as other forms of anonymous sexual interaction (e.g., telephone sex, use of prostitutes, pornography) are typically between the ages of 18 and 32, include both men and women, and are more likely to belong to socially stigmatized or marginalized groups (Pennington, 2002). These methods of sexual interaction are appealing to some people because they can disguise who they are and engage in fantasy rather than risking openness and self-disclosure to achieve intimacy. As with most addictive symptoms, behavioral counseling can develop healthier interpersonal patterns.

Chronic and Severe Mental Disorders

Counselors are assuming new roles in working with people who have chronic and severe mental disorders such as Schizophrenia, Dementia, Dissociative Identity Disorder, and recurrent Major Depressive Disorders and Bipolar Disorders. While the primary treatment for most people with disorders such as these is medication, many also benefit from traditional counseling as well as case management and advocacy services. In these roles, counselors integrate and oversee the various services being provided and help people to negotiate the health care delivery system so they can receive needed services. Counselors also may be involved in organizing social and leisure activities, job coaching, psychoeducation, and family counseling in order to provide a broad range of services to people with long-standing and incapacitating mental disorders.

Counseling Related to Medical Conditions, Health, and Wellness

Researchers such as Kobasa (1979) who studied the relationship between personal attributes and physical health, David Spiegel (1990) who found a connection between emotional support and the health and coping skills of women with advanced cancer, and many others have demonstrated the existence of a strong connection between emotional and physical health. Counselors are increasingly helping people cope with chronic and life-threatening medical conditions such as AIDS, cancer, heart disease, asthma, and arthritis. Counseling can help people make sound decisions about their medical treatment, cope more effectively with their conditions, obtain the support they need, and even reduce the severity of their symptoms (Seligman, 1996). Hill (1990) reported that as few as six sessions of psychotherapy could reduce medical bills by as much as 75% over 5 years. Techniques such as visual imagery and relaxation, creative therapies such as drawing and writing, and other cognitive and behavioral interventions are useful in counseling people with chronic and life-threatening illnesses.

Although many counselors have already learned these interventions, counseling people with serious physical illnesses probably requires some specific training. Particularly useful to counselors treating people with physical illnesses is information on the impact of chronic and life-threatening illness on individuals and families, the stages of coping with illness, stress management, expressive therapies, relaxation and visualization, ambiguous loss, fear of recurrence, the integration of medical and complementary psychological treatments, and standard medical treatments for HIV, cancer, heart disease, and other prevalent medical conditions.

Counseling also is assuming an important role in helping people without significant medical conditions maintain or improve their health. In 1989, the ACA passed a resolution entitled The Counseling Profession as Advocates for Optimum Health and Wellness that endorsed goals of promoting wellness and health development and preventing mental and physical illness (Myers, 1992). O'Donnell (1988, p. 369) stated, "Up to 90% of the patients seeking medical help are estimated to suffer from disorders well within the range of self-healing."

Behavioral medicine, a growing specialization for counselors, includes such areas as weight management, smoking cessation, promoting nutrition and exercise, stress management, and pain management. It usually entails psychoeducation, direct clinical service, family counseling, and consultation with medical personnel. Behavioral medication usually takes a holistic and comprehensive approach, helping people gain balance and fulfilment through physical and emotional health.

Career Concerns

Career concerns, including lack of direction, impaired motivation, diminished satisfaction, problems in decision-making, job-related stress, coping with technological change, harassment and conflict in the workplace, downsizing and unemployment, and other career-related issues are important areas of focus for counselors. These difficulties can lead to absenteeism, poor performance at work and school, and even substance misuse and family dysfunction. Some counselors specialize in helping people with career issues. Others address career concerns as part of their work at schools and colleges, in private practices, and in other mental health delivery programs.

The functions of counselors helping people with career concerns are many and varied. They help people clarify interests and abilities, choose careers or college majors, resolve interpersonal conflicts, cope with technological change, reduce stress and "workaholism," deal with relocation and job loss, facilitate resume writing and other job-seeking skills, and identify and balance personal and professional values. Knowledge of assessment, transferability of skills, stress management, team building, and conflict resolution are important skills for these counselors.

Other Issues

The previous section in this chapter highlighted some enduring as well as new and growing areas of attention for counselors. Counselors continue to help people with a broad range of other issues, not specifically mentioned here, including depression and anxiety, behavioral concerns, social skill deficits, loss and change, decision-making, goals and direction, and interpersonal concerns. Many of these are discussed further in Chapters 3 and 4. In addition, according to Kiselica and Robinson (2001, p. 387), the focus of counseling has expanded from the "intrapsychic concerns of clients to a broader focus on the many extrapsychic forces that adversely affect the emotional and physical well-being of people." Viewing the organization and community as clients, counselors are increasingly engaging in social action, advocacy, community organization, and other interventions to reduce social problems and promote justice.

EMPLOYMENT SETTINGS FOR MENTAL HEALTH COUNSELORS

Mental health counselors provide services to a challenging and diverse array of people, address a wide variety of concerns, and use a complex and innovative range of techniques and interventions. Correspondingly, counselors have an extensive and expanding array of employment options, discussed in this next section of this chapter.

Community Mental Health Centers

The movements of the 1950s and 1960s to reduce the psychiatric inpatient population (deinstitutionalization) and increase readily available mental health services led to rapid growth in community mental health centers (CMHCs) and in employment of mental health counselors. Offering preventive as well as clinical services, and treating people of all ages and economic circumstances, CMHCs were charged with providing 10 essential services: inpatient treatment, outpatient treatment, emergency services, partial hospitalization, consultation and education, diagnostic services, rehabilitation, pre- and aftercare, training, and research and evaluation (Bloom, 1983). CMHCs offer counselors a challenging and diverse client population and a broad range of opportunities for collaboration and intervention. However, high demand for services can lead to large caseloads and an emphasis on brief treatment and remediation rather than prevention. CMHCs are good places of employment for beginning counselors who want supervision, role models, and breadth of experience as they determine their areas of interest and specialization.

Couples and Family Counseling Agencies

The past 30 years have witnessed the rapid growth of family counseling. National attention has been paid to issues such as the high divorce rate; partner and child abuse; blended, single-parent, homosexual, and other nontraditional families; and the important part that family dynamics can play in the course of Schizophrenia, Mood Disorders, Attention-Deficit/Hyperactivity Disorders, and many other emotional and physical difficulties. Mental health agencies that specialize in family-related concerns are numerous, reflecting the belief that problems linked to family interaction respond best to treatment that involves the family as well as the person presenting the problem. Family counselors work with people of all ages and backgrounds. These counselors need to be knowledgeable about child development, family dynamics and structure, theories of family counseling (see Chapter 8), the impact of societal and environmental factors on families, gender issues, and intergenerational transmission. Some agencies that emphasize family counseling prefer their employees to have specialized training (e.g., play therapy, mediation, brief family therapy), but others provide employment to entry-level counselors, offering another setting where counselors can have a broad and rich experience.

Rehabilitation Counseling Agencies

Rehabilitation counselors work with people diagnosed with physical or medical conditions, mental retardation, substance-related (drug or alcohol) problems, and severe or chronic emotional disorders. They also work with people who have been incarcerated. Rehabilitation counselors seek to reduce disability and improve or restore people's functioning, life satisfaction, and independence (Corry & Jewell, 2001). Counseling tends to be goal-oriented, involving collaboration with other medical and mental health professionals. Strategies in the repertoire of rehabilitation counselors include behavioral change interventions to promote more effective coping; social and other life skills training; promoting self-esteem, independence, and feelings of competence; vocational rehabilitation; family education; cognitive therapy; and case management.

Originally, most rehabilitation counselors were employed in governmental agencies. Now, however, rehabilitation counselors have many options, including small private agencies, correctional programs, substance use treatment programs, public agencies, and medical facilities.

Counseling for People with Physical Disabilities

Many people have some type of physical condition or impairment that limits their choices. Livneh (1991) reported that 2 million Americans have significant visual impairment, 15–16 million have reduced hearing, 150,000 have spinal cord injuries, and as many as 5 million have epilepsy. Each year, one million people are diagnosed with cancer and 500,000 people incur traumatic head injuries. Many others have heart surgery, amputations, and other medical procedures that potentially have a negative impact on their physical functioning and emotional health. Rehabilitation counselors usually have specialized training in the medical aspects of their clients' disorders. The focus of counseling, then, is on both physical and psychosocial variables to facilitate clients' rewarding involvement in the community and the labor force. Counselors help people obtain appropriate training and employment, provide follow-up, and make referrals for additional help as needed in order to improve the quality of their lives (Livneh, 1991).

Hospitals, Nursing Homes, and Continuing Care Facilities

Because of their history of focusing more on developmental concerns than pathology, counselors once were unlikely to find employment in inpatient or psychiatric hospital settings. Now, however, mental health counselors have the diagnostic and intervention skills they need to counsel effectively in these settings and are increasingly working with an elderly, seriously disturbed, or physically ill population. In such settings, a team approach is typically used, with counselors promoting adjustment and providing family counseling while medication and other physical treatments are provided by physicians, psychiatrists, and other medical personnel. Counselors also play a rehabilitative role with people who are hospitalized for potentially life-threatening illnesses or surgery that has caused an alteration in appearance and functioning.

Counselors are finding a place for themselves in hospital emergency facilities. In those settings, counselors must make a rapid assessment and diagnosis of people with severe emotional symptoms and make recommendations for hospitalization or other treatment options.

Nursing homes and continuing care facilities are other medically related facilities that employ counselors. These residential programs provide care to people with serious mental or physical disorders such as Alzheimer's disease, head trauma, or advanced neurological disorders. A large percentage of people in these facilities are older adults, but younger people also may be found in these settings. The need for counselors in nursing homes and other primarily gerontological facilities is expected to increase because of the predicted growth in the numbers of older adults. The population of people age 65 and older in the United States is expected to grow by 75% to over 69 million people by 2030 (Ryan & Agresti, 1999). Family counseling and psychoeducation as well as consultation with medical personnel are important aspects of the counselors' role in these settings, although group and individual therapy to promote adjustment and improve functioning also are important.

Corrections and the Court System

Counselors with a special interest in corrections may find employment in prisons, pre-release programs, or parole settings. Sometimes counselors employed in corrections fill both counseling and supervisory roles, a difficult combination. Counselors in corrections usually have the opportunity for both group and individual counseling. They often deal with challenging and reluctant clients from diverse backgrounds who may have drug and alcohol problems, personality disorders, family dysfunction, abuse, and other issues.

Counselors also may become involved with the court system by providing assessment and testimony in child custody cases; through employment with juvenile and family courts; via agencies that specialize in treating people with behaviors that may lead to their arrest (e.g., partner abuse, pedophilia); and in serving as an expert witness. These counselors not only need to be skilled in group and individual behavioral counseling, but they also need to understand the legal system and the privileges and constraints it imposes on counselors.

Substance Abuse Treatment Programs

Substance abuse treatment facilities have been major employers of mental health counselors for many years. Counselors interested in helping people with drug or alcohol problems primarily provide group treatment, but often offer individual and family counseling, interventions for people who resist treatment, and education and information on substances and their impact. These counselors need to be knowledgeable about drug- and alcohol-related problems, their signs and negative effects, support groups such as Alcoholics Anonymous and Rational Recovery, and community resources that can help with job training and placement, public assistance, and continued treatment. Counselors specializing in the treatment of Substance-Related Disorders may be employed in inpatient settings where they work intensively with people who usually spend up to four weeks in treatment, or they may work in outpatient facilities where treatment is less intensive but broader and longer. Their goals in both settings are to help people stop abusing substances, avoid relapsing, and develop healthy and rewarding lives.

Treatment Programs for the Chronically Mentally Ill

Another area of increasing opportunity for counselors is programs for people with serious and chronic mental disorders such as Schizophrenia or severe personality disorders. Such programs often are affiliated with CMHCs and are funded primarily by government and insurance payments. The counselors' primary role is usually that of case manager, a multifaceted role that involves overseeing and coordinating clients' services, making referrals, collaborating with other professionals, providing family and individual counseling to promote adjustment, and perhaps making home visits.

Other Medical Services/Settings

Counselors have been working with medical personnel in outpatient settings in response to the growing awareness that attending to both physical and emotional concerns can facilitate decisions, adjustment, and recovery. Examples of such settings are programs to help people with problem pregnancies or infertility; programs to help people cope with cancer and its treatments; hospice programs to provide support and resources to people who are dying and their families; and genetic counseling facilities providing information on genetically transmitted disorders.

Residential Facilities

Counselors are employed at residential facilities such as group homes for troubled adolescents, apartments for mentally retarded adults, and halfway houses for people with substance-related problems or a recent history of incarceration. In such settings, counselors usually have small caseloads but work closely with their clients in flexible ways, perhaps teaching them life skills such as cooking and locating housing and employment. Work hours tend to be flexible but may entail weekend or evening commitments.

Day Treatment Programs

Day treatment programs serve people who have impaired functioning and who need a supervised and therapeutic daytime program. These programs have existed for many years for older people and for people who are chronically mentally ill. In recent years, day treatment programs for troubled children and adolescents have proliferated, partly in response to the high costs of inpatient treatment and partly due to the growing number of young people who present with dangerous conditions such as Conduct Disorders, suicidal ideation, and self-harming behaviors. Counselors in these settings provide psychoeducation, group and individual treatment, therapeutic activities, and family counseling. Day treatment programs typically simulate a community; they are structured, emphasize mutual support and behavior change, require residents to perform chores, provide activities, and have a system for earning rewards and penalties.

Crisis Intervention Settings

Counselors engaged in crisis intervention may focus on suicide prevention, may accompany the police to follow-up on reports of domestic violence, may be intake workers in a hospital or CMHC, may work in victim assistance programs, or may staff a telephone hot line. Crisis intervention counseling tends to be short term, perhaps only one contact, and typically requires counselors to make rapid decisions, intervene and mobilize clients' strengths quickly, and know and make use of referral sources.

Career Counseling and Employment Agencies

Increasing social acceptance of the lifelong nature of career development, the frequency of midlife career change, awareness of the impact of job satisfaction on work performance, and recognition of the relationship between career development to the rest of people's lives have led to growth in career counseling services. Career counselors may serve a general clientele or an identified group (e.g., women reentering the work force, high school students, military retirees). Career counselors also may serve as consultants to business, industry, and governmental agencies that are reducing the size of their staffs and need counselors to facilitate outplacement and retirement as well as help in maintaining organizational morale. Employment agencies, too, hire career counselors, but their focus is matching clients to job opportunities listed with the agency.

Agencies focused on career counseling typically offer a combination of services: counseling; assessment using computerized and paper and pencil inventories of interests, values, skills, and personality; information giving; and training in job-seeking skills such as networking, interviewing, and resume writing. They also may offer support groups for job seekers.

Employee Assistance Programs and Other Opportunities in Business and Industry

Employee assistance programs (EAPs) are generally affiliated with or retained by businesses, industries, and governmental organizations to provide counseling and referral to employees. Employers generally provide this service in order to maximize productivity, retain capable employees, and reduce absenteeism and accidents by helping employees address personal or job-related problems. Clients may be self-referred or supervisor-referred, although confidentiality is almost always guaranteed unless clients' continued employment depends on their cooperation with counseling.

Common concerns presented to EAP counselors are substance-related difficulties, family conflict and dysfunction, and employee–supervisor conflict. Counseling usually is brief and crisis- or problem-focused, with referrals made if extended counseling is needed. Counselors in EAPs not only provide individual or family counseling but also give workshops and seminars on such topics as stress management and career planning, conduct assessments, consult with supervisors and administrators, and market and evaluate their services. Prevention, referral, and remediation are important components of their role.

Additional opportunities for counselors in business and industry include executive coaching, team building, conflict resolution, mediation, organizational development, and leadership development (Morrissey, 1995). In addition, counselors in these settings may assume some of the responsibilities of career counselors, including promoting career advancement, administering interest inventories, and facilitating relocation, retirement, and outplacement.

Counseling in Schools and Colleges

Typical school counselors have large caseloads, often over 250 students, and a variety of responsibilities such as scheduling, assessment, and program development. Individual and group counseling and consultation with parents and teachers are also part of their role. The responsibilities of most school counselors generally do not include providing extensive counseling to students with serious emotional difficulties. When school counselors encourage parents to seek outside help for their children, only 11% of parents make and attend at least one appointment (Smith, 2002). However, when a mental health clinic is available at the school, 90% of children keep at least one appointment.

To provide children the help they need, many schools are forming partnerships with graduate schools and community agencies so that mental health counselors can be placed in schools for part of their work week. This increased availability of counselors trained to diagnose and treat serious mental disorders is expanding counseling services for children and adolescents.

Most school-based counselors emphasize prevention—helping people to avoid problems (primary prevention) or early identification and treatment of symptoms before they become serious (secondary prevention). Of course, treatment of mental disorders and significant problems also is provided. Such programs typically take a developmental–contextual approach to treatment, focusing on the reciprocal relationships between the students and the environment (e.g., school, teachers, administrators, policies, community) (Vondracek & Porfeli, 2002). Legislation, including the School Reform and Mental Health Reform Acts of 1994 and the No Child Left Behind Act of 2001, has encouraged the expansion of school-based mental health services.

Mental health counselors in schools need to have both knowledge of the school environment and clinical skills. They work closely with teachers and school counselors, need to be knowledgeable about the diagnosis and treatment of mental disorders that are common in children and adolescents, and have skill in techniques such as risk and violence assessment and prevention, cognitive restructuring, increasing self-esteem, stress management, teaching problem-solving and social skills, conflict resolution, and play therapy (Hall, 2002).

The availability of mental health services is increasing in elementary, middle, and high schools but not in colleges. According to Hayes (2002, p. 12), "Nationwide, counseling departments, especially those at smaller universities and community colleges, are increasingly in danger of being cut back or phased out altogether." The primary cause of this change is financial constraints and cutbacks. Unfortunately, at the same time, colleges are seeing more students with severe psychological difficulties, drug and alcohol problems, learning disorders, and eating disorders. High numbers of international students, people changing careers or beginning college in midlife, and students undecided about their majors or career goals also necessitate additional counseling services. The current curtailment of college counseling services is a serious concern, both for students and for counselors specializing in college counseling.

Military and Government Settings

Counselors are employed by a broad range of military and governmental agencies. Counselors affiliated with governmental agencies might work with people who are receiving public assistance, who are involved in foster care, or who are in funded programs to help people develop job skills. These counselors typically have a large caseload, see their clients on an irregular and as needed basis, and have case management, referral, and administrative responsibilities.

Counselors also are employed to help fire fighters, police, and others in stressful public service jobs. Critical incident response teams are especially useful in those settings.

The military, too, employs counselors. They are involved in addressing special problems among military personnel such as abuse, family relocation, and employment of spouses. Military counselors provide assessment and career counseling, work in schools for military dependents in the United States and overseas, and offer a broad range of services at inpatient and outpatient treatment facilities on military bases or connected with the Veterans Administration. Counselors in these settings need to be familiar with the diagnosis and treatment of the common problems found in these settings such as PTSD, partner abuse, substance-related problems, marital conflict, and Adjustment Disorders.

Religious/Spiritual Counseling Settings

Churches and other religious and spiritual settings increasingly are hiring counselors to supplement the work of the clergy, who may not have the time or expertise to offer mental health services. Counselors in these settings need to emphasize spiritual issues and understand and accept the diversity of beliefs and values held by their clients. These counselors also need to comprehend the difference between religion and spirituality. Although both involve finding a sense of meaning and purpose in life, religion involves adherence to the beliefs of an organized church or religious group while spirituality entails a sense of transcendence, a relationship with a higher power (Standard, Sandhu, & Painter, 2000). Both trained pastoral counselors and general mental health counselors are employed in religious and spiritual settings. Although some of their work entails helping people deal with religious and spiritual issues, most of their work is not much different from that of a general mental health counselor and involves primarily helping people with a broad range of interpersonal and adjustment problems.

Wellness and Prevention Settings

Particularly since the terrorist attacks of September 11, 2001, mental health professionals have recognized the importance of promoting resilience. As Newman (2002, p. 62) stated, "Resilience, the ability to adapt in the face of trauma, adversity, tragedy or even significant ongoing stressors, is receiving considerable attention of late." Resilience can be taught and is characterized by good relationships with others, a sense of belonging, a positive self-image, self-confidence, and an optimistic view of the world. People who are resilient still experience sadness, distress, and emotional pain, but they have effective ways to cope with adversity. Positive psychology, developed primarily by Martin Seligman (1999), is another important thrust in the wellness arena that similarly focuses on developing people's strengths. Positive psychology seeks to increase positive attitudes (e.g., optimism, sense of well-being), positive personality traits (e.g., forgiveness, courage, wisdom, sound interpersonal skills), and positive institutions (e.g., schools and agencies that promote altruism, tolerance, and improved relationships).

Wellness counseling not only encourages the development of resilience and positive personal assets, it typically endorses a holistic approach. For example, Myers, Sweeney, and Witmer (2000) identify five life tasks in their wellness model: Spirituality, Self-direction, Work and Leisure, Friendship, and Love.

Counselors' preventive and developmental skills are being put to especially good use in a variety of health and wellness settings. Counselors have found employment in fitness centers; in smoking cessation, weight control, and other behavioral change programs; and in programs that teach relaxation, meditation, and other wellness skills.

Specific Focus Agencies

A broad range of mental health agencies can be identified that specialize in treating a specific disorder, problem, or type of person. These agencies can be categorized according to the age group served (e.g., children, people over 65), the special population or problem addressed (e.g., people who recently have been bereaved, people from Latino backgrounds), or the advocated approach to treatment (e.g., Rational Emotive Behavior Therapy, biofeedback, hypnotherapy). Counselors with special areas of interest or training may seek employment in such settings. This may help them to develop strong skills in an area of specialization but usually will not provide them experience in counseling people with a broad range of disorders or concerns.

Consulting and Coaching

Counselors may be self-employed or employed by agencies to engage in the process of consulting, one of several roles for counselors that focus on effecting change in systems. Approximately 90% of master's degree programs in counseling offer coursework in consultation (Stoltenberg, 1993). Consultation usually involves a triadic relationship, including the consultant who is the expert or specialist, the consultee who is requesting help, and the client system that is the focus of the change efforts.

Typically, the counselor–consultant is hired by several different agencies on a short-term, fee-for-service contract to provide expertise in a specified area. Consultants might conduct assessments for a rehabilitation firm, provide training in communication skills for supervisors in business or government, offer stress management workshops for members of a professional association, or provide training for other mental health professionals in a particular skill or theory. The consultant role typically is an active, directive, and facilitative one, requiring skills and knowledge in needs assessment, evaluation, collaboration, organizational development, team building, conflict resolution, developing mission statements, interpersonal relationships, and communication. Chapters 9 and 10 provide additional information on this counseling role. While consulting may be an unpredictable and potentially stressful endeavor, many counselors enjoy part-time consulting in addition to full-time employment.

Coaching is one of the newest and fastest growing roles for counselors. According to the International Coach Federation, coaching is an ongoing relationship that focuses on people taking action toward the realization of their visions, goals, or desires. The coaching process helps people both define and achieve professional and personal goals. Coaches do not diagnose or address mental disorders or focus on pathology but, rather, assume their clients have the emotional resources they need to accomplish their goals. About 40% of the approximately 10,000 full-time coaches now in practice in the United States are former therapists, and 20% of therapists offer coaching as part of their practice (Naughton, 2002). Although certification for coaches exists, along with about 70 programs to train coaches, more research is needed to demonstrate the effectiveness of this approach and its methods.

Private Practice

The advent, in the 1970s, of state licensure and certification for counselors has led counselors to enter private practice in increasing numbers. Private practice is the most common work site for members of the American Mental Health Counselors Association (AMHCA), with close to half of its members in private practice (Messina, 1995). Private practices take many forms: they may be full-time or part-time, often in addition to teaching or another counseling position; they may be solo or group practices; and they may be general or specialized practices.

Private practice clearly is a viable option for counselors; state licensure allows them to practice independently and they are generally recognized by health insurance companies. Private practice has many rewards. Counselors can set their own hours, they can choose the clients or issues they want to address, and they have the potential to succeed financially. On the other hand, counselors in private practice, particularly those who practice alone, must assume responsibility for the diagnosis and treatment of their clients. Counselors in private practice often experience isolation and uncertain income. They must be actively involved in marketing, billing, and dealing with managed care and governmental requirements. In addition, MCOs exert an influence on the nature and duration of treatment provided by most counselors in private practice as well as on their income, with per session MCO payment to licensed professional counselors averaging about $60 (Davis, 2002).

Cybercounseling

Considerable professional debate in recent years has concerned the delivery of counseling services via electronic means, including the telephone (telecounseling) and the Internet (Webcounseling). These methods of counseling have both advantages and disadvantages. Benefits include lower cost, convenience, and flexibility; counseling can take place when clients or counselors are out of town or unable to travel. Some clients report they feel safer participating in distance counseling and, therefore, reveal more about themselves, participate more actively, and are more likely to experiment with new learning. On the other hand, most nonverbal cues are lost in distance counseling, technology can be unreliable, and ethical and legal guidelines are not yet fully clear. Giving clients complete information on encryption methods, providing links to credentialing bodies, determining ways to address technological failure, and giving the client the name of a local therapist to contact in case of an emergency can help to reduce the drawbacks of distance counseling. Perhaps with some additional experience and research, this approach will become a useful tool for most counselors. As Riemer-Reiss (2002, p. 189) stated, "Although telecounseling will not replace the conventional mode of service delivery, it could become an essential component to improve the accessibility of mental health counseling."

Overview of Opportunities

Counselors have a broad range of employment settings open to them. Beginning counselors should choose their initial work experiences carefully, starting with their internships. With each placement, skills are developed and opportunities are expanded. However, other opportunities become less available as counselors narrow their focus. A clear view of the path they hope their careers will take can help counselors to develop the competencies they need while still maximizing their marketability.

THE MENTAL HEALTH SERVICE PROVIDERS

In nearly all treatment settings, counselors increasingly are working collaboratively with other providers of mental health services. Counselors may be part of a treatment team or may consult with other providers to determine the best treatment for a client. To maximize the effectiveness of the collaboration as well as maintain their own roles, counselors need to be familiar with other mental health professionals as well as knowledgeable about how their own roles both differ from and resemble those of other mental health treatment providers.

The Mental Health Treatment Team

The diversity of training and areas of specialization of mental health professionals employed in CMHCs and other mental health facilities has led to the evolution of the mental health team. In this generic model of staffing, a mental health team is composed of two or more treatment providers with different areas of specialization. Such a team might include a psychiatrist, a psychologist, and a counselor or social worker. Depending upon the nature of the treatment facility, the team also might include recreation therapists, psychiatric nurses, and other specialists. Members of a team typically have some roles or duties they all perform, such as individual counseling, and some that are assigned only to certain members of the group based on their training and areas of expertise. For example, the psychiatrist determines the need for medication, the social worker may specialize in family therapy, and the counselor may focus on promoting behavioral change. Generally, the team will meet as a unit to develop treatment plans and will evaluate them regularly. One member of the team often serves as the case manager or primary therapist, ensuring that team members collaborate smoothly and that clients' needs are addressed.

The team approach offers many advantages. It allows mental health treatment providers to become experts in some areas while drawing on the knowledge and talents of others to supplement their skills. The collaboration afforded by the team approach can yield considerable information and insights about clients and often promotes sounder diagnoses and treatment plans.

Counselors, especially those in private practice, often develop their own informal treatment teams to reduce their isolation and increase the range of services they have available. For example, a counselor may meet with other counselors for weekly peer supervision, refer people who need medication to a trusted psychiatrist, suggest that clients with suspected learning disorders see a psychologist for testing, and consult with a social worker for information on subsidized housing and other social service programs. Networking can help mental health counselors provide the best possible treatment to their clients.

Although collaboration with other providers offers many benefits, it also may present challenges. Issues of competition, distribution of power, and manipulation by clients may arise. To maximize the likelihood of a smooth and productive collaboration, counselors should confer with their colleagues frequently; be sure they have compatible theoretical orientations, mutual understanding and appreciation of each other's skills; and share a cooperative orientation.

The Mental Health Treatment Specialists

The diversity of treatment providers can be confusing to clients as well as to the providers themselves. Counselors need to understand the differences and similarities among the various mental health professionals to know whom to consult when help is needed and how to facilitate productive communication and collaboration. The following section provides brief descriptions of the major categories of mental health treatment providers.

Psychiatrists

Psychiatrists have a medical degree, generally an M.D., and are qualified to assess physical conditions, diagnose medical problems, and prescribe medication. They have extensive education, including 4 years of medical school and at least several years of residency. However, the training that psychiatrists receive in psychotherapy varies; some have completed advanced training programs and additional residencies and have considerable expertise in psychotherapy while others concentrate on biochemical treatment of mental disorders and have relatively brief training and experience in psychotherapy. Counselors actually have more training and expertise in human development and psychotherapy than do some psychiatrists.

Although counselors, of course, cannot diagnose physical complaints or prescribe medication, they are often the first to hear of clients' medical complaints or their problems with medication. Consequently, counselors need to stay informed about their clients' medications and physical conditions and have a good understanding of what disorders and symptoms benefit from medication so that they can refer clients to a psychiatrist when warranted.

Psychologists

Doctoral-level psychologists can be categorized by their areas of specialization and their degrees. Most will have a Ph.D. degree (Doctor of Philosophy), some will have an Ed.D. (Doctor of Education), and others will have a Psy.D. (Doctor of Psychology). The Psy.D. is generally granted by programs focused on preparing practitioners rather than researchers. Ph.D. programs typically emphasize research as well as practice, and the Ed.D. is traditionally associated with teaching and employment in educational settings. However, considerable overlap exists among the requirements and course offerings for all three degrees.

Psychologists specialize in such areas as clinical psychology, counseling psychology, developmental psychology, experimental psychology, or industrial/organizational psychology. Psychologists in mental health settings are most likely to be clinical or counseling psychologists. Here, too, considerable overlap exists. However, clinical psychologists are typically more interested in abnormal behavior and severe emotional disturbance and their remediation while counseling psychologists tend to be more interested in normal development, prevention, and problems of adjustment.

Most practicing psychologists have completed 3–5 years of postbaccalaureate study, a 1-year internship, a thesis or dissertation, and 2 years of supervised postdoctoral experience. They are licensed by the states in which they practice. Doctoral-level clinical and counseling psychologists are trained in psychotherapy and typically also have considerable expertise in psychological testing, including the use of projective techniques.

Master's degree–level psychologists typically have received specialized training in a particular area of psychology (e.g., testing, counseling, industrial, or school psychology). They are often employed as psychometricians or school psychologists in settings where their primary function is assessment. Psychologists without a doctorate generally cannot be licensed or certified to practice independently as psychologists (although some states allow school psychologists to have independent practices that focus on educational psychology). Consequently, the role of the psychologist without a doctorate is limited. Some psychologists are circumventing this by taking extra coursework and seeking licensure as counselors.

Counselors who work with children and families often collaborate with school psychologists. They specialize in assessment of learning problems, developmental disorders, and other difficulties that may prevent children from performing well at school. School psychologists, in turn, work closely with school counselors to determine children's special needs and develop individualized educational plans to address them. Testing is emphasized in their work, although counseling is increasingly becoming part of the role of the school psychologist.

Social Workers

Practicing social workers typically have the master's degree in social work (M.S.W.) and credentials from state (LCSW) and national (ACSW) credentialing bodies. Requirements for credentialing are comparable to those for counselors: approximately 60 semester hours of graduate credit, including field work, followed by 2 years of supervised experience.

However, social workers have a longer history in the mental health field than do counselors. Initially, social workers often collaborated with psychiatrists, seeing the families of troubled clients. Over the years, they have acquired considerable independence and credibility. While overlap exists between the interests and training of social workers and mental health counselors, social workers tend to be more knowledgeable about public policy and organizational issues. However, they generally do not have counselors' expertise in testing and educational or career-related concerns. Social workers are particularly likely to be found in medical and social service settings although, like mental health counselors, they often work in private practices, family counseling, CMHCs, and other mental health treatment programs.

Psychiatric Nurses

Psychiatric nurses, sometimes known as clinical nurse specialists, generally have a master's degree in their field, with supervised experience in mental health settings. They are trained in counseling and human development as well as in medical diagnosis and treatment. Their work often emphasizes prevention, community health, and wellness. They frequently are part of a treatment team in hospital settings and in settings involving people with physical or medical concerns (e.g., detoxification programs, rehabilitation programs), but they also may be found in private practice, CMHCs, and other mental health settings.

Pastoral Counselors

Credentialed pastoral counselors generally have the same training and experience as other mental health counselors with additional or previous training in theology. Skilled pastoral counselors are not only interested in spiritual issues but also follow accepted principles of effective counseling such as offering advice sparingly and attempting to maintain objectivity.

Marriage and Family Therapists

National certification is available for marriage and family therapists through the American Association of Marriage and Family Therapy and through the IAMFC.

Some states also offer credentials for marriage and family therapists. These specific credentials are not required in order for counselors to do marriage and family therapy as long as they have state licensure or certification in counseling.

Marriage and family therapists may have had their training in programs especially for family therapists or may be mental health counselors, social workers, or other helping professionals with particular interest and special training in family counseling. They may be found in a broad range of mental health settings, including private practice, but of course, are likely to specialize in marriage and family therapy.

Certified Addictions Counselor

Certified addictions counselors (CACs) may have less education and training than other mental health professionals but more direct experience. Many CACs are recovering from their own addictions and want to use their experience to help others. The CAC credential requires a 2-year college degree with extensive coursework and experience in addictions and other mental health areas. As members of a treatment team, CACs may be able to establish rapport rapidly with clients and can offer special insights and information.

In recent years, the CAC credential has become very marketable because of the great need for counselors to have expertise in addictions. Consequently, many licensed mental health counselors also receive the specialized training they need to become CACs, a valuable combination of credentials.

Expressive Therapists

Expressive therapists specialize in the use of creative arts in counseling. They may focus on art therapy, music therapy, dance therapy, or other creative activities. They often have credentials as counselors or other helping professionals and use traditional counseling approaches as well as creative ones in their work. They can be especially helpful to people who have difficulty verbalizing their feelings, who have physical concerns, or who are very depressed.

Psychoanalysts

This term describes people who have received extensive specialized postgraduate training in psychoanalysis and who have generally undergone personal analysis. They may be psychiatrists, psychologists, social workers, or counselors. The term psychoanalyst does not indicate a degree but, rather, the nature of a person's training and practice (e.g., seeing clients multiple times a week for at least several years and using the ideas and techniques of Freud and his followers).

Psychotherapists

This is a general term that describes anyone who practices counseling or psychotherapy. It does not provide information about education, training, or techniques, but does imply an interest in treating people with mental disorders, rather than focusing on helping people with problems of adjustment or life circumstance.

Counselors

Definitions of mental health counselors have been provided earlier in this book. Considerable overlap and commonality exists between mental health counselors and the other helping professionals. A study by Falvey (1992) of 128 clinicians representing six mental health professions found that the clinicians were very similar in terms of the assessment criteria they used, the categories they addressed in their history taking, their treatment planning, and the goals they established for clients. Only their interventions showed much variability.

Mental health counselors are well trained to use a wide range of techniques and approaches to help people with developmental, social, emotional, family, and career-related concerns. Counselors conduct assessments, using interviews and standardized, objective tests; they make use of community resources and support systems to help people. They offer individual, group, and family counseling; diagnosis and treatment planning; supervision; program development and evaluation; training; consultation; staff development; community education and organization; referral; administration; fund raising and grant writing; and case management.

The work of mental health counselors also typically has a few clear limits. They cannot evaluate physical concerns or prescribe medication. Some states and test publishers limit their use of projective tests.

Despite these few limitations, the roles and skills of mental health counselors are broad, enabling them to effectively treat a wide range of clients and disorders. The rest of this book provides information on the essential skills of the mental health counselor.

Diagnostic Systems and Their Use

Diagnosis is an essential tool of the mental health counselor. According to Hinkle (1994b, p. 174), "At the foundation of effective mental health care is the establishment of a valid psychodiagnosis." The American Counseling Association Code of Ethics and Standards of Practice (1995, p. 36) states, "Counselors take special care to provide proper diagnosis of mental disorders." The message in these statements is supported by practice. In a nationwide survey of certified clinical mental health counselors (Mead, Hohenshil, & Singh, 1997, p. 394), 91% indicated that the *Diagnostic and Statistical Manual of Mental Disorders* (*DSM*) is their "most frequently used professional reference." Most of those surveyed viewed themselves as skilled in the use of the *DSM* and believed they were usually able to make an accurate diagnosis.

The purpose of this chapter is to familiarize counselors with the process of diagnosis, as well as its benefits and challenges. The overview of the *DSM-IV-TR* (fourth/text revision edition) (American Psychiatric Association [APA], 2000) presented here introduces that important reference and describes the mental disorders defined in the *DSM*. Appendix A at the end of this book helps readers make accurate diagnoses.

Benefits of Diagnosis

Based on a large systematic statistical random sample of the population of the United States, Kessler et al. (1994) estimated that 48% had met the *DSM* criteria for a mental disorder at some point in their lives; 21% had one mental disorder, 13% had two mental disorders, and 14% met the criteria for three or more mental disorders. Of the total group, 29% had experienced a mental disorder in the past year. Unfortunately, less than 40% had received treatment for their mental disorders. A great need exists for counselors to diagnose and treat mental disorders.

Knowledge of and skill in the use of diagnosis can enhance the counseling process and help the counselor in many ways including the following:

1. A diagnostic system such as the *DSM* offers a structured framework as well as a set of criteria for identifying and describing mental disorders.
2. Such a framework enables counselors to determine whether a particular person's symptoms meet the criteria for a mental disorder.
3. Having accurate diagnoses for their clients helps counselors determine those people who have the skills to counsel as well as those clients who need a referral for medication or other services that counselors do not provide.
4. Knowing a client's diagnosis helps counselors to understand better people's symptoms and how their disorders are likely to evolve and present themselves over time.
5. Probably the most important benefit of diagnosis is that it enables counselors to develop treatment plans that have a high probability of success.
6. Use of a standardized diagnostic system enables counselors to use the substantial and growing body of research on what interventions are most likely to ameliorate the symptoms of a given disorder to guide their treatment plans.
7. Standardized inventories (e.g., the Minnesota Multiphasic Personality Inventory, the Millon Clinical Multiaxial Inventory discussed in Chapter 4) can translate symptoms into diagnoses and suggested treatment interventions, thereby facilitating counseling.
8. Counselors are at less risk of malpractice suits if they have made a diagnosis and developed a treatment plan according to an accepted system.
9. Use of a standardized system of diagnosis such as the *DSM* is required for counselors to receive payments from management care organizations (MCOs) for their sessions, making counseling more affordable and available to more people.
10. Sharing diagnoses with clients, when appropriate, can promote self-awareness.
11. Knowing that others have experienced similar symptoms and that research is available on effective treatment of their disorders can reassure clients, reduce unwarranted blame and guilt, and increase their hopefulness and openness to change.
12. Diagnostic terminology is used by all mental health disciplines; knowledge of that terminology facilitates parity, credibility, communication, and collaboration.
13. If a person relocates or transfers from one counselor to another, communication of diagnostic information about that person can promote continuity of service.

14. Records of diagnoses, treatment interventions, and outcomes enable clinicians and agencies to research their practices, determine needed services, assess and refine the quality of their interventions, demonstrate accountability, and justify the work of the agency and its clinicians.

Controversies and Limitations

The process of diagnosing mental disorders is a challenging one. To maximize the accuracy of their diagnoses, counselors should be aware of the following questions, controversies, and limitations inherent in the diagnostic process as well as ways to address them effectively.

Should counselors diagnose mental disorders? Despite the many benefits inherent in the process of diagnosis, still some question whether diagnosis of mental disorders is an appropriate skill for counselors. As Johnson (1993, p. 236) wrote of this debate,

The field of mental health counseling is currently wrestling with at least two orientations toward carving out its unique role among the mental health professions. One orientation might be best described as placing an emphasis on a developmental-psychoeducational model ... A competing orientation suggests that, to take our place as another core mental health profession, we must engage in the practice of clinical diagnosis and treatment of mental and emotional disorders ... these orientations ... are not mutually exclusive.

Are counselors adequately trained and skilled in diagnosis? Although the great majority of graduate programs in counseling and psychology offer training in abnormal psychology and diagnosis of mental disorders, Benson (2002, p. 30) found that " ... even after years of experience with the *DSM*, clinicians still use their own theories to help them decide whether a patient belongs to a particular diagnostic group." McLaughlin (2002) echoed these concerns, identifying four sources of bias in diagnostic assessment: stereotyping, problems in data availability and clarity, self-confirmatory bias (focusing only on confirming information), and self-fulfilling prophecy.

Is multicultural competence compatible with diagnosis of mental disorders? D'Andrea (1999, p. 44), coming from a postmodern perspective, suggests that "psychological problems and discomfort are relative and culturally-determined concepts." He urges counselors to "avoid thinking about psychological problems primarily in terms of individual deficits or as various forms of psychological illnesses." Paniagua (2001, p. 14) has similar concerns and states, "Overdiagnosis, underdiagnosis, or misdiagnosis of psychopathology among clients from ... culturally diverse groups ... have been a critical issue ... for many years." However, Paniagua, McLaughlin, and others have identified ways to use the *DSM* that reflect multicultural competence. These will be discussed in the next section.

What other risks and limitations are involved in the process of diagnosis? Counselors can make the best use of the diagnostic process and avoid its pitfalls if they keep the following additional risks in mind (Seligman, 2001a):

1. Using a diagnostic label to characterize someone's symptoms can be stigmatizing and can lead to negative attitudes toward that person at school, work, or in the family.
2. In some cases, knowing the diagnostic term for a person's symptoms can be discouraging and threatening. For example, parents may be more comfortable dealing with a child they view as having high energy than with one who has an Attention-Deficit/Hyperactivity Disorder (ADHD).
3. Diagnosis can lead to viewing people as their mental disorders (e.g., a Schizophrenic, an Anorexic), rather than as people with a particular set of concerns, and can promote a focus on pathology rather than on health.
4. Although the linear process of diagnosis can facilitate information gathering and treatment planning, it can make it difficult to think about people in developmental and systemic terms and to maintain a holistic view of people and their difficulties.
5. Similarly, attaching a diagnostic label to one person may put the focus of treatment on that person rather than on a family or social context. This can reinforce a perception of that person as the problem and can make it more difficult for a family or community to work together on shared issues and concerns.
6. When a person's diagnosis is submitted to that person's MCO or insurance company, the diagnosis becomes a permanent part of the person's medical record. That sometimes can make it difficult for the person to obtain life insurance, disability insurance, health insurance, and security clearances.
7. In addition, the widely used *DSM* has been based primarily on disorders and conditions found in the United States, which stem from a Western perspective on mental illness, and may have limited relevance to people from other cultures.

Maximizing the Benefits of Diagnoses

Despite its limitations and challenges, the *DSM* is a valuable tool that can play an essential role in reducing people's suffering and developing their strengths and coping skills. Training, knowledge, insight, and caution can help clinicians maximize the benefits of the *DSM* and respond to the previous questions in constructive and helpful ways as described below.

Should counselors diagnose mental disorders? According to Hinkle (1994a, p. 34), "Just as mental health counselors 'cannot not communicate,' 'cannot

not influence,' and 'cannot not behave,' they cannot not diagnose or plan as part of the [counseling] context." Only if they know whether a person has a mental disorder and understand that mental disorder, if one is present, can counselors determine whether and what developmental, psychoeducational, or clinical interventions are likely to be effective.

Are counselors adequately trained and skilled in diagnosis? Research has shown that a high degree of agreement on diagnoses can be expected from experienced clinicians (APA, 2000). Mental health professionals agree on a given diagnosis 80% of the time (Pfeiffer, 1995). In order to make an accurate diagnosis, counselors should adhere to the specific criteria presented in the *DSM*. Hunches, based on clinical experience, may guide clinicians to the right diagnosis, but the accuracy of that diagnosis must be verified by a comparison of symptoms with *DSM* standards.

In addition, counselors must take a comprehensive and holistic approach to diagnosis, gathering information on people's presenting concerns, their backgrounds and history, and their current situations. Counselors then can organize and analyze this data. The *DSM* provides descriptions of mental disorders. However, other sources are needed to understand the development, nature, and impact of a mental disorder in a particular person and to determine helpful treatment approaches. Detailed information on intake interviews, assessment, and treatment planning, all part of the diagnostic process, is provided later in this book.

Is multicultural competence compatible with diagnosis of mental disorders? I agree with D'Andrea and Paniagua. "It is imperative that counselors acknowledge the validity of multiple perspectives and understand the story and viewpoints of each of their clients. Counselors also must promote ... the use of developmental, preventive, and culturally-sensitive intervention strategies" (Seligman, 1999, p. 6). However, I also believe that "barriers to effective counseling in the postmodern era lie more within the counselor than between the pages of a book. The *DSM*, when used properly, can enhance rather than detract from skilled and culturally sensitive counseling." The *DSM* supports this position and acknowledges, " ... the symptoms and course of a number of *DSM-IV-TR* disorders are influenced by cultural and ethnic factors" (APA, 2000, p. xxxiv). In defining a mental disorder, the *DSM* states, "this syndrome or pattern must not be merely an expectable and culturally sanctioned response to a particular event" (p. xxxi).

Awareness of the importance of multicultural factors is a first step in making culturally sensitive diagnoses. However, counselors must do more to determine whether, for example, a child's violent behavior reflects a Conduct Disorder or an appropriate response to growing up in a war-torn country and whether the self-effacing attitudes and circumscribed lifestyle of a Hispanic woman reflect a Dependent Personality Disorder or the cultural messages she received throughout her life. The *DSM* provides several tools to help counselors make distinctions such as these.

Most important is the Outline for Cultural Formulation, encouraging counselors to seek an in-depth and culturally relevant understanding of people's symptoms by assessing the following five areas: (1) the cultural identity of the individual, (2) cultural explanations of the person's symptoms and disorders, (3) the person's psychosocial environment, its stressors and supports, and how the person functions in that environment, (4) cultural aspects of the client–counselor relationship, and (5) how cultural considerations affect the person's diagnosis and treatment. In addition, the description of each major group of disorders presented in the *DSM* includes discussion of specific culture, age, and gender features that are important in understanding those disorders. The *DSM* also includes a description of culture-bound syndromes that provides information on disorders thus far found only in a limited geographic area. The *DSM* goes a long way toward promoting culturally sensitive diagnosis.

How can counselors address the other risks and limitations involved in diagnosis? The following guidelines should help counselors to make accurate and useful diagnoses and minimize the shortcomings of the diagnostic process:

1. View people in context, considering environmental, cultural, social, religious, gender, age, and other factors. Keep in mind that mental disorders should be diagnosed only if thoughts and behaviors are aberrant for the person's culture.
2. Be aware that the symptoms people present may change rapidly, depending on the time of day, their immediate stressors, the progression of the disorder, or the characteristics of and questions posed by the interviewer. Diagnosis is not an exact science and often requires considerable time and many samples of behavior, as well as information from records and other sources, before an accurate diagnosis can be made.
3. Do not be tempted to overdiagnose to maximize third-party payments or to underdiagnose to avoid stating that a person has a serious mental disorder. Both are unethical and can be illegal. Overdiagnosis can jeopardize a person's future insurance coverage and may prevent employment in some jobs; underdiagnosis suggests that the counselor failed to appreciate the severity of a person's difficulties.
4. Finally, always consider the whole person, with diagnosis being only one important piece of information about that person.

DIAGNOSTIC SYSTEMS

Two diagnostic systems are widely used. The *DSM-IV-TR*, now in its fourth/text revision edition (APA, 2000), currently is the accepted diagnostic system in the United States. In many other countries, however, the *International Statistical*

Classification of Mental and Behavioural Disorders (ICD-10) (World Health Organization, 1992) is the diagnostic system of choice. In addition, current HIPAA guidelines emphasizing *ICD* diagnoses will increase the use of that diagnostic system in the United States. The *DSM-IV-TR* and the *ICD-10* have a common numbering system and many similarities. The parallels between the two are outlined in appendix H of the *DSM-IV-TR*.

DEVELOPMENT OF THE *DSM*

At present, the *DSM* has been through six revisions. The first edition of the *DSM* containing 108 types of mental disorders (Hohenshil, 1993) was published in 1952. It was developed primarily by and for psychiatrists and presented a psychobiological view of emotional disorders. The *DSM-II*, published in 1968 and containing 185 categories of mental disorders, was strongly influenced by Freud and psychoanalytic theory. The *DSM-III*, published in 1980, with 265 varieties of mental disorders, can be viewed as the first of the modern generation of diagnostic manuals. A collaborative venture of the American Psychiatric Association and the American Psychological Association, the *DSM-III* was in preparation for several years and was field-tested by over 500 clinicians before it was published. A revision of the *DSM-III*, the *DSM-III-R*, was published in 1987. In 1994, the *DSM-IV* was published, describing over 300 mental disorders. Currently, the *DSM-IV-TR*, published in 2000, is in use and will probably not be replaced until 2008 or later. This latest edition of the *DSM* is viewed as a text revision because it included no significant changes in diagnostic criteria. However, many pages of new and revised narrative material were added to this edition of the *DSM*, most of it focused on multicultural aspects of mental disorders. The *DSM-IV-TR*, like the *DSM-III, DSM-III-R*, and *DSM-IV*, is deliberately atheoretical; it seeks to describe mental disorders in a way that is useful to clinicians of all theoretical orientations.

Three criteria have guided recent revisions of the *DSM*. The primary justification for change was compelling empirical support. Extensive literature reviews, clinical trials, and drafts with invited feedback provided the information to determine whether support was available for a suggested change. Clinical utility and compatibility with the *ICD* were other criteria for change.

Although the *DSM-IV-TR* does not provide information on treatment of mental disorders, this manual is the stepping-stone to determining effective treatment strategies. According to Hinkle (1994b, p. 182), "An understanding of this diagnostic system and its vast implications in counseling will be imperative to the effective and ethical delivery of professional mental health counseling services." Ivey and Ivey (1999) agreed, stating, "Counselors of all types need an understanding of and an ability to work with issues described by the *DSM*" (p. 484) and "Clearly, the *DSM-IV* is important for the future of the counseling profession" (p. 486).

For each disorder, the *DSM* generally provides information on the following:

- Diagnostic features
- Subtypes and/or specifiers relevant to the disorder
- Recording procedures
- Associated features and disorders
- Specific culture, age, and gender features
- Prevalence
- Typical course of the disorder
- Familial patterns
- Differential diagnoses or the differences between a particular disorder and similar ones.

DEFINITION OF A MENTAL DISORDER

The *DSM-IV-TR* defines a mental disorder as

... a clinically significant behavioral or psychological syndrome or pattern that occurs in an individual and is associated with present distress (e.g., a painful symptom), or disability (i.e., impairment in one or more important areas of functioning), or with a significantly increased risk of suffering death, pain, disability, or an important loss of freedom .... Whatever its original cause, it must currently be considered a manifestation of a behavioral, psychological, or biological dysfunction in the individual (APA, 2000, p. xxxi).

As indicated in this definition, mental disorders can only be diagnosed in individuals (rather than families or groups) and are characterized by significant distress or impairment or both. The *DSM* seeks to "enable clinicians and investigators to diagnose, communicate about, study, and treat people with various mental disorders" (APA, 2000, p. xxxvii).

MULTIAXIAL ASSESSMENT

Multiaxial assessment using the *DSM-IV-TR* involves the use of five axes or ways of viewing people. It is an approach to diagnosis that encourages clinicians to take a comprehensive and holistic view of their clients. Axis I, *Clinical Disorders and Other Conditions That May Be A Focus of Clinical Attention*, and Axis II, *Personality Disorders and Mental Retardation*, are the axes where mental disorders as well as other conditions are listed. Only two diagnostic groups are included on Axis II, encompassing long-standing and deeply ingrained disorders: all the Personality Disorders and Mental Retardation (including Borderline Intellectual Functioning). Defense mechanisms and personality traits also may be listed on Axis II. All other disorders and conditions are coded on Axis I.

Axis III is termed *General Medical Conditions*. Physical disorders that may be relevant to a person's emotional condition are listed on this axis. Although clinicians can informally list signs and symptoms of medical conditions on Axis III or indicate that a medical condition is reported by the client, an official multiaxial assessment should include on Axis III only medically verified physical conditions.

On Axis IV clinicians list *Psychosocial and Environmental Problems* that may be causing a person difficulty. These typically include external processes or events, such as living in poverty, getting divorced, or being incarcerated, that have occurred within the past year. Clinicians can simply list the stressors or organize them into categories provided in the *DSM*.

Axis V, the *Global Assessment of Functioning* (GAF) scale, is a 1–100 scale on which clinicians rate a person's current level of functioning. Higher numbers reflect better functioning and numbers below 50 indicate severe symptoms. GAF rating is determined by considering both symptom severity and functioning, with rating based on the more impaired of these two dimensions. In other words, someone who appears to function well but who is seriously considering suicide would receive a very low GAF rating.

Healthy, well-functioning people generally have GAF scores between 81 and 100. People with mild, transient symptoms usually have ratings between 71 and 80. Most people seen in outpatient settings, presenting concerns such as Mood Disorders, Anxiety Disorders, and Personality Disorders, typically are rated in the 50–70 range while people requiring inpatient treatment usually have GAF ratings below 50. GAF ratings are very useful in determining the nature and level of appropriate treatment and also in tracking progress over time.

The *DSM-IV-TR* assumes that a person's principal diagnosis is the first listed on Axis I. Only when another diagnosis is viewed as the principal diagnosis does that need to be specified. The *DSM-IV-TR* offers the optional use of the descriptor "Reason for Visit," most likely to be used if a presenting concern is listed but is not viewed by the clinician as the principal diagnosis. For example, a person who sought counseling for a Sleep Disorder (Reason for Visit) was found to have a Mood Disorder (Principal Diagnosis) that contributed to the sleep disorder.

Clinicians using the *DSM* generally specify the severity of a person's mental disorders as *Mild, Moderate,* or *Severe*. For a descriptor of Mild, a person must meet at least the minimal criteria for a particular disorder and manifest impairment that is mild relative to that disorder. The terms Moderate and Severe suggest greater impairment and more symptoms. Moderate suggests that a disorder could be presented with far worse symptoms than the client manifests.

Three descriptors also are available to describe past disorders. The descriptor *In Partial Remission* characterizes a mental disorder that once was present but is now manifested in more limited ways that do not meet the diagnostic criteria for the disorder. *In Full Remission* describes the presentation of disorders that are still clinically relevant but whose symptoms are no longer evident, perhaps because the person is receiving medication for the disorder. Another descriptor, *Prior History*, allows disorders to be listed that may have been absent or in remission for years but that are noteworthy, perhaps because they have a tendency to recur under stress.

EXAMPLE OF A MULTIAXIAL ASSESSMENT

The following is an example of a multiaxial assessment, reflecting the symptoms and concerns of Cathy, a 47-year-old woman.

Axis I.	296.23 Major depressive disorder, single episode, severe, without psychotic features.
	300.23 Social phobia, moderate.
Axis II.	301.6 Dependent personality disorder.
Axis III.	714.0 Arthritis, rheumatoid.
Axis IV.	Marital separation, change in residence.
Axis V.	GAF = 40.

The Principal Diagnosis for Cathy is Major Depressive Disorder. Specifiers indicate this is the first time she has had this disorder and that her symptoms are severe, although she is not out of touch with reality. In addition to presenting symptoms of incapacitating depression, unwarranted guilt, loss of appetite, and difficulty sleeping related to her Major Depressive Disorder, Cathy reported that throughout her life she had been uncomfortable in social situations that involved meeting new people in large groups. Much to her regret, she had avoided attending her children's school programs and her husband's office parties because of what she viewed as an irrational fear. Cathy experienced strong anxiety during her occasional involvement in large-scale meetings or social events. These symptoms suggest another Axis I diagnosis, Social Phobia, listed second because it has a lower treatment priority than does the Major Depressive Disorder.

Cathy also reported that she had low self-esteem and always tried her best to please others, regardless of her own feelings. She almost never disagreed with anyone and rarely took any initiative. Cathy lived with her parents until she was 27 and then married a man chosen for her by her father. She has spent the last 20 years caring for her home, her husband, and her children according to guidelines established by her husband. Although Cathy sometimes found her life rewarding, she usually felt bored and unfulfilled. However, she had never tried to make a change because she believed she was not capable of holding a job and felt she should always be available to meet the needs of her family. She reported great difficulty in decision-making and generally let her husband make all family decisions. Cathy also stated that she felt frightened and desperate when she was alone. These symptoms suggest a diagnosis of a Dependent Personality Disorder.

Cathy's physician made the diagnosis of arthritis on Axis III. Painful and sometimes disabling arthritis contributed to Cathy's fears and self-doubts.

Axis IV indicates the stressors in Cathy's life during the past year. Cathy's husband has asked for a divorce. They have sold their home and Cathy and her children now live with her parents.

The rating of 40 on Axis V reflects Cathy's depression, which includes some fleeting suicidal thoughts. Her counselor did not believe Cathy presented a danger to herself. However, close monitoring of her progress is needed in light of this GAF score.

This multiaxial assessment describes and promotes understanding of Cathy's difficulties. Counselors now could begin to plan Cathy's treatment based on this information.

THE 17 DIAGNOSTIC CATEGORIES

The *DSM-IV-TR* includes 17 broad categories, with multiple diagnoses included in each category. This section will present an overview of these diagnoses. Information on the treatment of these disorders will be provided in subsequent chapters.

DISORDERS USUALLY FIRST DIAGNOSED IN INFANCY, CHILDHOOD, OR ADOLESCENCE

The first category in the *DSM* is the most extensive and diverse. It includes disorders that typically begin before the age of 18, although most may persist into adulthood and may not be diagnosed until then. The following reflects the subcategories and their diagnostic features.

1. *Mental Retardation*—This category is typified by an IQ score below 70, accompanied by impairment in adaptive functioning (life skills). The *DSM-IV-TR* specifies four levels of severity: mild, moderate, severe, and profound. About 85% of people with this disorder meet the criteria for Mild Mental Retardation. By *DSM* definition, Mental Retardation begins before age 18. It is listed on Axis II, as is Borderline Intellectual Functioning discussed later.

2. *Learning Disorders*—These disorders reflect a pattern in which a person's achievement in a specific area is at least two standard deviations below that person's IQ score and interferes with academic or other functioning. The *DSM-IV-TR* identifies three specific areas of learning problems—*reading, mathematics, written expression*—as well as *Learning Disorder Not Otherwise Specified* (NOS) used

for other areas of learning. Standardized tests should be used to assess both achievement and intelligence. Problems of self-esteem, socialization, discouragement, and adjustment often accompany Learning Disorders. Approximately 5% of students in public schools in the United States have been diagnosed with a Learning Disorder, with reading being the most common. These students are at elevated risk of dropping out of school and of having Attention-Deficit and Disruptive Behavior Disorders (APA, 2000).

    3. *Motor Skills Disorder—Developmental Coordination Disorder*, the only disorder in this section, is characterized by motor coordination that is substantially below what would be expected, based on age and intellectual factors, and is severe enough to interfere with functioning. Coordination difficulties typically are reflected in crawling, sitting, walking, handwriting, and active play.

    4. *Communication Disorders*—This group includes four language disorders that interfere with academic and occupational achievement and socialization. *Expressive Language Disorder* is typified by a marked deficit in verbal skills (e.g., slow language development, limited vocabulary, errors in tense, use of only a few sentence structures). *Mixed Receptive/Expressive Language Disorder* describes symptoms that include difficulty with expressive as well as receptive language (understanding language). *Phonological Disorder* entails failure to use appropriate speech sounds (e.g., lisping, omission of certain sounds). Finally, *Stuttering* involves disturbances in verbal fluency and patterning. Communication Disorders are usually evident before age 5; early diagnosis and treatment can lead to a more rapid resolution of the difficulties. Care should be taken in diagnosing Communication Disorders in people who are bilingual, whose first language is not English, or who come from homes where the language of the person's current culture is not usually spoken. This diagnosis usually is not appropriate if the sole source of the communication problem is lack of adequate opportunity to learn the language.

    5. *Pervasive Developmental Disorders*—This section also includes four disorders: *Autistic Disorder, Rett's Disorder, Childhood Disintegrative Disorder*, and *Asperger's Disorder*. All are characterized by severe and pervasive impairment in one or more of the following areas: reciprocal social interaction, communication, and behavior (e.g., restricted activities, stereotyped behavior). These disorders begin in childhood and cause considerable impairment in functioning. Autistic Disorder begins before age 3 and involves impairment in all three of the above areas. It is often accompanied by mental retardation. Rett's Disorder, reported only in females, also involves pervasive impairment and mental retardation but is distinguished by a later onset (usually between 5 and 48 months, following a period of normal development) and by a deceleration in head growth. Childhood Disintegrative Disorder is evident between 2 and 10 years of age and involves deterioration leading to impairment in at least two of the three areas (social

interaction, communication, and behavior). Asperger's Disorder typically does not entail severe impairment in language, thinking, or self-help skills; problems focus on social interaction and behavior. Pervasive Developmental Disorders seem to be increasing for reasons not yet identified. Once considered very rare, approximately one million adults and children in the United States probably now have one of these disorders (Nash, 2002).

6. *Attention-Deficit and Disruptive Behavior Disorders*—This section includes what are probably the most common and important disorders found in children and adolescents: Attention-Deficit/Hyperactivity Disorder (*ADHD*), *Conduct Disorder*, and *Oppositional Defiant Disorder*. ADHD often coexists with one of the other two disorders. In addition, these disorders are often accompanied by depression, substance use, Learning Disorders, and impairment in academic functioning as well as peer and family relationships.

Three subtypes of *ADHD* are described in the *DSM*. (1) The *Predominantly Inattentive Type* is characterized primarily by inattention (e.g., forgetfulness, carelessness, disorganization, difficulty sustaining attention, distractibility). Girls are more likely to have this type of ADHD, harder to diagnose because of its less obvious symptoms. (2) Symptoms of the *Predominantly Hyperactive-Impulsive Type*, not surprisingly, include primarily hyperactivity and impulsivity (e.g., impatience, fidgeting, excessive talking, high level of motor activity). (3) The *Combined Type* encompasses symptoms of both of these types. To justify the diagnosis of ADHD, symptoms must be observed in at least two settings (e.g., school and home) and the onset must be before age 7. Estimates suggest that 3–7% of school-age children meet the criteria for ADHD (APA, 2000). Symptoms of excessive motor activity typically diminish in adolescence and adulthood, but attention difficulties can persist through adulthood and are often hereditary.

Conduct Disorder, more common in boys, entails a persistent and pervasive pattern of violating rules and the rights of others, including, in the past 12 months, at least three incidents of negative behaviors such as aggression toward people and animals, destruction or damage of property, serious violations of rules, lying, and theft. Subtypes of this disorder include *Childhood-Onset*, beginning before age 10, and *Adolescent-Onset*, with a later onset and generally better prognosis and peer relationships. Many children who exhibit bullying behavior meet the criteria for Conduct Disorder. If the symptoms of Conduct Disorder begin before age 15 and persist beyond age 18, the diagnosis usually is changed to Antisocial Personality Disorder (APD), on Axis II.

Oppositional Defiant Disorder is characterized by at least 6 months of negativistic, defiant, disobedient, and hostile behavior, particularly directed toward authority figures. Oppositional Defiant Disorder, usually evident by age 8, has a better prognosis than Conduct Disorder but it too can cause considerable impairment in family relationships and functioning at school. This disorder can evolve into Conduct Disorder.

7. *Feeding and Eating Disorders of Infancy or Early Childhood*—This group includes *Pica*, repeated eating of nonnutritive substances such as paint, clay, or leaves; *Rumination Disorder*, a disorder of early childhood involving persistent regurgitation and rechewing of food; and *Feeding Disorder of Infancy and Early Childhood*, beginning before age 6, and characterized by a refusal to eat adequately. All three disorders have a minimum duration of 1 month.

8. *Tic Disorders*—These disorders entail sudden, rapid, and recurrent involuntary motor movements or vocalizations that typically worsen under stress and last at least 4 weeks. *Tourette's Disorder*, a severe tic disorder, involves multiple motor tics and at least one vocal tic, sometimes including coprolalia (expression of socially unacceptable words such as obscenities or racial slurs). By definition, Tourette's Disorder begins by age 18 and lasts at least 1 year.

9. *Elimination Disorders*—This section lists disorders that entail repeated problems with bowel control (*Encopresis*) or bladder control (*Enuresis*) in children old enough to be toilet-trained (age 4 for Encopresis and 5 for Enuresis). Encopresis often has a physiological basis while people with enuresis usually have a first-degree biological relative who had the same disorder.

10. *Other Disorders of Infancy, Childhood,* or *Adolescence*—This section includes the remaining four diagnoses in this category of the *DSM*. *Separation Anxiety Disorder* is characterized by difficulty separating from home or caregivers as well as associated anxiety. It can involve refusal to go to school or to be alone as well as nightmares and multiple fears. Duration is at least 4 weeks. The primary symptom of *Selective Mutism* is a failure to speak in certain situations where speech is expected, despite speaking in other situations. Usually people with this disorder, which lasts at least 1 month, speak at home but not in other settings. The symptoms of *Reactive Attachment Disorder* begin before age 5 and involve problems in attachment or relatedness, stemming from a history of neglect or poor care. The *Inhibited Type* of this disorder is characterized by avoidance and ambivalence in interactions, while the *Disinhibited Type* is characterized by indiscriminate familiarity with others. *Stereotypic Movement Disorder*, the final diagnosis in this category, is typified by at least 4 weeks of repetitive and apparently driven motor behavior, such as rocking, hand waving, or head banging, that causes impairment and even self-injury. This disorder is often associated with mental retardation or physical disabilities such as blindness.

DELIRIUM, DEMENTIA, AMNESTIC, AND OTHER COGNITIVE DISORDERS ———

Disorders in this section, all due to brain damage or dysfunction, are referred to as Cognitive Disorders. Psychiatrists or neurologists have the primary responsibility for diagnosing and treating people with these disorders. Although counselors do need to know the signs of Cognitive Disorders so they can make appropriate referrals and support the work of the physicians, most will not need detailed diagnostic information on these disorders. Common symptoms of Cognitive Disorders include memory impairment, confusion, poor judgment, and decline in intellectual functioning. These disorders are more common in later life and stem from a medical condition, substance use, or a combination of these.

The Cognitive Disorders include the following diagnostic groups:

1. *Delirium*—This reflects a disturbance of consciousness and cognitive abilities, characterized by rapid development of symptoms such as disorientation, difficulty focusing, perceptual disturbance, and memory impairment.
2. *Dementia*—Multiple cognitive deficits with significant impairment in memory and executive functioning typify Dementia. Changes in personality and impulse control also are often reported. Common causes include drugs or alcohol, Alzheimer's disease, strokes (*Vascular Dementia*), and other medical conditions such as AIDS, Parkinson's disease, and head trauma.
3. *Amnestic Disorders*—Amnestic Disorders are cognitive disorders in which memory impairment is the primary or only symptom.

MENTAL DISORDERS DUE TO A GENERAL MEDICAL CONDITION

This section of the *DSM-IV-TR* includes the following disorders, directly caused by physiological or medical conditions: *Catatonic Disorder Due to a General Medical Condition* (such as encephalitis), *Personality Change Due to a General Medical Condition* (such as temporal lobe epilepsy), and *Mental Disorder Not Otherwise Specified Due to a General Medical Condition*. The medical cause of all these disorders should be listed on Axis III, while the mental disorder is listed on Axis I. These disorders, like the Cognitive Disorders, are diagnosed and treated primarily by physicians, although counselors may collaborate with them on treatment.

SUBSTANCE-RELATED DISORDERS

This section includes both the psychologically or behaviorally based *Substance Use Disorders* (*Substance Abuse* and *Substance Dependence*) and the physiologically based *Substance-Induced Disorders*, all resulting from misuse of drugs or alcohol. Examples of Substance-Induced Disorders include Intoxication and Substance-Induced Mood Disorder.

Of the two types of Substance Use Disorders, Substance Dependence typically is more severe than Substance Abuse. Substance Dependence is characterized by significant impairment resulting from drug or alcohol use, including at least three prominent symptoms (e.g., tolerance, withdrawal, unsuccessful efforts to control the substance use, reduction in occupational or leisure activities, continued use despite recognition of one's substance-related problems) occurring at any time during a 12-month period. The following specifiers can be used to describe the diagnosis of Substance Dependence: With or Without Physiological Dependence, In Remission, On Agonist Therapy (such as Antabuse or Methadone), and In a Controlled Environment (such as a prison or half-way house).

The diagnosis of Substance Abuse also can entail significant impairment. It includes one of the following criteria related to drug or alcohol use: continued use despite interpersonal problems related to the substance, failure to fulfill professional or interpersonal obligations, recurrent substance use in hazardous situations (e.g., while operating machinery), or recurrent substance-related legal difficulties (e.g., charges of driving while intoxicated).

The Substance-Related Disorders are listed alphabetically by substance in the *DSM* and include disorders stemming from use of alcohol; amphetamines; caffeine; cannabis; cocaine; hallucinogens; inhalants; nicotine; opioids; phencyclidine; sedatives, hypnotics, or anxiolytics; and others (such as steroids). Polysubstance dependence involves the use of at least three groups of substances with no single substance predominating.

SCHIZOPHRENIA AND OTHER PSYCHOTIC DISORDERS

The following psychotic disorders not caused by a medical condition but including delusions, hallucinations, and/or catatonic behavior are included in this section of the *DSM*:

1. *Schizophrenia*—This disorder is characterized by severe, pervasive loss of contact with reality, causing significant impairment and extending over at least 6 months. Common symptoms are hallucinations (usually auditory), disorganized speech or behavior, and delusions. Subtypes of Schizophrenia include *Paranoid Type, Disorganized Type, Catatonic Type* (usually characterized by agitation or motoric immobility), *Undifferentiated Type*, and *Residual Type* (characterized by the flat affect and lack of motivation that often remains between episodes of hallucinations and delusions). Schizophrenia sometimes has a genetic basis, usually has a gradual onset beginning in early adulthood, and causes considerable impairment.

2. *Schizophreniform Disorder*—This disorder is similar to Schizophrenia, except in duration. It has a minimum duration of 1 month and a maximum duration of 6 months. The specifier, With or Without Good Prognostic Features (including good premorbid functioning, rapid onset, perplexity regarding the symptoms and an absence of flat affect), provides information on the probable course of this disorder. About one third of people with this disorder recover while the rest develop Schizophrenia or Schizoaffective Disorder (APA, 2000).

3. *Schizoaffective Disorder*—This can be thought of as a hybrid diagnosis, including symptoms of Schizophrenia along with those of a Mood Disorder. Specifiers indicate whether a person has the *Bipolar Type* or the *Depressive Type* of Schizoaffective Disorder.

4. *Delusional Disorder*—This disorder is characterized by nonbizarre (possible even if unlikely) delusions of at least 1-month duration. The delusions tend to be egosyntonic or consistent with the person's personality and outlook and tend to focus on an area of stress or dissatisfaction. This disorder usually is less pervasive and incapacitating than the psychotic disorders discussed above. Types of Delusional Disorder include *Erotomanic Type* (characterized by an imagined romantic relationship, usually with someone of higher status), *Grandiose Type* (believing erroneously that one has a special gift or talent), *Jealous Type* (imagined infidelity), *Persecutory Type* (delusion that others are seeking to harm oneself), *Somatic Type* (delusions related to the body such as having a parasite or emitting a foul odor), *Mixed Type*, and *Unspecified Type*.

5. *Brief Psychotic Disorder*—This disorder encompasses symptoms of either Schizophrenia or Delusional Disorder, but with a briefer duration (at least 1 day but no more than 1 month) and a better prognosis. Brief Psychotic Disorder has the following specifiers: With or Without Marked Stressors and With Postpartum Onset, characterizing a psychotic disorder beginning within 4 weeks postpartum.

6. *Shared Psychotic Disorder*—This disorder involves the development of delusions in one person in a close relationship with another person who already has a Psychotic Disorder, usually Schizophrenia.

MOOD DISORDERS

These common disorders are characterized by a depressed mood and/or an elevated mood. Like Schizophrenia, Mood Disorders usually begin in late adolescence or early adulthood and often have a genetic component. The depressive disorders are particularly common in women. The following specifiers are available to clarify a person's experience of a mood disorder:

- *Melancholic Features* describes disorders characterized by loss of pleasure in almost all activities, as well as loss of reactivity.

- *Atypical Features*—strong mood reactivity, excessive sleeping and eating, and rejection sensitivity.
- *Catatonic Features*—motoric immobility or excessive activity.
- *Rapid Cycling*—at least four episodes of mood disturbance during 12 months of a Bipolar Disorder.
- *Seasonal Pattern*—a temporal relationship between mood disorder and season, usually reflected in winter depression.
- *Postpartum Onset*—prominent mood symptoms beginning within 4 weeks postpartum.
- *With or Without Interepisode Recovery*—recovery between episodes is associated with a better prognosis and the possibility of a seasonal pattern.

Included in the section on Mood Disorders are the following three mental disorders:

1. *Major Depressive Disorder*—Significant depression of at least 2 weeks duration characterizes this disorder. Suicidal ideation, hopelessness, loss of pleasure, and unreasonable guilt can be present as well as changes in appetite, weight, sleep patterns, and libido. This is probably the disorder most often treated in both inpatient and outpatient settings.

2. *Dysthymic Disorder*—This disorder is characterized by prolonged depression of moderate severity. It has a minimum duration of 1 year in children and adolescents and 2 years in adults. Sometimes people become so accustomed to this low-level depression that they are unaware that they are experiencing a significant mental disorder.

3. *Bipolar Disorders* involve mood fluctuations and include the following three diagnoses:

   a. *Bipolar I Disorder*—This includes at least one manic episode and may also include depressive, hypomanic, and mixed episodes. Manic episodes usually entail such symptoms as an elevated or irritable mood, inflated self-esteem, diminished need for sleep, rapid and pressured speech, loss of inhibitions, distractibility, poor judgment, and excessive pleasure-seeking and risk-taking behavior. Hypomanic episodes are similar to manic episodes but are less severe and incapacitating. Depressive episodes are like the mood episodes that characterize a Major Depressive Disorder. In a mixed episode, people meet the criteria for both manic and depressive episodes within one week.

   b. *Bipolar II Disorder*—This disorder is similar to Bipolar I but involves only hypomanic and depressive episodes; people with this disorder have never had a manic episode.

   c. *Cyclothymic Disorder*—This disorder is characterized by numerous episodes of hypomania and mild-to-moderate depression within a period of at least 2 years for adults and 1 year for children and adolescents.

In recent years, a considerable increase has been observed in adolescents presenting symptoms of Bipolar Disorders (Wilkinson, Taylor, & Holt, 2002). Symptoms tend to be more consistent than they are in adults and often include prolonged rage and tantrums, defiance of authority, disturbed sleep cycles, and impulsivity. Comorbid disorders, particularly Substance Use Disorders, are common as are suicidal ideation and academic, social, and family problems.

ANXIETY DISORDERS

Physical symptoms of anxiety (e.g., palpitations, sweating, trembling, dizziness, chills), subjective distress, and avoidance behavior characterize all the disorders in this section including:

   • *Panic Disorder With or Without Agoraphobia*—Hallmarks of these disorders are recurrent, brief, unexpected attacks of panic (usually as brief as 5 minutes and rarely longer than 30 minutes) as well as at least 1 month of concern about these attacks. Because the panic attacks have no obvious trigger, people with Panic Disorders often avoid any situations they believe might trigger a panic attack. This can lead to accompanying agoraphobia.
   • *Agoraphobia Without History of Panic Disorder*—Fear of crowded or other places from which escape might be difficult characterizes this disorder. To cope with their anxiety, people avoid fear-inducing places, especially when alone. People with severe forms of this disorder may not leave their homes for years.
   • *Specific Phobia*—This disorder involves a persistent and excessive fear of a stimulus. That fear markedly interferes with daily activities or causes significant distress even though people recognize that the fear is unreasonable. Subtypes include *Animal Type, Natural Environment Type* (e.g., heights, water, thunder), *Blood-Injection-Injury Type, Situational Type* (e.g., bridges, elevators, flying), and *Other Type*. Minimum duration in adults is 6 months.
   • *Social Phobia*—This disorder is characterized by a persistent and excessive fear of certain social or performance situations that pose the risk of embarrassment such as public speaking or parties. If the manifestation of this disorder extends to nearly all social activities, it is described as *Generalized Type*. As with Specific Phobia, although people recognize the excessive nature of their fears, they continue to experience distress or impairment resulting from the fears for at least 6 months.

• *Obsessive–Compulsive Disorder*—This disorder is characterized by recurrent unwanted thoughts (obsessions) and/or repetitive unwanted behaviors (compulsions) that cause distress and impairment. Washing, checking, counting, and repeating actions are particularly common compulsions; obsessions typically focus on violence, sinfulness, and contamination. The obsessive behaviors usually are designed to reduce anxiety and prevent negative situations. People with this disorder usually are aware that their thoughts and behaviors are excessive or illogical. If this is not the case, the specifier *With Poor Insight* is used.

• *Posttraumatic Stress Disorder* (PTSD)—This disorder has a minimum duration of 1 month and is triggered by an event that involves actual or threatened death or injury. PTSD is characterized by helplessness and horror upon witnessing the event, persistent reexperiencing of the event, avoidance and withdrawal, as well as increased arousal. Symptoms can be immediate or delayed for long periods of time. People with PTSD have undergone such experiences as war, rape, a serious accident, or a natural disaster. PTSD can also be found in police, fire fighters, and others who deal with or have observed life-threatening experiences and their aftermath. Specifiers include *Acute*, when the symptoms have lasted less than 3 months; *Chronic*, when they have lasted 3 months or longer; and *With Delayed Onset*, indicating that symptoms did not begin for at least 6 months after the traumatic event.

• *Acute Stress Disorder*—This diagnosis describes trauma-related reactions that do not persist as long as PTSD. Acute Stress Disorder can be viewed as a brief PTSD with rapid onset. This disorder begins within 4 weeks of a traumatic event; it lasts at least 2 days but no more than 4 weeks.

• *Generalized Anxiety Disorder*—This disorder is characterized by at least 6 months of excessive worry about multiple events and activities. Also present are physical symptoms of anxiety such as restlessness, irritability, tension, and sleep disturbance.

SOMATOFORM DISORDERS

People with Somatoform Disorders believe they have medical or physical diseases, illnesses, or abnormalities, and experience distress and impairment in functioning as a result. However, their complaints are not medically verified. Somatoform Disorders have been referred as psychosomatic disorders. People with these disorders seem to use their bodies as their vehicle for self-expression and often benefit from the secondary gains of their symptoms. However, they are not deliberately producing their physical symptoms and most are genuinely concerned about those symptoms. Care must be taken in diagnosing this disorder to be sure that a genuine medical condition has not been overlooked. The following mental disorders are included in this section:

- *Somatization Disorder*—People with this disorder (usually women) have a long history of multiple unverified physical complaints beginning before age 30. Criteria require a minimum of four pain symptoms, three gastrointestinal symptoms, one sexual symptom, and one pseudoneurological symptom.
- *Undifferentiated Somatoform Disorder*—This disorder, characterized by at least 6 months of distress or impairment in response to one or more medically unverified physical complaints, probably is more frequently used than Somatization Disorder. Clients' primary focus in both Somatization and Undifferentiated Somatoform Disorders generally is on the experience of the symptoms, not on the fear of disease.
- *Conversion Disorder*—This disorder typically is manifested in impairment in voluntary motor or sensory functioning such as paralysis of a limb, inability to see, or seizures, without medical cause. Subtypes include *With Motor Symptom or Deficit, With Sensory Symptom or Deficit, With Seizures or Convulsions*, and *With Mixed Presentations.*
- *Pain Disorder*—This disorder is characterized by a report of pain that either has no medical basis (*With Psychological Factors*) or is in excess of what would be expected, based on the existing medical problem (*With Both Psychological Factors and a General Medical Condition*). This disorder is *Acute* if it lasts less than 6 months; *Chronic*, if longer.
- *Hypochondriasis*—Hallmarks of this disorder include unwarranted preoccupation with having a serious disease and overinterpretation of physical symptoms, thereby causing significant distress or impairment. This disorder has a minimum duration of 6 months. The specifier, *With Poor Insight*, reflects a particularly treatment-resistant version of this disorder.
- *Body Dysmorphic Disorder*—This disorder involves preoccupation with an imagined or slight flaw in appearance, leading to significant distress and impairment. People with this disorder may have undergone many cosmetic surgeries; however, because their difficulty is emotional rather than physical, they are unlikely to feel much happier after their surgeries.

FACTITIOUS DISORDERS

Factitious Disorders differ from Somatoform Disorders in that Factitious Disorders involve intentional feigning of symptoms in order to assume the role of an ill person. This diagnosis has three subtypes, *With Predominantly Psychological*

Signs and Symptoms, With Predominantly Physical Signs and Symptoms, and *With Combined Psychological and Physical Signs and Symptoms.* The choice is based on whether the person presents with symptoms of a mental disorder or a medical condition. Sometimes people with this disorder attribute symptoms to, or even produce symptoms in, someone under their care, such as a child, an elderly person, or a disabled person, in order to receive attention and sympathy. This is known as *Factitious Disorder by Proxy* and is diagnosed as *Factitious Disorder NOS.*

DISSOCIATIVE DISORDERS

Dissociative Disorders involve a "disruption in the … functions of consciousness, memory, identity, or perception" (APA, 2000, p. 519) not caused by substance use or by a general medical condition. Consideration of multicultural variables is essential in diagnosing these disorders; sometimes their symptoms reflect culturally sanctioned responses. The *DSM-IV-TR* includes the following four Dissociative Disorders as well as Dissociative Disorder NOS, which can include trance states.

1. *Dissociative Amnesia*—This disorder involves inability to recall extensive and important information about one's identity or past, leading to significant distress or impairment. Usually the forgotten information is stressful or traumatic.
2. *Dissociative Fugue*—A sudden decision to travel away from one's home, along with confusion or memory loss related to one's identity, characterize this disorder. Often, it reflects an underlying wish to escape a current situation.
3. *Dissociative Identity Disorder* (DID)—DID is the current name for what used to be called Multiple Personality Disorder. DID is a more accurate term to describe people whose personalities have dissociated or fragmented. Such people may report having a range of diverse personalities of both genders, various ages, and widely differing abilities and presentations. This disorder, like Dissociative Amnesia and Fugue, usually entails inability to remember important information and can cause considerable distress and impairment. A history of abuse is common in people with this disorder. DID currently is a controversial diagnosis, with some people questioning the plausibility of so-called repressed memories which often typify DID and others reporting detailed cases of people with these symptoms.
4. *Depersonalization Disorder*—This disorder involves persistent, distressing experiences of feeling detached, in a dreamlike state, or outside one's body observing oneself. Transient symptoms of this disorder are common; the disorder should only be diagnosed if marked distress or impairment accompanies the symptoms.

SEXUAL AND GENDER IDENTITY DISORDERS

This category includes three groups of disorders: Sexual Dysfunctions, Paraphilias, and Gender Identity Disorders, along with Sexual Disorder NOS and Sexual Dysfunction NOS.

1. *Sexual Dysfunctions*—Disorders in this section describe sexual difficulties that are due either to psychological factors or to a combination of psychological factors and medical conditions. Specifiers indicate whether the symptoms are *Lifelong* or *Acquired, Generalized* or *Situational*. Sexual Dysfunctions include:

   a. *Sexual Desire Disorders*, including *Hypoactive Sexual Desire Disorder* (little or no desire) and *Sexual Aversion Disorder* (fear or disgust related to sexual intimacy);
   b. *Sexual Arousal Disorders*, including *Female Sexual Arousal Disorder* and *Male Erectile Disorder*;
   c. *Orgasmic Disorders*, including *Female Orgasmic Disorder, Male Orgasmic Disorder*, and in men *Premature Ejaculation*;
   d. *Sexual Pain Disorders*, including *Dyspareunia* (genital pain associated with intercourse) and *Vaginismus* (involuntary vaginal contractions which make intercourse painful if not impossible).

2. *Paraphilias*—Disorders in this section all involve a period of at least 6 months in which a person has a source of strong sexual arousal that involves nonhuman objects, suffering and humiliation, or children or other nonconsenting persons (APA, 2000). These urges and behaviors cause interpersonal difficulties and can also cause distress. People with these disorders are often resistant to treatment and may enter treatment via the court system or under pressure from another person. Paraphilias include:

   a. *Exhibitionism*—inappropriate exposure of one's genitals;
   b. *Frotteurism*—touching and rubbing against a nonconsenting person;
   c. *Fetishism*—sexual activity with objects such as a shoe or garment;
   d. *Pedophilia*—sexual activity with children 13 or younger;
   e. *Sexual Masochism*—deriving pleasure from experiencing suffering and humiliation during sexual activities;
   f. *Sexual Sadism*—deriving pleasure from sexual activities that entail inflicting suffering and humiliation;
   g. *Transvestic Fetishism*—cross-dressing;
   h. *Voyeurism*—observing others unclothed or engaged in sexual activities.

3. *Gender Identity Disorders*—These includes *Gender Identity Disorder in Children* and *Gender Identity Disorder in Adolescents and Adults*.

Both are characterized by significant distress or impairment related to discomfort with one's anatomical gender, accompanied by a strong identification with the other gender.

The Not Otherwise Specified diagnoses in Sexual and Gender Identity Disorders can include a broad array of symptoms related to sexual attitudes and functioning. Examples are marked distress about one's sexual orientation, feelings of sexual inadequacy, and overinvolvement with Cybersex, telephone sex, pornography, or multiple anonymous partners.

EATING DISORDERS

Two prevalent eating disorders, both most often found in young women, are in this section. Both can have serious medical consequences and Anorexia Nervosa, in particular, may even lead to death.

Anorexia Nervosa is characterized by refusal to maintain a healthy body weight, a weight that is 85% or less than what is expected based on the person's build, a strong fear of becoming overweight, a distorted body image, and absence of at least three consecutive menstrual cycles (in postmenarcheal females). Perfectionism and depression also often accompany this disorder. Specifiers for Anorexia Nervosa include *Restricting Type* if the low weight is due to limited eating and *Binge-Eating/Purging Type* if it is due to a pattern of excessive eating and purging.

Bulimia Nervosa is a disorder that entails recurrent binge eating (an average of two times a week for 3 months). Specifiers include *Purging Type*, if compensatory behaviors such as self-induced vomiting or excessive use of laxatives are present, and *Nonpurging Type*, if those behaviors are not manifested. Bulimia Nervosa also is often associated with depression.

Eating Disorder NOS can be used if people have symptoms of the above disorders but do not meet the full criteria for a specific eating disorder. For example, they may engage in purging without bingeing or significant weight loss.

SLEEP DISORDERS

In diagnosing Sleep Disorders, clinicians must determine whether other disorders are causing or related to the sleeping difficulties. Sleep Disorders that stand alone are called *Primary Sleep Disorders*, while those related to other diagnoses are classified under *Sleep Disorders Related to Another Mental Disorder* or *Sleep Disorders Due to a General Medical Condition*. Diagnosis of a Sleep Disorder often requires overnight assessment in a sleep clinic.

The *DSM-IV-TR* includes the following Sleep Disorders, all of which cause marked distress or impairment:

1. *Insomnia*—This disorder is characterized by difficulty initiating or maintaining sleep for at least 1 month and is often associated with depression.
2. *Hypersomnia*—Excessive sleepiness and difficulty awakening, with symptoms extending over at least 1 month, are the hallmarks of this disorder.
3. *Narcolepsy*—This diagnosis is characterized by uncontrollable attacks of sleep, occurring daily over at least 3 months, associated with rapid eye movements (REM) and sudden loss of muscle tone. The attacks are most likely to occur under conditions of high arousal or boredom.
4. *Breathing-Related Sleep Disorder*—This disorder, reportedly more common in men, involves a breathing condition that interferes with restful sleep and can lead to serious physical problems. Loud, sudden snoring following a period of silence when breathing has stopped can signal the presence of this disorder.
5. *Circadian Rhythm Sleep Disorder*—This diagnosis involves a mismatch between a person's circadian sleep–wake cycle and that person's lifestyle, leading to sleep disruption, fatigue, difficulty awakening, and reliance on substances to promote sleepiness or wakefulness. Types include *Delayed Sleep Phase Type*, *Jet Lag Type*, *Shift Work Type*, and *Unspecified Type*.
6. *Nightmare Disorder*—Frightening dreams are the hallmark of this disorder, usually occurring during REM sleep in the second half of the night and usually recalled upon awakening.
7. *Sleep Terror Disorder*—This disorder also involves frightening dreams, typically during the first third of a major sleep period, from which the person awakens terrified and disoriented.
8. *Sleepwalking Disorder*—Repeated walking while asleep characterizes this disorder.

IMPULSE-CONTROL DISORDERS NOT ELSEWHERE CLASSIFIED

Typically, people with Impulse-Control Disorders experience a buildup of tension that they release through dysfunctional impulsive behavior. Pleasure, relief, and sometimes regret follow the discharge of tension. This section encompasses the following disorders:

1. *Intermittent Explosive Disorder*—This disorder is characterized by episodes of violent and aggressive behavior out of proportion to the stimulus. The aggression can be expressed through assault or destruction of property. Substance-Related Disorders and Mood Disorders often accompany this disorder.

2. *Kleptomania*—Impulsive theft of objects that are not needed is the hall-mark of this disorder. It, too, often is accompanied by other disorders, especially Mood and Anxiety Disorders.

3. *Pyromania*—Recurrent fire setting, accompanied by a fascination with fire and fire fighting, is the primary symptom of this disorder, which is more prevalent in males than females.

4. *Pathological Gambling*—Persistent and self-destructive gambling charac-terizes this disorder, also more common in men. Depression, anxiety, deception, illegal efforts to obtain funds, and impaired relationships and careers are commonly associated with Pathological Gambling.

5. *Trichotillomania*—This disorder involves pulling out the hairs on one's own head or body, leading to noticeable hair loss. It is more common in females and is often associated with Mood, Anxiety, or other Impulse-Control Disorders.

6. *Impulse-Control Disorder Not Otherwise Specified*—Other impulsive symptoms, causing marked distress and impairment, can be included here. Examples are impulsive spending, repeated cutting or burning one-self, and picking one's skin.

ADJUSTMENT DISORDERS

Adjustment Disorders entail mild to moderate distress or impairment that develops within 3 months of a stressor (e.g., divorce, serious illness, abuse, relocation, school problems, retirement, job loss). This diagnosis can be maintained for a max-imum of 6 months after the end of the stressor and its consequences. This affords clinicians some flexibility in their use of this diagnosis, particularly when the stres-sor is an enduring one such as an illness or abuse. Subtypes of this disorder include *With Depressed Mood*, *With Anxiety*, *With Mixed Anxiety and Depressed Mood*, *With Disturbance of Conduct*, *With Mixed Disturbance of Emotions and Conduct*, and *Unspecified*. This disorder is described as *Acute* if the symptoms last less than 6 months or *Chronic* if the symptoms persist for a longer period of time.

PERSONALITY DISORDERS

Personality Disorders all involve long-standing deeply ingrained, pervasive, and maladaptive behaviors. People with these disorders typically have poor social skills, difficulty with impulse control, inflexibility, and impairment in most or all areas of their lives. Some people with these disorders experience distress while others externalize responsibility for their difficulties. Personality Disorders are usually evident by adolescence or early adulthood; symptoms must be present for at least a year before they can be diagnosed in a child. Personality Disorders are listed on Axis II of the multiaxial assessment and are very prevalent.

The following list includes the ten Personality Disorders, divided into three clusters, along with their primary characteristics:

Cluster A—characterized by odd or eccentric features:

1. *Paranoid Personality Disorder*—Pervasive distrust and suspiciousness characterize people with this disorder. They typically expect others to criticize, betray, or harm them and so share little with others and often hold grudges. This Personality Disorder is described as *Premorbid* if it precedes the onset of Schizophrenia.
2. *Schizoid Personality Disorder*—Indifference to other people, detachment, involvement primarily with solitary and non-people-oriented activities, lack of close relationships, and emotional restriction are all typical of people with this disorder.
3. *Schizotypal Personality Disorder*—Impaired social skills, poor awareness of reality reflected in symptoms such as ideas of reference and magical thinking, personal oddities and eccentricities, and restricted affect are hallmarks of this disorder.

Cluster B—characterized by emotional, dramatic, and egocentric features:

1. *Antisocial Personality Disorder (APD)*—Disregard for the laws and the rights of others, impulsivity, irresponsibility, and lack of remorse characterize this disorder. APD is not diagnosed until age 18 and must be preceded by Conduct Disorder beginning before age 15. A large percentage of people who are incarcerated have APD, which is more common in men.
2. *Borderline Personality Disorder*—Low self-esteem, feelings of emptiness, instability, problems with impulse control, dependence on others, inappropriate anger, and depression are primary features of this disorder. Borderline Personality Disorder is more common in females and is often associated with a history of abuse as well as self-injurious and suicidal behavior.
3. *Histrionic Personality Disorder*—High emotionality, attention seeking, excessive focus on physical appearance and intimate relationships, egocentrism, and suggestibility are characteristic of people with this disorder.
4. *Narcissistic Personality Disorder*—Egocentrism, high need for power and admiration, and a sense of entitlement and specialness are features of this disorder. People with this disorder are usually male and often appear arrogant and grandiose, with little empathy for others.

Cluster C—characterized by anxiety, fearfulness, and self-doubts.

1. *Avoidant Personality Disorder*—Social discomfort and avoidance, low self-esteem, and hypersensitivity characterize people with this disorder. They often desire more social contact but are fearful of criticism and inhibited about socializing.

2. *Dependent Personality Disorder*—Lack of initiative, deference to the wishes of others, difficulty making decisions, submissiveness, a need to be taken care of, and overinvestment in relationships are typical of people with this disorder. Although it seems to be more common in women than in men, this diagnosis should not be applied inappropriately to women who follow traditional paths but do not manifest the pathology associated with this disorder.

3. *Obsessive–Compulsive Personality Disorder*—Perfectionism, inflexibility, self-righteousness, rigidity, and a tendency to be controlling characterize people with this disorder. Their devotion to work and adherence to rules can bring some occupational success, but difficulty completing tasks often undermines their efforts. People with this disorder typically have considerable difficulty as partners, parents, and supervisors.

Personality Disorder NOS can be used for Personality Disorders that are mixed (include elements of two or more Personality Disorders but do not fully meet the criteria for any one) or for pervasive patterns that resemble Personality Disorders. Examples are Depressive Personality Disorder and Passive–Aggressive Personality Disorder.

Personality Traits—These are milder than Personality Disorders, perhaps less pervasive, enduring, or disruptive. Personality Traits come in the same varieties as Personality Disorders (e.g., Dependent Personality Traits, Avoidant Personality Traits). Although they have no code numbers and are not considered mental disorders, they are listed on Axis II and can provide useful descriptive information about a person's patterns of behavior and thinking.

OTHER CONDITIONS THAT MAY BE A FOCUS OF CLINICAL ATTENTION

The terms in this section identify areas that may be a focus of attention in counseling but are not considered mental disorders. These terms may stand alone if they are used to describe a person who does not have a mental disorder or they may be used along with one or more mental disorders on a multiaxial assessment to indicate essential issues to be addressed in treatment.

This section is comprised of the following conditions:

1. *Psychological Factors Affecting Medical Condition*—This condition is reflected by the presence of a personality, behavioral, or emotional condition

that has a negative impact on a general medical condition, such as anxiety worsening high blood pressure or the impact of persistently eating high-fat foods on cholesterol. The medical condition is listed on Axis III.

2. *Medication-Induced Movement Disorders*—This section contains conditions such as *Neuroleptic-Induced Tardive Dyskinesia* and *Medication-Induced Postural Tremor* that reflect the adverse physiological effects of neuroleptic or other medications.

3. *Relational Problems*—This section encompasses *Relational Problem Related to a Mental Disorder or General Medical Condition, Parent–Child Relational Problem, Partner Relational Problem, Sibling Relational Problem*, and *Relational Problem Not Otherwise Specified* that are used to refer to problems with friends, in-laws, coworkers, or others not named here.

4. *Problems Related to Abuse or Neglect*—This section includes *Physical Abuse of Child, Sexual Abuse of Child, Neglect of Child*, and *Physical Abuse of Adult*. These conditions can be used to describe either the survivor or the perpetrator of abuse.

5. *Additional Conditions that may be a Focus of Clinical Attention*—Included in this final miscellaneous group of conditions are the following:

   a. *Noncompliance with Treatment* entails refusing needed treatment for either a mental disorder or a medical condition.

   b. *Malingering* is deliberately feigning or exaggerating symptoms, perhaps to obtain financial gain, prescriptions for drugs, or diminished responsibilities.

   c. *Adult, Adolescent,* or *Childhood Antisocial Behavior* encompasses antisocial behavior not due to a mental disorder. Usually it is manifested by isolated acts rather than persistent patterns.

   d. *Borderline Intellectual Functioning*, listed on Axis II, is characterized by an IQ between 71 and 84, as measured by standardized tests.

   e. *Age-Related Cognitive Decline* includes memory impairment within normal limits.

   f. *Bereavement* identifies grief reactions to the recent death of a loved one.

   g. *Academic Problem, Occupational Problem, Identity Problem, Religious or Spiritual Problem*, and *Acculturation Problem* describe distress or difficulty related to such areas as academic achievement, career development, sense of self, religious beliefs and affiliation, and adjustment to cultural change.

   h. *Phase of Life Problem* includes issues linked to a particular age or life stage, such as problems related to graduation from school, marriage, entering a new occupation, parenting, divorce, retirement, and many others.

ADDITIONAL CODES

Of course, not every client has a mental disorder or condition on Axis I and Axis II. When a diagnosis is not appropriate, the phrases No Diagnosis or Condition on Axis I and No Diagnosis on Axis II can be used. Diagnosis or Condition Deferred or Unspecified Mental Disorder can also be written on either axis to indicate diagnostic uncertainty. In addition, as already mentioned, at the end of each major category in the *DSM* is an NOS diagnosis (e.g., Sexual Disorder Not Otherwise Specified, Mood Disorder Not Otherwise Specified). The NOS diagnoses are sometimes useful in labeling symptoms that do not exactly match a specific diagnosis but clearly represent a mental disorder.

MAKING A DIAGNOSIS

When symptoms are prominent and clinicians are astute, mental disorders can be immediately apparent. At other times, clinicians can use some tools to help them make diagnoses.

Decision Trees

Appendix A of the *DSM-IV-TR* includes six decision trees to facilitate the process of diagnostic discrimination. Each tree consists of a series of boxed descriptive statements that act as yes-or-no questions. To use these tools, the clinician begins at the upper left box in each tree and then follows the arrows determined by responses to the items in the boxes until the clinician arrives at a diagnosis. The six decision trees include:

1. *Mental Disorders Due to a General Medical Condition*—This tree lists mental disorders that are caused by a medical illness or condition.
2. *Substance-Induced Disorders*—This tree includes disorders that are a direct consequence of drug or alcohol use such as Substance-Induced Sexual Dysfunction and Substance Withdrawal. The tree does not include Substance Dependence or Substance Abuse.
3. *Psychotic Disorders*—Schizophrenia, Schizophreniform Disorder, Schizoaffective Disorder, Delusional Disorders, Brief Psychotic Disorder, and other disorders that entail loss of contact with reality are included in this tree.
4. *Mood Disorders*—This tree encompasses Major Depressive Disorder, Dysthymic Disorder, Bipolar I and II Disorders, and Cyclothymic Disorder, all characterized by depression, irritability, expansiveness, and/or an elevated mood.

5. *Anxiety Disorders*—Panic Disorders, Agoraphobia, Specific and Social Phobias, PTSD, Acute Stress Disorder, Obsessive–Compulsive Disorder, Generalized Anxiety Disorder, Separation Anxiety Disorder, and other disorders with anxiety, fear, increased arousal, and avoidance as their hallmarks are included in this tree.

6. *Somatoform Disorders*—Disorders characterized primarily by physical complaints that do not have a verified medical explanation are listed in this tree. This includes all the Somatoform Disorders (e.g., Somatization Disorder, Conversion Disorder, Pain Disorder, Hypochondriasis, Body Dysmorphic Disorder), the Factitious Disorders, Psychological Factors Affecting Medical Condition, and other disorders and conditions. Although physical complaints may produce anxiety, when the physical complaints are the person's primary concern, this tree, rather than the Anxiety Disorders tree, should be consulted.

<hr>

Key Questions for Diagnosis

Although the decision trees are very useful, they do not include all mental disorders. A more comprehensive approach to diagnosis is the use of the following four key questions:

1. *What are the primary symptoms?*—This question should be answered in nontechnical terms, with typical symptoms including anxiety, depression, acting out, excessive consumption of alcohol, medically unverified physical pain, or pervasive dysfunction.

2. *What is the approximate duration of the disorder?*—Responses might include number of days, weeks, months, or years, or indicate that the disorder is of indefinite and long-standing duration.

3. *How severe are the symptoms?*—Assessment of severity is comparable to Axis V, the Global Assessment Scale of the Multiaxial Assessment, but uses verbal descriptors rather than numerical ratings. Severity is assessed by considering both distress and impairment. Adjustment Disorders typically are mild, while a Dysthymic Disorder is in the mild-to-moderate range. Disorders of moderate severity include many of the Personality Disorders and most of the Mood and Anxiety Disorders. A Borderline Personality Disorder might be described as moderate-to-severe. Disorders that cause great impairment and loss of contact with reality, such as most of the Psychotic and Cognitive Disorders, are severe.

4. *Has a specific cause or precipitant for the symptoms been identified?*— This yes-or-no question often provides important diagnostic information.

Application of the Key Questions

Appendix A provides a series of tables, applying the key questions to the most common mental disorders. Using those tables in conjunction with the *DSM* facilitates the diagnostic process. Table A1 divides the mental disorders into seven broad categories: Adjustment Disorders and Conditions; Behavior and Impulse-Control Disorders; Mood Disorders; Anxiety Disorders; Somatoform Disorders, Factitious Disorders, and Malingering; Personality Disorders; and Cognitive, Dissociative, and Psychotic Disorders. Readers can identify the broad category in which a client's symptoms fall by responding to the Key Questions and comparing those responses with those on Table A1. A note under the name of each of the seven categories on Table A1 suggests additional tables in the A3 series that readers should review to make a precise diagnosis.

Another approach to making a diagnosis based on the Key Questions is provided in Table A2. This table is organized according to primary symptoms (Key Question 1). Once primary symptoms have been located on Table A2, additional tables in the A3 series can help readers make a specific diagnosis.

Next, readers should progress onto the suggested tables in the A3 series, comparing responses to the Key Questions to the key descriptions for each diagnosis in those tables. This process should lead to the correct diagnosis.

Finally, the *DSM* or earlier sections of this chapter can be used to identify appropriate specifiers for the diagnosis. Incorporating additional client information can help integrate this diagnosis into a multiaxial assessment.

The following example illustrates the application of the key questions:

Case. A 28-year-old single female lawyer sought counseling 3 weeks after she discovered that the man she had been dating and hoping to marry was already married. She reacted with bouts of sadness and crying, slightly diminished performance at work, and some withdrawal from friends and leisure activities, although she maintained a demanding work schedule and reported no suicidal ideation. She stated that she had never experienced similar feelings in the past. She was optimistic that, with some help, she could put this disappointment behind her, learn from this experience, and resume an active social life.
Primary symptoms: Sadness, crying, some impairment in coping with a stressful situation
Duration: Brief/several weeks
Severity: Mild
Precipitant: Yes

Table A1 identifies this client's diagnosis as an Adjustment Disorder (brief, mild–moderate, including a precipitant, involving problems in coping). Table A2 indicates that disorders characterized by depression (sadness) are in Table A.3.I; that table confirms the diagnosis of Adjustment Disorder.

SUPPLEMENTS TO THE *DSM*

Several worthwhile resources have been developed to help people refine their diagnostic skills. The *DSM-IV-TR Casebook* (Spitzer, Gibbon, Skodol, Williams, & First, 2002) is a compendium of interesting case vignettes with their appropriate diagnoses. This book acquaints its readers with a broad range of mental disorders. Other books that provide further clarification of the *DSM* include *DSM-IV Made Easy* (Morrison, 1995a), the four-volume *DSM-IV Sourcebook*, published by the American Psychiatric Association, and *Study Guide to DSM-IV-TR* (Fauman, 2002).

CASES FOR DIAGNOSIS

Assess your diagnostic abilities. Do a multiaxial assessment for the following five cases before looking at the answers that follow the last case.

Case 1. June is a 38-year-old elementary school teacher. Several months ago, while watching her students in the playground, she became extremely anxious; she felt her heart pounding and thought she might faint. Although she recovered within 20 minutes, she experienced these same symptoms a few weeks later in the school cafeteria and, not long after, while teaching her class. Since then, June has become apprehensive and is fearful about going to work each day. She has been taking so many sick days because of this fear that her job is now in jeopardy.

June's life over the past year has been difficult. Her mother died and she has been caring for her elderly father. She has tried to maintain an active social life but has found that difficult because of work and family demands. In addition, she has been diagnosed with endometriosis. Before this year, June functioned well, had several friends, and was involved in many activities. She had received high ratings at work.

Case 2. Fred is a 7-year-old boy who was brought to counseling by his mother. Fred's parents divorced about 2 years ago and Fred has seen little of his father since then. Two months ago, Fred's father remarried and moved to South America. Since the divorce, Fred has been sad and listless, although he is occasionally irritable. He had little appetite and often has difficulty falling asleep. He no longer had much enthusiasm, even for his favorite activities and friends. When he learned of his father's marriage and relocation, Fred's symptoms worsened considerably. His mother has great difficulty getting Fred out of bed in the morning. Two weeks ago, Fred's mother found him with a pillow over his head, trying to stop his breathing. Fred told her that he didn't want to live anymore because he felt so sad. Fred is in a special class because of his intellectual level (IQ score in the 73–77 range). Fred's mother also reports that Fred has never been fully toilet trained and continues to wet the bed at least twice a week. Fred has no apparent or reported medical conditions.

Case 3. Marcy, age 12, was brought to counseling by her parents. They reported that for the past 2 months, since the birth of her baby brother, Marcy has been difficult. She has a quick temper and is hostile and argumentative, she frequently disobeys her parents, she blames her teachers for her poor grades but will not ask them for help, and she has even been teasing her 6-year-old sister, whom she used to adore. Although Marcy has never been a strong student because of the great difficulty she has in writing, she is a bright girl who once welcomed help with her writing difficulty. Now, however, her attitude has changed; family as well as teachers report that she is difficult and uncooperative. A physical examination revealed no medical problems other than chronic asthma, diagnosed about 7 years earlier.

Cases 4 and 5. Peter and Doris came for counseling at the urging of Doris's oncologist. Peter and Doris, both age 44, have been married for 22 years and have three children, aged 17, 14, and 9. Doris had always focused her energies on her family, cooking, cleaning, and sewing for long hours each day, in part to help her deal with her fear of being alone. She had few friends or outside interests and tended to cling to her husband and children, frequently asking their advice, rarely voicing her own opinion, and constantly seeking their approval. Recently, Doris had a hysterectomy because of a cancerous tumor. Her recovery has progressed slowly, partly because Doris insists on doing more than she should, although her physician has advised her to rest and recuperate for the next month. Doris expresses guilt about her illness and blames herself because the house is not as clean as it used to be. She is also very worried about the impact of her surgery on her family relationships, fearing that Peter will reject her and her children will no longer think she is a good mother.

In fact, Peter has hinted that if Doris is not back to normal soon, he will have to look elsewhere for gratification. Peter blames Doris for her medical condition, insisting that she should have seen a physician earlier, and expresses the belief that Doris is enjoying her illness because she is "getting a free ride" and "doesn't have to do anything around the house." This attitude is typical of Peter's behavior both at home and at work, where he often suspects that others are taking advantage of him and are untrustworthy. He has long-standing grudges against several of his coworkers and has been referred to the employee assistance program at work several times because of conflicts with others. When asked about these difficulties, Peter accuses the counselor of trying to make him look like a fool. However, Peter does report that he is concerned about his own health. For several years, he has believed that he has stomach cancer and cannot understand why Doris is getting so much attention when he is even sicker than she. He has consulted many physicians, both oncologists and specialists in gastrointestinal problems, but none could find a medical explanation for his intestinal discomfort.

Case 1. *June*
Axis I.   300.21 Panic Disorder With Agoraphobia, Moderate
Axis II.   V71.09 No Mental Disorder on Axis II
Axis III. 617.9 Endometriosis
Axis IV.   Death of mother, caretaking of father
Axis V.   55

Case 2. *Fred*
Axis I.   296.23 Major Depressive Disorder, Single Episode, Severe Without
           Psychotic Features
           300.4 Dysthymic Disorder, Moderate, Early Onset
           307.6 Enuresis, Nocturnal Only
Axis II.   V62.89 Borderline Intellectual Functioning
Axis III. None reported
Axis IV   Parents' divorce, little contact with father
Axis V.   20

Case 3. *Marcy*
Axis I.   309.4 Adjustment Disorder With Mixed Disturbance of
           Emotions and Conduct
           315.2 Disorder of Written Expression, Mild
Axis II.   V71.09 No Mental Disorder on Axis II
Axis III. 493.20 Asthma, Chronic Obstructive
Axis IV.   Family conflict, academic difficulties
Axis V.   63

Case 4. *Peter*
Axis I.   300.7 Hypochondriasis, With Poor Insight, Moderate
Axis II.   301.0 Paranoid Personality Disorder
Axis III. Deferred—reports intestinal discomfort
Axis IV.   Wife diagnosed with cancer, conflict at work, intestinal discomfort
Axis V.   55

Case 5. *Doris*
Axis I.   309.24 Adjustment Disorder With Mixed Anxiety and Depressed Mood
Axis II.   301.6 Dependent Personality Disorder
Axis III. 183.0 Neoplasm, Malignant, Uterus, Primary
Axis IV.   Diagnosis and treatment of cancer, conflict with husband
Axis V.   55

Now that you have some knowledge of and skill in diagnosis, you can build on that knowledge by acquiring tools for information gathering and approaches to treating mental disorders. Chapters 5 and 6 focus on information gathering using inventories, intake interviews, and the mental status examination. Chapters 7–11 focus on treatment planning and delivery.

The Use of Assessment in Diagnosis and Treatment Planning

"The meaning of diagnosis is 'to know' the client in terms of both internal and external perspectives" (Blocher & Biggs, 1983, p. 186). The process of diagnosis can be approached in a comprehensive way that enables counselors to develop a good understanding of people and their environments and, through the process of assessment, formulate a diagnosis and treatment plan as well as enhance the counseling relationship. This chapter builds on the information provided in Chapter 3 by expanding your knowledge of the assessment process and describing many tools and procedures to facilitate assessment.

Most people who seek counseling are in pain and are eager for help. They generally respond well to a caring and empathic counselor. The assessment process should reflect these attitudes and affirm the importance and uniqueness of each person. It is a way of saying to a client, "You are special and I want to get to know and understand you so that I can determine the best way to help you." This message helps clients feel optimistic and committed to the counseling process. Ideally, assessment is a collaboration between counselor and client in which both gain in knowledge and understanding while enhancing their working relationship.

Historical Overview of Assessment

Formal study of individual human differences began in the late 19th and early 20th centuries (Walsh & Betz, 2001). Initial focus of this effort was on measurement of intelligence. Milestones occurred in 1905, when Alfred Binet and Theodore Simon developed the first widely used intelligence scale and in 1938, when David Wechsler developed the Wechsler–Bellevue Intelligence Scale. These are the precursors of today's widely used Stanford–Binet Intelligence Scale and the Wechsler Intelligence Scales.

Development of inventories to assess aptitudes and achievement, personality, and interests was not far behind. The Stanford Achievement Test, a comprehensive measure of scholastic abilities, was published in 1923; Carl Seashore's inventory, Measures of Musical Talent, was issued in 1918. Personality assessment began with the development of projective tests such as the Rorschach Inkblot Test (1921) and Henry Murray's Thematic Apperception Test (1938), both still used for in-depth personality assessment. The Minnesota Multiphasic Personality Inventory (MMPI), published in 1943, sought to provide a standardized and objective assessment of personality. Landmark interest inventories appeared at about the same time; the Strong Vocational Interest Blank was issued in 1934 and the Kuder Preference Record in 1934. Many of those early inventories proved their value over time; although much revised, they remain the prototypes for effective assessment.

The inventories of the early 20th century laid the groundwork for the assessment field of today. Assessment during the late 20th and early 21st centuries encompasses both the well-established inventories of the early 20th century and many new tools and approaches, such as those focusing on family dynamics and social environments.

Conducting an Effective Assessment

A structured assessment can occur at several points in a counseling relationship (although ongoing assessment is inherent in effective counseling). Some sort of assessment almost always occurs at the outset of the counseling process. Typically, an intake interview is conducted, perhaps accompanied by psychological testing, so that an initial diagnosis and treatment plan can be developed. Chapter 5 discusses the intake process in detail.

Structured assessment also can occur later in counseling. Assessment at that time can be occasioned by the counselor or client wanting to measure progress or recognizing that new issues and dynamics have come to light, requiring a reconceptualization of the original diagnosis and treatment plan. Such an assessment also can occur when an agency or managed care organization requests a review and progress report. Midcounseling assessments may be global, a way to provide an overview of the client's development and level of functioning, or they may be specific, seeking information on a particular aspect of the person's life (e.g., career development, intellectual ability, substance use). Assessments also may be conducted toward the end of the counseling process to measure goal attainment and determine the appropriateness of termination.

According to Shertzer and Linden (1979), assessment has four overriding purposes: classification, evaluation, selection, and prediction. All four may be involved in diagnosis and treatment planning. *Evaluation* and *classification* generally are most important as the counselor explores the cognitive, behavioral, emotional, interpersonal, and environmental aspects of a person and classifies the findings according to some framework (e.g., biopsychosocial, the *DSM*, developmental stages, levels of intellectual ability). Assessment for *selection* may be used to choose people for certain therapeutic programs (e.g., counseling groups, day treatment centers). *Predicting* the likelihood of events such as a person's succeeding in a particular educational program or engaging in violent or suicidal behavior also plays a part in treatment planning.

Benefits of Assessment

Assessment can enhance the counseling process in the following ways (Seligman, 1994):

1. Streamline and structure the information-gathering process.
2. Enhance the credibility and validity of that process.
3. Assess and promote motivation toward positive change and client–counselor collaboration.
4. Identify and measure the severity of people's symptoms and assess change in those symptoms.
5. Promote insight into a person's self-concept and self-esteem.
6. Clarify whether pathology is present and help determine the client's diagnosis.
7. Identify intellectual and academic strengths and weaknesses, as well as learning style.
8. Clarify leisure and career interests, needs, and values.
9. Provide information on personality style, affect, interpersonal skills, and overall personal strengths and difficulties.
10. Assess and quantify habits and behaviors.
11. Translate interests, abilities, and personality into occupational terms.
12. Provide information on environment, family constellation, social and multicultural background and context.
13. Determine a person's suitability for a particular program or treatment.
14. Facilitate development of a treatment plan that is likely to be effective.
15. Simplify goal setting.
16. Promote more relevant and focused counseling and discussion.
17. Generate options and alternatives.
18. Facilitate planning and decision-making.
19. Indicate likelihood of certain events (e.g., success in occupational or academic endeavors).
20. Determine whether and how much progress has been made.

Areas of Assessment

The assessment process may focus on any or all of the following areas:

1. *Cognitive Attributes*—Assessment may be comprehensive or specific, focusing on areas such as thinking and learning style, intellectual abilities, achievement, aptitude, problem solving, and awareness of reality.
2. *Behaviors*—Inventories look at overall behavioral patterns as well as specific behaviors such as eating, sleeping, substance use, attention, violence, assertiveness, and communication style.
3. *Personality and Affect*—Assessment may provide a comprehensive picture of personality or assess emotional states and traits such as mood, values, self-esteem, and anger.
4. *Interpersonal Relationships and Context*—Possible areas of focus include family background and dynamics, relationship patterns, interpersonal conflicts and strengths.
5. *Physical/Biological Attributes*—Often assessed are appearance, size and shape, physical abilities and disabilities, and medical conditions.
6. *Social and Multicultural Environment*—Assessment in this area may focus on socioeconomic level, cultural beliefs and values, support systems, and other variables.

Setting the Stage for Assessment

Assessment is an integral part of counseling. It should be planned and conducted with the same care as the overall counseling process. According to the ACA's ethical standards (1995, June, p. 36), "Counselors promote the welfare and best interests of the client in the development, publication, and utilization of educational and psychological assessment techniques." Increasingly, mental health professionals are recognizing that the counselor, not the test, is the key ingredient in effective assessment. As Anastasi (1992, p. 610) stated, "Most popular criticisms of tests are clearly identifiable as criticisms of test use (or misuse), rather than criticisms of the tests themselves. Tests are essentially tools. Whether any tool is an instrument of good or harm depends on how the tool is used."

Assessment should contribute to the development of rapport, advance the goals of counseling, and take account of the client's preferences and areas of difficulty. Both counselor and client should understand the purpose and nature of the assessment process and should be involved in its planning and implementation. Results should be shared in a timely and helpful way. Assessment may be formal or informal, ongoing or time-limited, and use any of a broad range of quantitative or qualitative tools. The rest of this chapter discusses the assessment process as well as the approaches and tools that are available for conducting an assessment.

PLANNING THE ASSESSMENT

The intake interview, discussed further in Chapter 5, is usually the core of the process of diagnosis and treatment planning. Often, however, the intake interview is not enough to give counselors a sound understanding of their clients. People who have difficulty with self-expression and insight, who are hostile or resistant, who are confused or severely disturbed, or present ill-defined or unusual symptoms are likely candidates for a structured assessment. Even when none of these characteristics is present, testing can enhance counseling. It can provide new ideas and perspectives, lend depth and clarity to available information, and promote discussion and exploration. However, assessment also can be threatening and arduous for clients and harmful to the client–counselor relationship. Counselors should ensure that the assessment process is both effective and expeditious; testing should not be routine or gratuitous, but should only be used to answer questions or fill in important gaps that cannot be resolved in less obtrusive ways.

Formulating Assessment Questions

Before deciding to use tests or inventories, counselors should ask themselves the following questions (Seligman, 1994):

1. What are the goals of the counseling process?
2. What information is needed to accomplish those goals?
3. Have available sources of information such as the client's own experiences and self-knowledge as well as previous records and tests been used effectively and fully?
4. Does it seem likely that testing and other forms of assessment will provide important information that is not available from other sources?
5. What important questions can be answered by the testing?
6. How should testing be planned and integrated into the counseling process to maximize its benefits?

Counselors should know what further information is needed before testing begins. Especially if the client is being referred elsewhere for testing, counselors must clarify the reasons for the assessment and communicate them as specifically as possible to the examiner. This is particularly likely to yield the needed information. Precise questions, such as the following, are typical of those asked during assessment:

- Does this person have a mental disorder? If so, what is the diagnosis?
- Does this person need hospitalization or is outpatient treatment adequate?
- What interpersonal patterns seem to undermine this person's social relationships?

- Is this child likely to perform satisfactorily in a regular classroom?
- What is the severity of this person's depression?
- What is this person's intellectual level?

Sometimes, such specific questions cannot be formulated because of a lack of clarity about a person's development and difficulties. In such cases, a general psychological assessment, involving a battery of tests combined with an interview, is typically used to provide a comprehensive picture of the person.

Selection of Inventories

Selection of assessment tools depends primarily on the purpose of the assessment. Other factors, however, also guide the choice of particular inventories out of the many that are available. Clinicians need to consider the stated purpose of the inventory, the qualifications and time required for its administration, the reading level of the inventory, the ages for which it is appropriate, the group on which its norms are based, the inventory's validity and reliability, efforts to minimize culture and gender bias in the inventory, the format of the inventory (e.g., computerized, true–false), the ways scores are obtained and presented, and the cost of the inventory. Catalogs of test publishers, test manuals, and references such as *Tests in Print, Tests, Test Critiques, Measures for Clinical Practice*, and *Mental Measurements Yearbook* can help counselors obtain this information and locate inventories that meet their needs. Websites such as the ERIC Clearinghouse on Assessment and Evaluation (http://ericae.net/), Association of Test Publishers (http://www.testpublishers.org/), and Buros Institute of Mental Measurements (http://www.unl.edu/buros) also are useful. Additional information on specific and commonly used inventories is provided later in this chapter.

Some examples of batteries of tests and inventories are:

1. General assessment conducted by a counselor of a person going through a midlife transition: California Psychological Inventory, Strong Interest Inventory, Lifestyle Assessment Questionnaire, Profile of Mood States, Values Scale.
2. General assessment conducted by a psychologist: Rorschach Test, Thematic Apperception Test, Projective Drawings, Bender–Gestalt, Wechsler Adult Intelligence Scale, Minnesota Multiphasic Personality Inventory.
3. Assessment of an adolescent with career confusion: Strong Interest Inventory, Differential Aptitude Test, Career Maturity Inventory, Hall Occupational Orientation Inventory.
4. Assessment of a person with significant depression and interpersonal concerns: Millon Clinical Multiaxial Inventory, Beck Depression Inventory, Myers–Briggs Type Indicator.

Preparing People for an Assessment

To maximize client motivation and reduce anxiety, counselors should work collaboratively with their clients to determine the questions they hope testing will answer and in planning the assessment process. Counselors should provide information on the purpose of the assessment, clarifying how it will benefit the client. They should provide details on the testing site, the length of the assessment process, the nature of the inventories to be administered, the name of the examiner, and what information the person can expect to receive from the assessment. (Of course, clients also should be informed in advance if they will not receive detailed information on their assessment, as often is the case with projective testing.) Clients should have an opportunity to ask questions and express their ideas about how to plan the testing as well as the selection of tests.

TOOLS OF ASSESSMENT

Assessment tools can be qualitative or quantitative. Qualitative tools are typically more subjective in nature, their interpretation being more ambiguous and challenging. They yield information that may have limited reliability and validity but can provide important insights that perhaps cannot be obtained in any other way. Quantitative tools, on the other hand, yield numerical data, thereby facilitating comparisons and providing a useful measure of change. The combination of qualitative and quantitative approaches to assessment can provide a picture with depth and richness as well as adequate reliability.

Qualitative Approaches

Qualitative methods are gaining credibility, both for assessment and research in counseling. Ponteretto (2002, p. 394) characterized qualitative research methods as the fifth force in psychology (following psychoanalysis, behaviorism, humanism, and multiculturalism).

   Interviews are the most important qualitative approach to assessment. They are nearly always part of the process of diagnosis and treatment planning and tend to be the first method used to gather information and build rapport with a client. The primary goals for the interviewer are having a clear purpose and direction in mind and conducting an interview that will achieve that purpose. However, interviewer bias, client resistance, and other factors can affect interviews, as well as other forms of qualitative data. Interviews are discussed further in Chapter 5.

   Counselor-made questionnaires often are combined with intake interviews and also can be useful in gathering information. Most mental health agencies use questionnaires as a way of gathering demographic and background information on clients. Counselors often supplement those with either general or specific questionnaires on people's concerns or on aspects of their development (e.g., marital adjustment, career development, social history). Providing written rather than oral responses is easier for some people and can promote self-disclosure.

Observational data provide another source of qualitative information and may be gathered in systematic or informal ways. In *systematic* observation, the person is observed during a predetermined period or event. For example, a student with an Attention-Deficit/Hyperactivity Disorder might be observed for the first 15 minutes of school every day in order to assess frequency of disruptive and inattentive behaviors. Systematic observation often involves counting behaviors, which makes the observation a quantitative as well as a qualitative measure. *Informal* observations are conducted in casual and unobtrusive ways. Data obtained typically will be anecdotal rather than numerical. Counselors might gather such data by observing a person in the waiting room, making a home visit to a client, or observing a child engaged in play. Teachers and school counselors sometimes keep *anecdotal records* on students as a way of observing patterns and changes in behavior. Of course, throughout the counseling process, clinicians also are gathering observational information in informal ways.

Observations provide insight into people's environments and can help counselors understand how people behave outside the counseling setting. They also provide baseline information that facilitates assessment of subsequent change. In structuring observations and collecting observational data, however, counselors may damage the counseling relationship if deception or embarrassment is involved. Observations should be carefully planned to ensure that they are beneficial for clients as well as counselors.

Reports or information provided by others are another source of qualitative data. These might be provided to counselors by clients' teachers, employers, friends, or family members as well as by other mental health professionals. Information on previous diagnoses and treatment of someone with a long-standing or prior mental disorder is essential to sound treatment planning. Sometimes counselors seek out such data. For example, counselors working with young children almost always interview their parents and perhaps also their teachers.

Counselors should exercise caution in obtaining information from third parties. Of course, with mentally competent adults, counselors must secure the client's permission before seeking information from another person. This is also advisable but not mandatory when counseling children. Legal and ethical guidelines, as well as the client's best interest, should guide decisions to obtain outside information about that person. In addition, when interpreting and evaluating second-hand reports, counselors should take into account the possible bias and personal needs of the observer. Used cautiously, such sources can provide important and otherwise unavailable material.

Autobiographies or life histories written by clients can provide useful information, especially with people who are uncomfortable with discussion. These tools also can be used to promote self-exploration. People may be given some direction in writing the narrative (e.g., "Write an overview of your life in no more than 10 pages") or the person may be given guidelines or questions to direct the development of the autobiography. A comparison of interview and autobiography can be fruitful; the counselor can take note of similarities and differences in content, tone, emphasis, and organization. Errors and distortions may come to light as well as areas of consistency and repetition.

Products made by a person can be another valuable source of information as well as a way of promoting discussion, especially with withdrawn or hostile clients. These products might include drawings, poems, photographs, crafts projects, letters, essays, songs, and other items that are important to the person and reflect an investment of time and energy. Suggested products also can be useful in resolving impasses or conflicts in treatment. For example, a client was asked to write a letter to her deceased father who had sexually abused her; a client who was enraged because his counselor had been out of town when he had a crisis was asked to draw a picture of his anger; and a client who was a skilled weaver was asked to create a wall hanging that reflected her relationship with her mother. Discussion of the creation of these items and the meaning they have for the person can reveal much about values, experiences, feelings, and abilities.

Time lines are yet another way of obtaining information. A line can be drawn, representing a person's life to date as well as his or her future. Ages might be indicated on the time line to provide guidance. The client then is asked to add developmental milestones or significant events, writing them next to the age at which they occurred. Projections also can be made of future happenings or realization of goals. Discussion of this information can give counselor and client a good sense of the person's hopes and history.

Early memories, according to Alfred Adler (1931), are a rich source of information on how people perceive and deal with their world. Adler suggested eliciting at least three memories that people perceive as among their earliest, looking for shared themes among those memories, and determining whether those themes shed light on people's current lifestyles.

Daydreams, dreams during sleep, and fantasies are other sources of qualitative information that can provide insight. These can be explored via their images and can give a perspective on people that is quite different than what might be elicited in other ways.

Nonstandardized Quantitative Approaches

Nonstandardized quantitative approaches to acquiring information yield a number, score, or rating but do not have established validity and reliability. Consequently, such instruments do not allow predictions to be made with any confidence nor do they permit a meaningful comparison of one person to another. However, they do provide a frame of reference and a convenient method of obtaining data. These approaches can be useful for measuring changes in a person's behavior, thoughts, or feelings; for clarifying areas needing further exploration; and for promoting discussion. This information can be gathered via commercially available questionnaires and rating scales or through informal tools developed by the counselor.

Checklists typically present an array of symptoms, problems, or concerns; people mark those that affect them. This can provide a useful starting point for an intake interview and can be especially valuable in couples or family counseling with family members independently completing the checklists and then comparing their self-reports.

Like checklists, *semantic differentials* are a common format for inventories that may have only face or content validity. These typically consist of pairs of items placed on a bipolar, 7-point continuum for measuring variables such as potency (strong–weak), activity (fast–slow), or quality (good–bad). An example is:

Cheerful   1   2   3   4   5   6   7   Depressed

People indicate where on the scale they would place themselves or some aspect of their lives. Counselor-made semantic differential scales are useful in assessing client self-image and attitudes. Several administrations of the same scales over time can provide an indication of change.

Rating scales are useful not only for an initial assessment but also for setting goals and measuring progress. Once difficulties have been identified, people indicate the severity of their concerns on a 1–10 scale (e.g., how troubled are you by the conflict you are having with your sister? how fearful are you of dogs?) Goals can then be set, using the rating scale (e.g., what number on the scale would you realistically like to reflect your comfort with dogs?) Progress can be tracked via periodic use of the rating scales. Despite the imprecise nature of this scale, most people have little difficulty providing meaningful ratings.

Numerical rating scales can be made more specific by providing five to seven graduated descriptions for the rater's use. The following example describes frequency of behavior:

I am able to assert myself with authority figures:

5—almost always
4—usually
3—often
2—sometimes
1—rarely

A similar rating tool is the *visual or linear analog*. People are presented with a line of a consistent length (10 cm is common) with descriptive statements at each end reflecting the extremes of the construct being assessed. They are asked to make a mark on the visual analog line to indicate their level of the construct. An example would be:

Not at all tired _____ Extremely tired

Measurement of the distance between the left end of the line and the mark a person has made on the line provides a baseline and allows comparison with subsequent administrations of this tool. This instrument is easy to create, administer, and score. It has demonstrated good test–retest reliability and is strongly correlated with longer paper-and-pencil measures (Cella & Perry, 1986).

Card sorts are another tool that can be developed or adapted to meet the needs of a particular client. The client is presented with a set of cards containing descriptors, pictures, statements, or other stimuli such as a different occupation written on each card. The person then divides the cards into a predetermined number of stacks according to their relative standing on a particular criterion (e.g., importance, interest). The number of cards to be sorted into each pile usually is specified. This can promote self-awareness and facilitate decision-making.

Rank ordering can serve similar purposes. In this approach, people are asked to organize a list of variables (e.g., goals, tasks, losses, interests) in a hierarchical way according to a guiding principle such as importance or urgency.

Frequency logs are used to assess how often events occur, as well as their nature. People might be asked to keep daily logs of negative behaviors such as drug or alcohol consumption, dysfunctional eating behaviors, suicidal thoughts, or angry outbursts, as well as of positive behaviors such as initiating a conversation, getting to work on time, and playing with their children. Affect can be tracked by asking people to rate their levels of depression or anxiety at 1-hour intervals. Concurrent behaviors, thoughts, or life events also can be listed in the log to facilitate understanding of precipitants of dysfunctional behaviors.

All of the formats described in this section (checklists, semantic differentials, numerical rating scales, rank orders, linear analogs, card sorts, and frequency logs) have been widely used. They can be found in both standardized inventories with high reliability and validity and for nonstandardized or counselor-made inventories used for exploration and discussion.

Standardized Quantitative Approaches

Standardized inventories that demonstrate a satisfactory degree of validity and reliability can enhance the counseling process by providing an objective source of data, allowing comparison of the client with others, facilitating the uncertain process of prediction, and providing access to new information. The process of administering and interpreting standardized tests and inventories requires some skills and knowledge. Counselors should be knowledgeable about the types of available tests and inventories and should be comfortable using *Mental Measurements Yearbooks, Tests in Print,* and other references designed to facilitate test selection. Some knowledge of the statistical aspects of assessment also is needed when counselors evaluate the appropriateness and worth of a standardized inventory and when counselors are interpreting people's inventoried scores. In addition, counselors should be aware of optimal procedures for test administration and should become accustomed to observing people's test-taking behaviors, another source of information on their adjustment, attitudes, motivation, and work habits.

TYPES OF INVENTORIES

A survey of members of the ACA engaged in community-based counseling indicated that over 50% used standardized testing in their work (Bubenzer et al., 1990). Most used several instruments on a regular basis and found testing helpful primarily to assess personality, intelligence, and career-related interests. Inventories used by counselors, in order of frequency reported, included the Minnesota Multiphasic Personality Inventory, the Strong Interest Inventory, the Wechsler Adult Intelligence Scale, the Myers–Briggs Type Indicator, and the Wechsler Intelligence Scale for Children. In addition, counselors also make considerable use of the 16 Personality Factor, the Thematic Apperception Test, the Bender–Gestalt Visual-Motor Test, the Wide Range Achievement Test, the Millon Clinical Multiaxial Inventory, the Beck Depression Inventory, and the Beck Anxiety Inventory.

Standardized inventories can be divided into three categories, depending on whether they were designed to measure abilities, interests, or personality. Although it is beyond the scope of this book to provide extensive information on specific inventories or on the statistical aspects of assessment, an overview of the categories of inventories is provided to help counselors determine when testing is in order and what types of inventories might be most useful.

Measures of Ability

Tests of ability measure a combination of innate capacities and learning acquired through formal and informal education. These tests can be threatening to some people because they raise the possibility of poor performance. The impact of such instruments on the client–counselor relationship should, consequently, be considered carefully before they are administered. In addition, charges of gender as well as racial and cultural bias have been levied against measures of ability, necessitating extreme caution in their selection and interpretation. Inventories should be viewed as only one of many sources of information on a person's abilities; the information they yield should be combined with other data to yield the most meaningful and accurate knowledge. With proper use, however, such tests can provide important information on people's abilities, their academic needs, and their suitability for particular educational or occupational endeavors.

Achievement, intelligence, and aptitude tests all are measures of ability. The three types of tests may appear indistinguishable, since all consist of a series of questions or tasks with predetermined correct answers. However, the development, scoring systems, and normative samples of the inventories usually differ, depending on their specific purpose.

Achievement tests measure previously attained mastery or ability in a particular area. These tests generally are used to assess the impact of educational experiences, to indicate academic strengths and weaknesses, to provide an objective measure of learning, and to indicate the relative standing of a person's level of learning in a sample or normative group (class, school, nationwide sample). Tests given as part of college courses are almost always achievement tests.

Achievement tests typically are of limited interest to most mental health counselors but are of considerable interest to school, employment, and career counselors. However, students' records may include performance data on achievement tests such as the Iowa Tests of Basic Skills (Riverside), the Stanford Achievement Series and the Metropolitan Achievement Tests (both published by Psychological Corporation) that need to be understood and interpreted by the mental health counselor. Many high schools require satisfactory performance on proficiency or achievement tests as a prerequisite for graduation. Counselors dealing with adolescents may consequently become involved in the process of assessing achievement. Also, counselors may make use of a comprehensive achievement test such as the Wide Range Achievement Test (WRAT), published by Jastak Associates, as part of a test battery. The WRAT, which evaluates achievement in spelling, arithmetic, and reading, is a much used inventory, designed to measure the basic academic skills of young people and adults. Both the Scholastic Aptitude Tests (SAT) and the Graduate Record Examination (GRE), published by Educational Testing Service, include achievement tests in selected subject areas. Other well-known achievement tests are the Tests of General Educational Development (GED), used by adults to earn a high school diploma, and the College-Level Examination Program (CLEP), enabling people to earn credits by examination.

Intelligence tests are more likely than achievement tests to become part of the diagnostician's repertoire, although they, too, are not widely used by mental health counselors. Nearly 100 years of debate have addressed the question of exactly what intelligence is and how it can best be measured. Recent writings have broadened the definition and conceptualization of intelligence. Howard Gardner's Multiple Intelligence Theory (2003), for example, proposes seven types of intelligence: visual/spatial intelligence, musical intelligence, verbal intelligence, logical/mathematical intelligence, interpersonal intelligence, intrapersonal intelligence, and bodily/kinesthetic intelligence. Robert Sternberg's (2003) Triarchic Theory divided intelligence into three components: a cognitive factor dealing with information processing; an experiential or creative factor that enables people to deal with new situations and access high levels of information processing; and a conceptual or contextual factor that includes practical and social intelligence. Daniel Goleman (1995) and others broadened the concept of intelligence even further by introducing the construct of emotional intelligence. Intelligence is now widely viewed as an attribute that has multiple components that evolve and change throughout the life span.

Although few tests have as yet been developed to assess multiple intelligences, most measures of intelligence have been modified in recent years to reflect new definitions of that construct. Intelligence tests are used primarily during career or academic counseling. They can be very informative when counselors suspect that a person's academic experiences have not accurately reflected his or her academic achievement (i.e., a so-called underachiever) or when mental retardation is suspected. Group and individual tests of intelligence are available.

Most counselors are qualified to administer group tests of intelligence. Frequently used examples of these tools include the Otis-Lennon School Ability Test (Psychological Corporation), the Slosson Intelligence Test (Slosson Educational Publications), the Kaufman Brief Intelligence Test (AGS Publishing), and the Wide Range Intelligence Test (Wide Range, Inc.).

Some counselors have specialized training in administering individual intelligence tests such as the Stanford–Binet Intelligence Scale (Riverside) and the Wechsler intelligence scales (the Wechsler Preschool and Primary Scale of Intelligence, the Wechsler Intelligence Scale for Children, and the Wechsler Adult Intelligence Scale, all published by Psychological Corporation). Counselors without this specialized training will need to make a referral to a psychologist when a highly reliable measure of a person's intellectual functioning must be obtained.

Several innovative measures of intelligence also are available, although they are not currently in wide use. Raven's Progressive Matrices (Psychological Corporation), Culture Fair Intelligence Test (IPAT), and the Test of Nonverbal Intelligence (Pro-Ed) are examples of intelligence tests developed specifically to reduce cultural bias in assessment. Another example is the BarOn Emotional Quotient Inventory (MHS), designed to assess five major domains of emotional intelligence: intrapersonal, interpersonal, stress management, adaptability, and general mood scale.

Aptitude tests are designed to evaluate a person's potential for learning or profiting from a given educational experience or the probability of that person succeeding in a particular occupation or course of study. Aptitude test scores tend to be highly correlated with school grades and scores on other inventories of ability.

Therefore, counselors often can infer information on people's aptitudes without administering these inventories. However, counselors do need to understand the aptitude test scores in a person's record and may decide to include an aptitude test as part of a battery of tests administered to a person contemplating a career change or experiencing academic difficulties. Aptitude, as well as achievement and intelligence tests, also can aid in the diagnosis of developmental and learning disorders.

Two types of aptitudes have been identified: *simple or specific aptitudes* and *complex aptitudes*. Inventories have been developed to measure each type. Specific aptitudes often assessed include motor abilities, clerical ability, and language ability. Complex aptitudes usually are measured by using a multiple aptitude battery that consists of a group of tests of specific aptitudes that can be given either singly or together. Combining scores from a group of tests in the battery can yield an overall measure of aptitude.

Complex aptitudes are difficult to define, although many inventories have been developed for their assessment. The Differential Aptitude Tests (Psychological Corporation), the Armed Services Vocational Aptitude Battery (U.S. Department of Defense), the Tests of Adult Basic Education (CTB/Macmillan), and the General Aptitude Test Battery (U.S. Employment Service) are examples of widely used multiple aptitude test batteries. The Scholastic Aptitude Tests, the Graduate Record Examination (Educational Testing Service), and the Miller Analogies Test (Psychological Corporation) are multiple aptitude tests required for admission to many colleges and universities.

Interest Inventories

Interests can be defined as constellations of likes and dislikes, manifested through the activities people pursue, the objects they value, and their patterns of behavior. Information on people's interests can be gathered through discussion (expressed interests), an examination of behaviors and activities (manifest interests), and scores on questionnaires (inventoried interests). Interests typically are the primary determinant of both college major and occupational choices. Congruence of interests and career choice is significantly correlated with enjoyment of, and persistence in, an occupation (Betz, Fitzgerald, & Hill, 1989).

Identification of interests is important not only in career and rehabilitation counseling but also in counseling focused on emotional difficulties such as Somatoform Disorders, depression, anxiety, and relationship problems. Often, people with concerns such as these are withdrawn, maintain a low activity level, and have a lifestyle that does not mesh well with their interests. Planning activities that are pleasurable, are congruent with people's interests, and provide feelings of competence can contribute to improvement in mood, coping skills, and interpersonal relationships.

A large variety of interest inventories are available. They range from self-administered and self-scored inventories such as the Self-Directed Search (Psychological Assessment Resources) to the Strong Interest Inventory (Consulting Psychologists Press), an extensive computer-scored questionnaire measuring people's interest in over 200 occupational areas. Other well-known interest inventories include the Campbell Interest and Skills Survey (Pearson Assessment), the Harrington-O'Shea Career Decision-Making System (AGS), and the Kuder family of inventories (Science Research Associates). Comprehensive assessment tools such as the COPSystem Career Guidance Program (EdITS) and the Differential Aptitude Test Career Planning Program (Psychological Corporation) assess interests as well as aptitudes and values.

Interest inventories, which have no right or wrong answers, are typically less threatening to people than are tests of ability. However, scores on interest inventories also tend to be less clear-cut and more difficult to interpret than those of ability tests. A high interest score in the occupation of musician, for example, should not immediately be interpreted to mean that the person should become a musician. Exploration is needed to determine the person's preparation for and talent in the field, the degree of congruence between the lifestyle of a musician and the person's preferred lifestyle, and the attraction of that occupation for the person. Related occupations that involve music, creativity, and the experience of performing also should be explored, as well as the option of satisfying the person's interests through leisure rather than occupational activities. Client–counselor dialog, then, is critical to the effective interpretation of interest inventories.

Successful career development depends on more than matching interests and occupation. Consequently, a variety of other inventories are available to enhance the career counseling process. Examples include the Jackson Vocational Interest Survey (Sigma Assessment Systems), which focuses on work styles; the Career Factors Inventory and the Career Beliefs Inventory (Consulting Psychologists Press) designed to identify factors that inhibit effective career decision-making; the Career Maturity Inventory (Careerware); and the Learning Styles Inventory (Western Psychological Services). Inventories such as these combine elements of both interest and personality inventories.

Personality Inventories

Personality inventories can be global in scope, designed to provide an overall picture of a person's emotional style, or they may be specific, focusing on particular aspects of personality (e.g., self-concept, mood, behavior). Measures of personality can help counselors develop accurate diagnoses and effective treatment plans. Inventories can provide a clear and well-organized picture of a person's personality, highlight strengths and weaknesses, and yield information a person may be unwilling or unable to provide directly. Personality inventories that measure states (short-term changes), rather than traits (underlying personality dimensions), are useful in assessing progress. These inventories also are useful in career and family counseling.

Types of Personality Inventories

Nearly all counselors are trained to use standardized measures of personality. These generally consist of a series of descriptive statements; respondents indicate whether the items are true of them or which of several items best describes them. Scoring is standardized, and numerical values, related to predetermined aspects of personality, are provided when the inventory is scored. Little skill is involved in the administration and scoring of these inventories. However, their interpretation can require considerable skill and knowledge of both behavior and personality.

Standardized personality inventories can be divided into General Personality Inventories, Clinical Personality Inventories, and Specialized Personality Inventories. *General personality inventories* are designed to provide a broad-based picture of the personalities of people who are not assumed to have significant emotional difficulties. Well-established general personality inventories available for counselor use include:

1. *Adjective Checklist* (ACL)—This inventory, published by Consulting Psychologists Press, consists of 300 adjectives. People can indicate on this inventory how they perceive their real selves and their ideal selves, as well as how they believe they are perceived by others.

2. *California Psychological Inventory* (CPI)—The CPI, also published by Consulting Psychologists Press, consists of true/false items that yield scores in five areas: Interpersonal Behavior, Social and Personal Values, Cognitive Needs and Performance, Personal Characteristics, and Work-Related Characteristics. The CPI is useful for assessing personal style, goals, motivation, and drives of both adolescents and adults.

3. *Myers–Briggs Type Indicator* (MBTI)—The MBTI, published by Consulting Psychologists Press and based on Carl Jung's theory of personality, is one of the most widely used personality inventories for general populations. It is useful in promoting personal growth, self-awareness, leadership skills, team building, career development, and improved interpersonal skills. Important to its appeal is its assumption that all personality types are equally valuable. The MBTI yields scores on four bipolar dimensions: introversion–extroversion, sensing–intuition, thinking–feeling, and judging–perceiving. Combinations of these scores describe 16 personality types. The MBTI can be computer analyzed to provide information on the interaction of the personality types of two people, which is useful in

couples counseling. A children's version of the MBTI, the Murphy–Meisgeier Type Indicator for Children, is available for grades 2 through 8. The MBTI can be taken and scored in combination with the Strong Interest Inventory to clarify the relationship of a person's personality and interests.

4. *Sixteen Personality Factor* (16 PF)—The 16 PF, published by IPAT, measures 16 basic bipolar dimensions of personality as well as five global factors (extraversion, anxiety, tough-mindedness, independence, and self-control). Versions of this inventory measure the personalities of adults, adolescents, and children as young as 6.

Many *clinical personality inventories* also are available. These provide information on the diagnosis and treatment of mental disorders and are of great use to mental health counselors. Three widely used comprehensive and standardized clinical personality inventories are:

1. *Minnesota Multiphasic Personality Inventory* (MMPI)—First published in 1942 and revised in 1989, the MMPI (now published by MHS) is probably the most widely used and researched personality inventory (Duckworth & Anderson, 1995). Consisting of 567 true-false items designed to identify symptoms and diagnose pathology, the MMPI scales assess such areas as depression, anxiety, psychosis, and physical complaints. Many special scales have been developed, making the MMPI a very flexible and useful inventory. The MMPI is computer scored. Its interpretation is complex, however, and requires special training and experience.

2. *Millon Clinical Multiaxial Inventory* (MCMI)—Published by National Computer System, the MCMI was developed by Theodore Millon, an expert on personality disorders. The MCMI is linked to the *DSM* and provides information on the diagnosis and treatment of personality and other mental disorders. Like the MMPI, it is a lengthy inventory that is best scored by machine. An adolescent version of this inventory also is available.

3. *Profile of Mood States* (POMS)—The POMS, published by EdITS, consists of 65 5-point rating scales. Respondents indicate on these scales the extent to which they experienced specified feelings during the past week. Completion of the inventory yields scores on six mood states (Tension-Anxiety, Depression-Dejection, Anger-Hostility, Vigor-Activity, Fatigue-Inertia, and Confusion-Bewilderment) as well as a total mood disturbance score. This inventory is easy to administer and score and can be used repeatedly to assess change.

Specialized personality inventories also can be useful in mental health counseling to assess particular variables and to track progress. The following list includes important types of these inventories:

1. *Specialized Clinical Inventories*—A broad range of specialized inventories has been developed to assess specific emotional or behavioral difficulties.

These are important to counselors involved in diagnosis and treatment planning. Even if counselors believe they have made an accurate diagnosis, an inventory can serve as a double-check on the counselors' conclusions. These inventories also quantify and provide descriptive information on symptoms, thereby facilitating treatment planning, goal setting, and assessment of progress. Widely used examples of these inventories include the Beck Depression and Anxiety Inventories (Psychological Corporation), the Eating Disorder Inventory (Psychological Assessment Resources), the Tennessee Self-Concept Scale (Western Psychological Services), and the Maslach Burnout Inventory (Consulting Psychologists Press).

2. *Inventories of Behavior*—These inventories are especially important to counselors working with children and adolescents. Examples of such inventories include the Behavior Assessment System for Children (AGS), which includes rating scales for youth, parents, and teachers; Connors Rating Scales (MHS) for measuring level of attention in children and adults; and the Achenbach System of Empirically Based Assessment (Riverside) to measure children's behavioral and emotional difficulties.

3. *Values Inventories*—These inventories probably are used most by career counselors but also can be used by other mental health counselors to promote client self-awareness, to facilitate decisions and transitions, and to help people with religious or spiritual concerns. Examples of values inventories include the Salience Inventory and the Values Scale (Consulting Psychologists Press), based on the research of career-development pioneer Donald Super, and the Hall Occupational Orientation Inventory (Scholastic Testing Service).

4. *Wellness and Leisure Inventories*—These inventories, too, can promote self-awareness and help people make their lifestyles healthier and more rewarding. The Lifestyle Coping Inventory, published by the National Wellness Institute, is typical of these and yields information on the following 10 dimensions: physical fitness, nutrition, self-care, drugs and driving, social-environmental, emotional awareness, emotional control, intellectual, occupational, and spiritual.

5. *Other Personality Inventories*—Inventories are available to assess thinking and decision-making style (e.g., the Decision Making Inventory, Marathon Consulting Press); marital satisfaction and adjustment (e.g., The Marital Satisfaction Inventory, Western Psychological Services); and assessment of environment (e.g., Moos' Social Climate Scales, Consulting Psychologists Press).

Projective Personality Tests

Projective tests present people with a series of relatively unstructured and ambiguous stimuli such as inkblots or pictures and allow them to project themselves into the inventories by describing their perceptions, making up stories, drawing, or providing other types of responses. The administration and interpretation of projective personality tests require specialized training and supervised experience. Such training generally is not a part of counselor education programs and most counselors, therefore, are not qualified to administer projective tests. Whether or not they have training in projective testing, counselors still need to become familiar with these tools since they may want to refer clients to psychologists for projective testing and often will receive client records and intake reports that contain an analysis of projective material.

Projective personality tests are intended to provide a global picture of people's emotional makeup. These tests seek to bypass people's defense mechanisms and reflect unconscious feelings and motives, as well as pathology that may be controlled on the conscious level. The most widely used projective personality tests are:

1. *Rorschach Inkblot Test*—Developed by Hermann Rorschach in 1921, this test consists of 10 inkblots. People are asked to report what they see and where it is located on the blot. Analysis yields information on their wishes, attitudes, and perceptions of the world.

2. *Thematic Apperception Test* (TAT)—The TAT, developed by Murray and Morgan in 1938, consists of 30 black and white pictures and a blank card. Usually, 10 pictures are selected by the examiner for relevance. The person tells a story to explain each picture. Responses provide information on needs, conflicts, relationships, experiences, and overall personality.

3. *Sentence Completion*—Best known is the Rotter Incomplete Sentences Blank consisting of 40 sentence stems (e.g., I like …). The person completes each stem with the first words that come to mind. Information is provided on concerns, feelings, and attitudes.

4. *Projective Drawings*—Typically, people providing projective drawings are instructed to draw a house, a tree, and one or more whole people, sometimes an entire family. The drawings offer insights into people's self-images and perceptions of their families as well as their overall emotional development and intelligence.

5. *Bender Visual–Motor Gestalt Test*—This is primarily a measure of visual-motor development and learning disability. However, it also has been widely used and studied as a projective personality test. The Bender–Gestalt consists of nine designs (each on a separate card) that the person copies. Analysis of the designs for accuracy, size, placement, and other variables offers data on people's relationships, areas of concern, and emotional development.

A complete psychological assessment is likely to include most or all of the above inventories as well as an individual intelligence test. It also might include the MMPI, discussed previously. Giving a person several tests reduces uncertainty.

The examiner can then base interpretations on recurring patterns and themes rather than on isolated responses, yielding a more detailed and reliable report.

Other Sources of Assessment

Assessment of abilities, interests, and personality is within the range of skills of most counselors. However, sometimes clients present symptoms and concerns that require assessment tools and skills that are outside the repertoire of most counselors. At such times counselors should refer the client to a trusted colleague in another field and collaborate with that person in developing a diagnosis and treatment plan. Examples include referral to an urologist or gynecologist for a person with sexual difficulties, referral to a neurologist for someone with symptoms of cognitive impairment, and a referral to a pediatrician for a child with problems in bladder or bowel control or a troubling tic. Counselors should be familiar with and make good use of outside sources of appraisal to ensure they obtain a clear understanding of their clients' difficulties. Of course, clients' written permission should be obtained before sharing their information with anyone.

FRAMEWORKS FOR UNDERSTANDING PEOPLE

Once data have been gathered, the counselor has the sometimes challenging task of organizing and analyzing the information. Interpretation of assessment data generally involves comparing patterns evidenced by the client in interviews and inventories with preestablished or common patterns. This lends structure and confidence to the interpretations.

Which framework to use depends on several factors: the theoretical orientation of the counselor, the nature of the client's difficulties, and the approaches to treating emotional difficulties advocated by the agency where treatment is taking place. A variety of frameworks are considered here and illustrated later in this chapter. This list is by no means exhaustive and counselors should feel free to use alternate frameworks or develop frameworks that are helpful to them in assessing their clients.

Developmental Framework

Perhaps the most basic frameworks for assessment are developmental ones. Classic and well-established developmental frameworks include those of Sigmund Freud (Brill, 1938), Piaget (1963), and Erik Erikson (1963). Such frameworks enable counselors to assess people's psychosocial, psychosexual, and cognitive development, with particular emphasis on the early years. Many more recent books on human development provide additional information and models for assessing the development of children, adolescents, and adults.

Models also are available to help counselors assess special areas of development. For example, Super (1957) and Ginzberg (1972) developed enduring and well-supported theories of career development. *The Expanded Family Life Cycle* (Carter & McGoldrick, 1999) provided a framework for examining the growth and history of a family.

Multicultural Frameworks

Another way to view people is through a multicultural lens, looking at gender, age, context, socioeconomic status, religion, culture, and ethnicity. This provides a structure for exploring means for comparing clients' individual patterns. Extensive literature on multiculturalism is available to help counselors draw comparisons. Most counselors also have some awareness of common views and experiences of multicultural groups and can draw on their own knowledge. Such information should be used with caution, however, and counselors should seek verification in the literature of any guidelines or patterns that they use.

Psychological Frameworks: Strengths and Difficulties

Of particular importance to counselors and clients is the analysis of people's coping skills and symptoms of emotional disorders. The *DSM* (2000), discussed in Chapter 3, provides useful standards for determining whether a person has one or more mental disorders. Textbooks on psychology offer information on healthy emotional development and coping skills. The mental status examination, discussed in Chapter 5, provides another perspective on the assessment of psychological functioning. Additional psychological frameworks, which target specific aspects of personality, include the following.

Psychological Frameworks: Suicidal Ideation and Behavior

Approximately 30,000 suicides occur annually in the United States. Most of these are people experiencing depression who have given some warning of their intent and who might have been prevented from committing suicide. Suicide is particularly common in men age 45 and older, employed in professional or skilled areas, living alone, experiencing unusual stress or threat of financial loss, and abusing drugs or alcohol (Motto, Heilbron, & Juster, 1985). Factors such as confusion about sexual orientation and a family history of alcoholism, depression, or suicide (especially by one's mother) also predispose people toward suicidal ideation. Common warning behaviors of people contemplating suicide include social withdrawal, giving away important possessions, persistent insomnia, weight gain or loss, a decline in occupational or academic performance, previous suicide attempts, unsuccessful efforts to obtain help, ideas of persecution, and feelings of hopelessness, failure, defeat, shame, and guilt. Whenever counselors note symptoms such as these or believe a client may be considering suicide, counselors should explore the person's potential for self-destructive behavior.

Assessment of suicidal thoughts should explore the following areas:

1. *Motivation*—Whether it is escape from pain, revenge, attention seeking, or another motive, people have a reason for considering suicide.
2. *Nature of the Plan* and the availability of the means are of great importance. People who have a clear plan for suicide, including the use of a lethal weapon, are at high risk for suicide.
3. *Triggering Events* such as a loss, a perceived humiliation or failure, or rejection can prompt a suicide.
4. *Symptoms* such as depression, psychosis, anxiety, impulsivity, guilt, hostility, hopelessness, helplessness, emotional disregulation, and misuse of drugs and alcohol are associated with an elevated incidence of suicidal thinking and behavior. Counselors should pay particularly close attention to people with suicidal thoughts when their depressions begin to lift. People in the depths of depression may not even have the energy to commit suicide; an increase in energy, coupled with continuing depression, can precipitate a suicide attempt.
5. *Behaviors*, especially a history of suicide attempts, verbalized suicidal ideation, and high-risk behaviors are strongly associated with suicide.
6. *Family History and Support Systems* are other important factors; people with few supports and a negative family history have a higher likelihood of suicidal behavior.

Although all suicidal thoughts and actions should be taken seriously because of their potential lethality, people who are contemplating suicide almost always are conflicted or ambivalent. Consequently, counseling—including empathy, a safe-keeping contract, encouragement of coping skills and hopefulness, use of support systems, and sometimes medication and hospitalization—often can prevent a suicide.

Suicidal ideation can be frightening to counselors. However, the assessment of suicide risk and prevention of suicide is a critical aspect of counselors' roles. Consultation with colleagues or supervisors can help counselors deal with decisions about suicide prevention.

Psychological Aspects: Violence

Although most clients are more likely to harm themselves than others, counselors should be alert to the possibility that clients might engage in physically harmful or destructive acts against others. The most important predictor of violent behavior is a past history of violence. Therefore, history-taking is of great importance whenever destructive or harmful behavior is suspected. People who are accident prone and who drive recklessly also have an elevated risk of engaging in self-destructive or violent behavior. People who commit violent acts against others are typically male, abuse drugs or alcohol, and have feelings of failure, low self-esteem, and psychological and neurological difficulties. Paranoid thinking also is associated with violent client behavior.

Psychological Aspects: Defense Mechanisms

All people use defense mechanisms. These are unconscious psychological processes that help people balance their instinctual drives and the demands of daily life. Defense mechanisms assist people in coping with reality, deferring gratification, and meeting their needs in socially acceptable ways.

A broad range of defense mechanisms has been identified. People's preferred defense mechanisms provide important information on the nature of their difficulties, their styles of interaction, and their likely response to counseling. The following classification and description of defense mechanisms can be useful to mental health professionals (Kaplan & Sadock, 1994; Perry & Cooper, 1989; Vaillant, Bond, & Vaillant, 1986).

1. *Narcissistic or Psychotic Defenses*—Especially evident in children and people with psychotic disorders, and often reflected in dreams, these defenses include *delusional projection* of one's own characteristics onto others, *denial* of reality, and *distortion*, involving reshaping of external reality to meet inner needs.

2. *Immature Defenses*—Common in adolescents as well as in people with addictive, personality, and depressive disorders, these include *acting out* (socially unacceptable expression of sexual or aggressive wishes and impulses), *blocking* (inhibition of feelings, thoughts, or impulses), *devaluation* (attributing exaggerated negative characteristics to another person), escape into *fantasy, idealization* (exaggeration of another's virtues), *introjection* (internalization of characteristics of a loved or feared person), *passive–aggressive behavior* (indirect expression of anger and hostility), *projection, regression* (returning to an earlier situation or previous stage of development to avoid anxieties or concerns), *somatization* (converting feelings or impulses into physical, sensory, or

neuromuscular symptoms), *splitting* (viewing oneself or others as being all good or all bad), and *turning inward* a hostile thought about another person.

3. *Neurotic Defenses*—Common in most people, these include *controlling* (extreme attempts to direct one's environment), *displacement* (changing the object of an impulse or feeling to a less threatening object), *dissociation* (avoiding stress by cutting off one's experiences, feelings, or thoughts), *externalization* (perceiving aspects of one's own personality in the environment and in external objects), *inhibition* (limiting or renouncing specific behaviors such as sexual involvement to avoid conflict and anxiety), *intellectualization* (controlling feelings and impulses by thinking and analyzing rather than experiencing), *isolation* (splitting off emotion from content and experience), *rationalization* (justification of attitudes or behaviors by focusing on favorable motives and ignoring others), *reaction formation* or *overcompensation* (managing unacceptable feelings by expressing their opposites), *repression* (excluding thoughts, impulses, and memories from consciousness), *sexualization* (attributing unwarranted sexual significance to an object, person, or activity to ward off anxiety), and *somatization* (defined earlier).

4. *Mature Defenses*—Common in normal, healthy adults, these include *altruism* (directing energies toward constructive and gratifying service to others), *anticipation* (realistic, goal-directed planning to deal with difficulties), *compensation* (overemphasizing one area to balance disappointment in another or overcorrecting for a limitation), *humor* (using non-hurtful wit to make uncomfortable feelings more tolerable), *sublimation* (modifying unacceptable urges into acceptable ones by changing the object or vehicle of expression), and *suppression* (conscious or semiconscious postponement of gratification or exclusion from awareness of an impulse).

People engaging in immature, narcissistic, or neurotic defenses are more likely to be seen in counseling than are people using predominantly mature defenses. Analysis of the nature of people's defense mechanisms can facilitate understanding and help counselors to promote increased use of mature defense mechanisms.

Medical and Neurological Frameworks

Even though counselors hardly ever receive extensive training in identifying and understanding medical and neurological symptoms and disorders, often those are the underlying causes of apparent emotional difficulties. According to Pollak, Levy, and Breitholtz (1999, p. 350), "Misdiagnosis of a medical illness or a neurodevelopmental disorder as a primary mental disorder is relatively common." Tools such as the Mini-Mental Status Examination and the Adult Neuropsychological

Inventory can help counselors make a preliminary assessment of cognitive functioning and determine when a referral to a neurologist, psychiatrist, or other physician is indicated. In addition the following symptoms should prompt counselors to consider the possibility of a medical or neurological cause for a person's difficulties: acute onset of symptoms in the absence of relevant stressors, initial onset after age 40, onset temporally linked to change in physical health or medication, memory loss, confusion and disorientation, language deficits, impairment in motor functioning, feelings of depersonalization, headaches, feelings of weakness, problems in breathing, and nonauditory hallucinations.

Individualized Frameworks

People can serve as their own frameworks for analysis. Through interviews and inventories, counselors can identify typical patterns of emotions, thoughts, and behaviors that characterize particular clients. Once the counselor has a sense of a person's history and past patterns, future patterns can be anticipated and modified. For example, a person who has consistently responded to any threat of rejection or disapproval through flight and avoidance is likely to persist in that behavior without alternative responses. Exceptions to dysfunctional patterns, as well as introduction of new modes of response, can promote positive change

PROCESS OF ANALYSIS AND INTERPRETATION

Analyzing and interpreting the information gathered on a person probably is the most challenging and creative aspect of diagnosis and treatment planning. The process involves developing and checking hypotheses about the significance and importance of the information in order to provide insight into the person and facilitate decisions about diagnosis and treatment. Frameworks such as those discussed in this chapter help counselors to develop and organize their ideas.

Questions to Guide the Process

Assume an intake interview has been conducted, inventories have been administered and scored, and any records or other information have been reviewed. The counselor now can begin the process of analysis by asking the following six questions about the accumulated information:

1. *What underlying themes or repeated issues are present in the information?* These may be obvious, such as a person's repeated negative references to men

(e.g., a demanding and critical father, an abusive first husband, projective testing showing negative feelings toward men, and job losses stemming from conflict with male supervisors). Often, however, patterns are subtler. For example, the person may describe two recent car accidents and a series of errors at work and may omit many items during the testing process. Such a person may be prone to self-destructive behavior or dissociation, may have attentional difficulties, or may be so confused and anxious he feels overwhelmed and out of control.

2. *What items or issues were given greatest importance by the person?* Counselors tend to focus on aspects of a person's narrative that they believe to be of particular relevance in understanding people. These might include the person's family situation, thought processes, or previous emotional difficulties. While this process of selective attending and exploring provides counselors a structure for information gathering, counselors also should step into the client's shoes and determine what that person perceives as important. The client, for example, may talk at length about home repair projects. The counselor should take note of this and try to determine what the projects mean to the person. Do they represent a source of stress, a gratification, or the person's feeling that all aspects of his life, the house included, are falling apart?

3. *What unusual pieces of information, reactions, or thoughts does the person present?* If a person simply reports that he owns a dog, that piece of information might not be worth mentioning in an intake report. If, however, the person talks at length about her 5 dogs, 14 cats, 6 gerbils, and pet hyena and states that she wishes she didn't have to work full-time so that she could be with her animals all day, this certainly is noteworthy and should be explored.

4. *What omissions or contradictions appeared in the person's presentation?* In reviewing an intake interview, the counselor may note that a person said almost nothing about her mother, although she talked extensively about her father. Another person might report that he has a wonderful marriage but then verbalizes only criticisms of his wife's behavior. Counselors should attend to these contradictions and omissions and, if possible, explore them with the person.

5. *How does a given piece of information fit in with what else is known about the person and his or her environment?* Interpretations should rarely be made on the basis of a single piece of information. Rather, the counselor should seek to develop a comprehensive and coherent picture of a person that integrates and makes sense of the presented information.

6. *What frameworks help make sense of this information?* This chapter previously discussed frameworks for analysis. Relevant frameworks provide a baseline or structure for analyzing and evaluating the information clients present. A developmental framework, for example, can help a counselor determine whether to be concerned about a 6-year-old who cannot speak in complete sentences while a multicultural framework reminds counselors to assess clients from multiple perspectives.

GUIDELINES FOR INTERPRETATION

Interpretation of assessment and other information gathered on a client can be useful in promoting self-awareness as well as the counselor's understanding of that person. Interpretation can facilitate the process of diagnosis and effective treatment planning, clarify important issues and coping skills, and guide formation of a sound therapeutic alliance.

At the same time, making skillful and accurate interpretations can be challenging and may be mishandled. Counselors sometimes become judgmental and draw unjustified conclusions. Interpretations should not condemn, criticize, or stigmatize the client; they should be well substantiated and should generally be cautious and tentative. It is preferable to talk in terms of possibilities and likelihoods rather than absolutes. Having a relevant framework for an interpretation provides a structure for assessing the client and focusing attention on important aspects of the client and the counseling process. Sharing interpretations with clients in appropriate ways can promote self-awareness and involvement in the treatment process.

EXAMPLES OF FRAMEWORKS FOR INTERPRETATION

The following paragraphs illustrate brief interpretations made about a client from five different perspectives or frameworks: testing, multicultural, developmental, diagnostic, and defenses. The client Kahing is a 24-year-old man who sought counseling because of depression and career indecision.

Testing Framework

Kahing's profile on the Myers–Briggs Type Inventory was ISTP (introverted, sensing, thinking, perceiving). He prefers being alone or with a small number of close friends and family members to being in large groups. He tends to be concrete and practical in his approach to life, rarely looking for deeper meanings. Making plans and decisions is uncomfortable for Kahing; he prefers to leave his options open and await new possibilities.

On the Strong Interest Inventory, Kahing had a relatively flat profile, although his scores were somewhat elevated on the Engineer and Accountant scales. Results suggest he prefers to work alone, is not interested in continuing his education, and tends to avoid risks.

Kahing achieved a score of 16 on the Beck Depression Inventory. This suggests he is moderately depressed. Responses suggest high levels of guilt and discouragement.

As he reported, Kahing is experiencing some moderate clinical depression. His depression, his negative feelings about himself, and his difficulty in making decisions all have combined to make it difficult for him to identify a clear career direction.

Multicultural Framework

Kahing was born in mainland China. He is the youngest child in his family and has five older sisters. When he was 12, his family immigrated to the United States, where his father found more favorable employment opportunities. This was a difficult transition for Kahing. He spoke no English and was often teased by his peers. His school grades were initially low and he never developed much interest in school.

Kahing has a special role in his family as the youngest and the only son. His mother and sisters reportedly dote him on, and the entire family has very high expectations for him. Not surprisingly, Kahing feels that he has let his family down by his low academic achievement, his decision to leave college after his sophomore year, and his current employment as a data entry clerk. Although he wants to better his situation, he is afraid of making a mistake, does not have a clear career direction, and feels stuck. His limited socialization and his unmarried status are additional sources of disappointment to both Kahing and his family; they frequently hint that he should soon marry and carry on the family name.

Developmental Framework

Kahing is a 28-year-old man who completed 2 years of college and has been working in a series of data entry positions. He continues to live with his parents and a married sister and her two children. His sister prepares Kahing's meals and he is not expected to participate in household chores. However, he is expected to contribute financially to his parents, now retired.

Kahing and his family immigrated from China to the United States when Kahing was 12. Since that time, he has continued to feel isolated and different from his peers. He has not experienced many of the usual developmental milestones of adolescence and young adulthood. He has no close relationships with men or women outside of his family. He has never lived away from his family and has rarely made decisions for himself. His dependency on his family stems, in part, from multicultural factors but developmental lags also have contributed greatly to Kahing's current lack of direction and his depression.

Diagnostic Framework

Kahing's symptoms of guilt, sadness, difficulty with decision-making, and impaired sleeping and eating patterns, along with his elevated score on the Beck Depression

Inventory, suggest that he is experiencing a moderate depression. The duration of his depression is at least 5 years, meeting the criteria for a Dysthymic Disorder. When asked, Kahing expressed some vague suicidal ideation, stating that he often wished he could "just disappear." However, he does not have a suicide plan or readily available means and stated strongly that he would never commit suicide. He does not seem to be in imminent danger.

Defensiveness Framework

Kahing manifests several immature defenses that he uses in an effort to avoid addressing his negative feelings and situations in which he believes he might fail. Maintaining a dependent role in his family is an important protection for him. Although he did live in a college dormitory for 2 years, his poor performance in college led him to return to the safety of his family and avoid independence. In addition, Kahing engages in considerable blocking by inhibiting feelings, thoughts, and impulses. He minimizes the severity of his depression, denies that he would like rewarding friendships and activities, and suppresses impulses toward breaking out of his narrow world. Instead, he assumes a bland demeanor and expresses primarily indifference about his situation. Only occasional flashes of anger and references to sometimes feeling trapped reveal his underlying wish for change.

Discussion

These five examples each illustrate a different approach to interpretation of information about Kahing. While none of them is perfect, some are both more useful to the counselor and more helpful to the client. Which interpretation would be most helpful to you if you were Kahing's counselor? Perhaps you would want to develop your own interpretation, integrating information provided in the five examples above. The theoretical orientation of the counselor, the personality and presenting concerns of the client, and the goals of the treatment process all contribute to determining the most useful interpretation. When formulating interpretations, counselors should make use of their special skills: their knowledge of human development and behavior, their empathy and sensitivity, their insight into people, and their multicultural competence. By drawing on these skills, counselors can maximize the effectiveness of their assessments, interpretations, diagnoses, and treatment plans. They also can present their clients as full human beings whose lives and experiences have coherence and importance.

The next chapter focuses on information gathering through an intake interview, an essential tool in the assessment process. It also includes the transcript of an interview and an accompanying analysis that further clarifies many of the points presented in this chapter.

Intake Interviews and Their Role in Diagnosis and Treatment Planning

In most mental health agencies, clients are seen for an intake interview before treatment begins. Counselors in private practice also typically conduct a comprehensive initial interview, although this process may not be labelled as a formal intake procedure. Initial interviews serve the following purposes:

1. *Determining suitability of person for agency's services*—Generally, clients (or their referral sources) are knowledgeable enough about mental health services to seek treatment from a person or agency that can meet their needs. Sometimes, however, the person or agency they consult cannot provide appropriate help. For example, a man with severe depression seeks help from a career-counseling program. In cases such as these, counselors should make a referral (discussed in Chapter 7).

Sometimes people request a specific form of treatment (e.g., eye movement desensitization and reprocessing, psychoanalysis) not available at the chosen agency. The reasoning behind the person's preference should be explored to be sure the requested treatment is a sound and carefully chosen one. If so, a referral can be made; if not, the counselor can describe alternative and potentially more helpful approaches.

2. *Assess and respond to urgency of person's situation*—A person in a crisis, perhaps having suicidal thoughts, needs help as soon as possible. Similarly, a severely disturbed person, perhaps one who is hallucinating or spending money impulsively during a manic episode, also needs immediate attention. A goal of the intake process is assessing the urgency of people's concerns and providing immediate intervention if warranted.

3. *Familiarize person with agency and counseling process*—Many people are apprehensive and unsophisticated about counseling. They may view counseling as being only for people who are weak or defective in some way. Preconceptions of counseling that clients have expressed to me include having to "lie on a couch and dredge up terrible dreams and memories," being "forced to tell the truth," and being given "shock therapy."

People's expectations of the counseling process should be explored and any fears or distortions alleviated by a clear, concise description of that process. Information should be provided on relevant agency policies such as scheduling, fees, confidentiality, and emergencies. In addition, people should receive information on the steps in the treatment process, their next appointment, and whether they will meet again with the intake interviewer or someone else.

4. *Begin to engender positive client attitudes toward counseling*—Part of the process of helping people to feel comfortable with counseling is the development of some counselor–client rapport and a sense of optimism. Clients should leave the initial interview feeling that they have been heard, that counseling is likely to help them, and that they have already begun to make progress. Intake interviews are pivotal in determining whether people will return for counseling, ready to make a commitment to that process.

5. *Gather sufficient information on presenting problem, history, and dynamics to allow formulation of a diagnosis and treatment plan*—The focal task of the intake interview is gathering enough information on the client to allow the formulation of at least a provisional diagnosis and treatment plan. Although many agencies have recommended procedures and forms for intake interviews, the interviewers are responsible for determining what information is needed, conducting an interview that provides that information, and concluding the interview when they have achieved the goals of the intake process.

OVERVIEW OF THE INTAKE PROCESS

The intake process itself can vary considerably depending on several variables. These include the personnel involved in the process, the approaches to gathering information, the intake schedule and format, the client, and the relationship of the intake process to treatment.

Intake Personnel

In some agencies, one person is responsible for gathering data on and evaluating a client's mental status, the nature and dynamics of that person's presenting concerns, and relevant history. However, in other agencies, clients meet with several mental health professionals as part of the intake process. A mental health counselor might gather information on presenting problems and background. A psychiatrist might conduct a physical and mental status examination. A referral also might be made to a psychologist for projective testing and an assessment of intelligence, or to a social worker who will interview family members and make a home visit. The nature of the intake process can vary considerably, depending on who is involved in that process.

Information Gathering

The manner in which data are gathered is another aspect of the intake process. Nearly all agencies have a standard intake procedure. Some agencies rely exclusively on information provided by clients through unstructured interviews and demographic questionnaires. Others include structured interviews such as the Brief Symptom Inventory or the Behavior and Symptom Identification Scale and might also use inventories such as the Beck Depression Inventory to assess symptom severity. Still other agencies advocate a broad-based approach to collecting information and, with the client's permission, interview family members and close friends of the client, request academic and medical records, and contact teachers or employers for information. Sample formats and procedures for intake interviews are provided later in this chapter.

Depth and Duration of Intake Process

Intake interviews may be as brief as 20 minutes in an emergency room where people who are suicidal or actively psychotic can be seen for immediate treatment. On the other hand, intake procedures can take 4 hours or more, especially if psychological testing is involved, and can span three or more sessions, scheduled on different days with different mental health specialists. However, most counselors devote 1–2 hours to the intake process.

Agency policy and practice largely determine the depth of the interview. In some agencies, intake interviewers function as selective and intelligent tape recorders. They gather information, sort important from unimportant, and write up relevant material in a concise format. They do little interpretation or analysis, viewing that as more appropriate in treatment than during intake—or not part of the counseling process at all. Other agencies advocate a more analytical role for the interviewer, viewing that person's goal as understanding the dynamics of people's concerns.

Nature of Client

At the outset of an intake interview, counselors should rapidly assess their client in order to meet urgent needs quickly and appropriately structure the intake interview. To facilitate their efforts in quickly understanding a client, counselors should consider the source and stated purpose of the referral, the client's presenting concerns, and the apparent level of that person's motivation and functioning.

The reason for a referral can provide essential information. Referral sources may be transferring responsibility for the person's treatment to a second agency, as in the case of most court referrals and referrals from employee assistance or managed care programs. On the other hand, the referral source may be seeking only a specific form of treatment for a person (e.g., career counseling, hypnotherapy for weight loss) while the referring agency continues to provide and oversee the person's treatment. Generally, the counselor has contact with the referring agency to determine the reason for the referral and whether collaboration is indicated.

Sometimes clients are encouraged to seek counseling by family or friends who want the client to change. Clients such as these may be resistant and have little motivation to change or they may be highly motivated to maintain their relationships and lifestyle. Attitudes toward treatment should be addressed early to promote productive counseling.

Externally motivated clients represent only one type of client who may prove challenging to the intake interviewer. Others include the severely depressed person, the person who is psychotic, the hostile person, the seductive or manipulative person, and the person expressing suicidal ideation. With such people, the interviewer's efforts to follow a standard format and develop a comprehensive picture of the client may be frustrated. Intake interviewers must take into account the nature of people's presenting concerns and their attitudes toward counseling so that the interview can be appropriately individualized. With people who are depressed, for example, interviewers usually assume a more active role, relying on clear and concrete questions and interventions that facilitate self-expression. Hostile clients might require limit-setting and confrontation as a part of the interview, while the person in crisis may require immediate assistance and only a minimal intake process. Counselors must adapt their standard procedures so that, at the completion of the intake process, the client is motivated and optimistic and the counselor has a useful understanding of the person's difficulties and is ready to plan the treatment.

Relationship of Intake Process to Treatment

Following the intake interview, one of several things may happen. The client might begin counseling with the intake interviewer or another counselor, the client may be placed on a waiting list or presented at a case conference, or the client may decide not to begin treatment. Whichever of these outcomes occurs, the interviewer should ensure that the following procedures occur:

1. Urgent client needs are met quickly.
2. The process of diagnosis and treatment planning is under way.
3. Both client and intake interviewer have a sense of closure and comfort at the end of the intake process and are aware of the next step in the treatment process.

4. The intake interviewer ensures that referrals and follow-up are accomplished. If people need time to decide whether to continue treatment or want to delay treatment, the intake interviewer arranges for contact at a later date. If clients sever interaction with the agency unexpectedly, further contact usually is made to offer another opportunity to receive help and ensure that the intake process did not discourage or alienate the clients.

CONDUCTING AN INTAKE INTERVIEW

Intake interviewers generally have little background or preparatory information on the people they interview and so must be flexible, resourceful, and experienced enough to handle a broad range of clients and presenting concerns. Sometimes new counselors at an agency conduct many of the intake interviews as a way of learning about agency procedures and clients. This also helps them build up a caseload and can enable more experienced counselors to concentrate on treatment. This does not mean that conducting intake interviews is easier than counseling. Rather, the intake interview often is challenging and demanding because it involves dealing with an unknown client who may not be motivated or comfortable with counseling.

At some agencies, appointments for intake interviews are scheduled in advance. At other agencies, intake interviewers cover predetermined blocks of time. For example, a counselor may interview any new clients who arrive on Mondays between 9 a.m. and 1 p.m. That enables an agency to provide immediate service, but can be more taxing for the counselor who may see no clients one week and five on another week.

Interventions

Counselors have many ways to begin an intake interview. Some start with an ice breaker or a series of social amenities: "How's the weather out there? ... Did you have any trouble finding a parking place? ... It's nice to see you today." Others go to an opposite extreme and begin with, "Tell me what your problems are." The social approach usually is counterproductive because it fails to set the proper tone for a counseling interview, can mislead the person as to the nature of the counselor-client relationship, and might increase clients' anxiety since they have come to see an expert, not a friend. On the other hand, the problem-focused approach also can clash with people's perceptions of why they are seeking counseling and may promote resistance if they are reluctant to see themselves as having problems. An approach that is professional, businesslike, and relatively nonthreatening seems ideal. The counselor might open the interview with a neutral question such as, "What brings you in today?" or "What sort of help were you seeking?"

Once the counselor–client dialog is under way, the counselor orients the client to the purpose and nature of the intake interview. If the interviewer will not be providing the person's treatment, this should be stated at the outset, lest the client feels misled. After establishing the ground rules for the intake process, the counselor then spends most of the interview exploring the person's presenting concerns, gathering information on history and life circumstances, and gaining insight into the dynamics of the person's difficulties. According to Morrison (1995b), the time spent in a typical initial interview is divided as follows: 15%, general conversation and presenting concern; 30%, diagnostic inquiry including exploration of suicidal and violent thoughts and actions, other prominent symptoms; 15%, medical history, social context, and family history; 25%, personal and social history, functioning and impairment; 10%, mental status examination; and 5%, summarization of session, feedback to client, and planning for next meeting. Detailed information on the mental status examination, categories of inquiry, and the process and analysis of initial interviews is provided later in this chapter.

Techniques used by the intake interviewer do not differ greatly from techniques used in other counseling sessions: open and closed questions, reflection of feeling, restatement, paraphrase, encouragers, and summarization are likely to be the primary modes of intervention. However, the percentage of each type of intervention used in initial interviews probably does differ from its percentage of use in other sessions. Counselors typically take more control of intake sessions than they do of other sessions; they tend to be relatively structured and intervene frequently. Usually more questions are used because information gathering is a primary focus.

Interviewers should select interventions that encourage meaningful responses, engage clients in the process of self-discovery, and initiate the development of rapport. Open questions are important tools for accomplishing these goals. For example, the intake interviewer might ask, "How do you feel about your work?" rather than "Do you like your work?" Questions evolve out of both predetermined topics and information provided by clients.

Although sensitivity to the client and timing are important, part of the role of the interviewer is exploring relevant issues that may seem very personal, such as inquiries about hallucinations, suicidal ideation, sexual experiences, and financial circumstances. Most clients expect such questions and respond openly to direct and clear questions such as, "Have you ever thought about hurting or killing yourself?" or "Do you ever see or hear things that seem strange or that other people do not see or hear?" Questions of this nature should be phrased carefully so that they do not suggest or encourage specific responses. For example, asking, "Tell me about any use you have made of drugs or alcohol in the past week" usually will elicit more information than asking, "Do you have a drinking problem?" While beginning counselors, in particular, may feel they are intruding by asking such questions, they should bear in mind the difference between counseling and socializing. Most people seeking counseling are relieved to have these difficult areas discussed in an open and nonjudgmental fashion.

SEQUENCE OF TOPICS IN AN INITIAL INTERVIEW

Because most people seek counseling due to their presenting concerns, counselors generally begin intake interviews by exploring those issues. However, in order to obtain background information, part of the intake interview usually focuses on the client's history. To help clients understand and become comfortable with this shift in focus, counselors might say something like, "We've spent some time exploring the concerns that brought you in for help and we will certainly talk more about those. However, I find it useful to put those concerns in context, so I would like to spend some of our time taking a broader view and talking about your background as well as other aspects of your life. How does that sound to you?" With this explanation, nearly all clients agree to expanding the focus of the initial interview beyond their presenting problems. To further reassure clients that the counselor recognizes the importance of the presenting concerns, the counselor should be sure to bring the focus of the interview back to the target concerns before the end of the session. Suggesting a relevant task or new perspective on those concerns at the conclusion of the session is yet another way to convey to clients that the primary purpose of the treatment process will be to address the client's issues.

Recording Information

Because a great deal of information is gathered in a short time, most intake interviewers use either note taking or tape recording to assist recall. Both approaches have pros and cons.

The client's permission must be obtained before a session is tape recorded. Although few people object to being recorded, this can be viewed as a violation of privacy and makes some people uneasy, despite assurances of confidentiality. Counselors also may need as much time to review a tape recording as they do to conduct an intake interview. However, tape recording has the important advantage of preserving the intake interview with minimam distortion. Also, once the mechanics of discussing and starting the recorder are completed, most people become oblivious to that process. During the session, then, it is less obtrusive than note taking.

Note taking generally is less threatening than tape recording and usually requires little discussion beyond an explanation of why the counselor is taking notes and how the security of the notes will be maintained. However, note taking has several possible disadvantages. It can prevent counselors from giving clients their full attention. Notes are inevitably incomplete, possibly leading to significant omissions or distortions. Also, clients are sometimes distracted by note taking and may attribute significance to the instances of note taking, perhaps even focusing more on topics that seem to precipitate note taking. If note taking is used, counselors should minimize its impact on the interview while still capturing in writing the essence of the interview.

Combining note taking and tape recording is yet another option, allowing counselors to listen to all or part of the recording while having notes available for quick review. Whether to tape record or take notes on sessions is an individual decision determined by counselor preference and the nature of a particular client. However, few counselors today rely exclusively on memory; most use note taking rather than tape recording.

Concluding the Intake Interview

Particularly when the intake interview is not a predetermined length, the interviewer must decide when to end the interview and inform the client that the conclusion of the interview is imminent. The counselor should do this in a positive way, allowing at least a few minutes for client additions and questions. A typical closing to an initial interview might be:

> Counselor: You've certainly told me a great deal about yourself. I think I have the information I need so that we can move ahead and plan your counseling. Is there anything you'd like to add?
>
> Client: No, I don't think so.
>
> Counselor: All right. Let me fill you in on just what will happen now and how long that will take. You will have some time to ask any questions you might have before we wrap up for today.

The interview then draws to a close, with the counselor informing the client about the steps for continuing treatment and the timetable that will be followed. The counselor also should be sure that the person is familiar with any necessary procedures before leaving the agency (e.g., making payments, completing forms, scheduling an appointment).

THE COMPREHENSIVE INTAKE INTERVIEW

This section of the chapter familiarizes readers with the content and process of a typical comprehensive intake interview, including the categories of inquiry, the mental status examination, a transcript of a comprehensive intake interview, and a report based on that transcript. A subsequent section of this chapter provides examples of brief intake reports.

The interviewer has a multifaceted role: establishing rapport, orienting the client to the counseling process, assessing the urgency of the client's concerns, obtaining information needed to initiate diagnosis and treatment planning, and analyzing the intake interview.

Such interviews have both overt and covert agendas. The overt agenda involves gathering useful information on people's concerns and on their relevant history. Most of the questions aimed at acquiring this material will be direct and their goals apparent. At the same time, the counselor also is gathering information on a client's mental status. This process is subtler and involves using observational or inferential information as well as factual material provided by the clients.

Sometimes, as mentioned earlier, the interviewer uses checklists, inventories, or questionnaires to supplement, focus, and standardize the interview process. These might be comprehensive inventories designed to help the interviewer gather a broad range of information on a person's level of functioning, presenting problems, and history. Specific questionnaires also are available to assess problem areas such as phobias, depression, anxiety, use of drugs and alcohol, and eating behaviors. Whether such instruments are used depends on agency policy, counselor preference, and client concerns.

MENTAL STATUS EXAMINATION

The purpose of a mental status examination (MSE) is obtaining information on how people are feeling, thinking, and acting. Emphasis is on identifying areas of impairment, along with strengths, to provide a clear picture of people's functioning. An MSE facilitates diagnosis and effective treatment planning. In addition, managed care organizations frequently require an MSE as part of the documentation required for authorization of treatment.

When drawing conclusions about people's mental status, intake interviewers rely heavily on their knowledge of healthy functioning as well as on their observations and information provided by clients. A formal examination generally is not involved. However, checklists or specific questions can help ensure counselors' accuracy. Because of the relatively subjective nature of the MSE, interviewers must be aware of and sensitive to multicultural norms and should consider clients' functioning in their culture of origin as well as in their current culture.

Mental status can be conceptualized in terms of the following 12 categories (Morrison, 1995b; Seligman, 2004; Wiger & Solberg, 2001):

1. *Appearance*

   a. General impression
   b. Nature and appropriateness of clothing for weather and occasion

    c. Cleanliness and self-care

    d. Noteworthy physical characteristics

2. *Behavior*

    a. Social functioning (e.g., eye contact, willingness to respond to questions)

    b. Habits (e.g., smoking, rocking, nail biting)

    c. Movement retardation or agitation and hyperactivity

    d. Tremors, tics, or other unusual mannerisms

    e. Sensory difficulties (e.g., visual, motor, auditory)

    f. Attitude toward counselor and counseling process (e.g., motivated, domineering, meek)

3. *Speech and Language*

    a. Clarity of articulation and communication

    b. Rate and volume of speech (e.g., slow, pressured, or fluid; loud, quiet, or appropriate)

    c. Speech or word usage reflective of cultural background or unusual in some way

4. *Emotions*

    a. Observable emotions, including immediate as well as underlying long-standing emotional states (e.g., depression, anxiety, elation, irritability)

    b. Range and lability (amount of change) of emotions

    c. Quality of emotions (e.g., flat and blunted, highly charged)

    d. Congruence of emotions and content

5. *Orientation to Reality*

    a. Aware of time (hour, day, month, year)

    b. Aware of place (where interview is being conducted)

    c. Aware of person (who client and counselor are)

    d. Aware of situation (what is happening)

6. *Concentration and Attention*

    a. Ability to focus well, maintain attention (sometimes assessed by asking people to repeat a sequence of at least five digits or repeat three words in reverse order)

    b. Ability to sustain attention (can be assessed by asking people to subtract by 7s from 100)

    c. Ability to provide clear and relevant responses

    d. Alert and responsive, lethargic, or distracted

7. *Thought Processes*

   a. Capacity for abstract thinking (sometimes assessed by asking people to explain several proverbs such as, "The early bird catches the worm" and "Strike while the iron is hot")
   b. Coherence, clarity, and continuity in thoughts, "flight of ideas," and loose associations
   c. Repetitions, perseverations
   d. Responses produced quickly or delayed, relevant or confused and tangential
   e. Capacity for logical thinking and sound reasoning

8. *Thought Content*

   a. Suicidal ideation
   b. Violence, aggression, rage
   c. Fears and phobias
   d. Obsessions and compulsions
   e. Thoughts of reference, suspicion, and persecution
   f. Delusions
   g. Intrusive traumatic recollections or other prominent thoughts

9. *Perception*

   a. Hallucinations (auditory, visual, tactile, olfactory, gustatory)
   b. Illusions and other unusual experiences, beliefs, or perceptions

10. *Memory*

    a. Adequacy of immediate memory (less than 1 min)
    b. Adequacy of short-term memory (e.g., information provided at beginning of interview)
    c. Adequacy of recent past memory (e.g., events occurring weeks or months ago)
    d. Adequacy of remote memory (e.g., person's educational background, historical events)

11. *Intelligence and Knowledge*

    a. Educational level
    b. Level of vocabulary
    c. Knowledge about the world (fund of information)

12. *Judgment and Insight*

    a. Ability to make decisions
    b. Ability to solve problems

    c. Ability to take appropriate responsibility
    d. Ability to delay action and control impulses
    e. Awareness of and insight into own difficulties
    f. Self-image, including strengths and weaknesses

This comprehensive outline of an MSE is much longer than a typical written MSE. In most cases, a few paragraphs, perhaps a page at most, are sufficient to describe mental status. An example is provided later in this chapter.

OUTLINE OF AN EXTENDED INTAKE INTERVIEW

The following is an outline of the categories of inquiry in a typical comprehensive intake interview. Suggested questions and topics can help counselors conduct such an interview. Although this outline can be useful in providing structure and important areas of inquiry for in-depth interviews, this outline should be viewed as a guide. Each interview, like each client, is unique, and effective interviewers conduct intake sessions with flexibility and sensitivity to the clients' needs. Questions and topics are individualized to suit the concerns, age, background, functioning, and motivation of each client.

1. *Identifying Information*

    a. Gender
    b. Age
    c. Ethnic and cultural background, religion, languages spoken
    d. Partner/marital status
    e. Family composition
    f. Educational background and level
    g. Place and nature of residence and cohabitants

2. *Presenting Problem(s)*

    a. Chief complaints and difficulties
    b. Source of referral, reason for referral, or how client selected this clinician
    c. Immediate precipitant for seeking counseling at this time
    d. Symptoms and impact on functioning
    e. Duration
    f. Previous efforts to obtain help

3. *Other Current Problems and Previous Difficulties*—For all problem areas explored, interviewers should obtain information about the following:

    a. Nature of concern
    b. Circumstances and time of onset

   c Symptoms

   d. History of concerns (initial or recurrent, frequency, duration)

   e. Dynamics of concern (What seems to cause it to develop, change, or abate? What does the person do to address the concern? How do others react to the concern?)

   f. Previous treatment for concern and effect of treatment

   g. Impact of concern on person's lifestyle, activities, relationships, eating, sleeping, mood

4. *Present Life Situation*

   a. Family relationships

   b. Other important interpersonal relationships

   c. Occupational/educational activities

   d. Social and leisure activities

   e. Typical day in person's life

   f. Sources of stress and satisfaction

5. *Family of Origin*

   a. Composition of family and description of each family member

   b. Family constellation and subsystems

   c. Client's birth order

   d. Social, economic, ethnic, cultural, religious and spiritual origins and influences

   e. Genetic and historical patterns

   f. Patterns of physical or emotional dysfunction in the family (especially substance misuse, depression, suicide, neglect, sexual or physical abuse, violence, incarceration)

   g. Significant crises, events, changes, losses

   h. Power structure in family

   i. Patterns of communication, closeness, and distance

   j. Family values, norms, and messages

   k. Parenting and discipline style

   l. Client's role models in the family

   m. Current and past relationships with father, mother, siblings, other important family members

6. *Current Family*

   a. Composition of family and description of each family member

   b. Family constellation and subsystems

   c. Social, economic, ethnic, cultural, religious, and spiritual influences

   d. Patterns of dysfunction and problems in the family

e. Significant crises, events, changes, losses
f. Power structure in the family
g. Patterns of communication, closeness, and distance
h. Family values, norms, messages
i. Client's current and past relationships with family members

7. *Developmental History*—Interviewers focus on times of greatest relevance to the person's age and current situation. The following comprehensive outline should be used to give direction rather than as an exact
list of topics to be explored. For each age group, counselors should ask
about important events and memories, difficulties, and successes. For
young people, information can be obtained from parents and guardians
as well as from clients themselves

8. *Infancy*

a. Birth history—parents' circumstances, ages, health; reactions to child's
birth and gender; child's health at birth
b. Early development—family relationships, child care, feeding, toilet
training, overall development, health, discipline, any habits, fears, or
early problems

9. *Early Childhood (Preschool Years)*

a. Living conditions
b. Family composition
c. Child's roles and relationships in the family
d. Early social relationships outside of the family
e. Liked and disliked activities
f. Child's personality

10. *Middle and Late Childhood*

a. Early educational history, reactions to school, relationships with
teachers, level of achievement, favorite and disliked subjects
b. Relationships with other children
c. Liked and disliked activities
d. Changes, patterns, or problems in family relationships during these
years
e. Any behavioral problems
f. Sense of initiative, level of self-confidence, and capacity for
accomplishment.
g. Personality and emotional development

11. *Adolescence*

    a. Timetable of physical maturation and reaction to physical changes
    b. Peer relationships and interactions, especially close friendships
    c Patterns of sexual activity and interest
    d. Reactions to authority figures
    e. Academic performance
    f. Family relationships
    g. Liked and disliked social and leisure activities
    h. Career and education aspirations
    i. Any emotional, physical, or behavioral problems

12. *Adulthood*

    a. Academic abilities, accomplishments, and areas of difficulty
    b. Career and educational history
    c. Nature of and time spent on leisure and cultural activities
    d. Relationships with family, friends, others—nature, number, duration, and intensity (consider changes in relationships with family of origin; relationship patterns with partner, children, in-laws, friends, colleagues, associates)
    e. Sexual orientation, sexual and intimate relationships
    f. Current financial situation
    g. Religious and spiritual beliefs and values
    h. Any arrests, incarcerations, or lawsuits
    i. Use of drugs and alcohol
    j. Any abuse or mistreatment
    k. Primary sources of satisfaction and disappointment
    l. Self-image
    m. Important goals and future dreams, vision of life in 5 and 10 years

13. *Medical and Counseling History and Treatments*

    a. Current and past illnesses and accidents of significance
    b. Past and current medical treatments or medications and their side effects
    c. Previous treatment for emotional difficulties (nature, duration, outcome)
    d. Expectations for current counseling (nature, duration, outcome)

14. *Additional Information Important to the Client*

TRANSCRIPT OF EXTENDED INTERVIEW —————————————————————

The following pages include a transcript of an extended initial interview, a report written on that interview, and two additional brief intake reports. This illustrates how such an interview might be conducted and subsequently analyzed. Client is Maria Sanchez, a 36-year-old woman, born in El Salvador, who sought counseling at a community mental health center.

Interviewer: What brings you in for counseling today, Maria?

Maria: I've been feeling very depressed lately and haven't been able to get the things done that I need to do. I don't know what's wrong with me. This should be the happiest time in my life.

Interviewer: You seem very worried. Tell me more about what you are feeling.

Maria: As you can see, I'm pregnant; the baby is due in about 3 months. This will be my fourth child. I have three sons who are each about 2 years apart; the oldest is 7. Now I'm going to have a little girl. I always dreamed of having a big family and my dreams are coming true. This has been a difficult pregnancy, but I don't understand why I feel so bad.

Interviewer: What are these depressed feelings like for you?

Maria: I feel pretty hopeless about the future. I think about what is happening in the world and I feel guilty that I am bringing children into such a world. I have trouble sleeping and just think about all the awful things that can happen to my children. Being pregnant and having pain in my back and my legs don't help either. And I seem to eat all the time. The doctor told me I've already gained more than enough weight for the whole pregnancy but I just keep eating. I eat with the kids, I eat with my husband, and then I eat alone. The first time I was pregnant, I felt so beautiful but now I feel fat and ugly. I know this is crazy but I feel like I'm useless and nobody cares about me. I feel like I'm letting them all down.

Interviewer: I can hear that this is a very hard time for you in many ways. Have you ever felt so bad that you have thought about hurting or even killing yourself?

Maria: No, I would never do that to my family. I know what it is like to grow up without a mother. My boys are my life. I'll bring you a picture of them. They are so cute, like stair steps when they stand together. And so smart! The oldest one reads chapter books, the middle one reads words and does addition, and even the little one knows his letters. They're like their father.

Interviewer: You sound so proud of both your sons and your husband. Tell me about your husband and the relationship you two have.

Maria: We met about 10 years ago. I was a legal assistant in a downtown law firm and he was already a partner in the firm. He's 10 years older that I am; I'm 36 and he's 46. I thought he was the most brilliant lawyer in the firm, and very handsome too. I never thought he would be interested in me. But then we started going out for coffee, then lunch, then a movie, and after a while I realized we were falling in love. You know, I'd never had a serious relationship before and I couldn't believe this was really happening to me. We went out together for about 2 years and then one day he said, "When do you think we should get married?" Just like that! I wasn't so ready to rush into things; I wanted to be sure I didn't make a mistake. So we talked a lot and we both said we wanted a big family and wanted to have children soon so here we are.

Interviewer: It sounds like a dream come true for you.

Maria: It really is. If I could have written a story about how my life would turn out, this would be it. I can't understand the way I feel. My husband tries so hard to help but nothing works.

Interviewer: How has he tried to help?

Maria: He sees how hard it is for me to take care of the boys. He said we should get a nanny, but I don't want to leave the boys with anyone but him or me. And he has to work very long hours at the law firm. When he comes home, the boys are already in bed and he usually leaves before they get up in the morning. We try to do things as a family on the weekend but I need him to watch the children while I do the grocery shopping and other errands so there isn't much family time.

Interviewer: I can hear that you are very busy. Besides feeling depressed, what other changes have you noticed in yourself that bother you?

Maria: I'm tired all the time, even if I go to bed when the boys do. And I don't seem to concentrate well. Sometimes one of the boys asks me something and I'm so distracted, I don't even hear him. They ask me to read them a story and I lose my place in the book. And I have trouble making decisions, even silly things like what color to paint the nursery for the new baby. When I was at the law firm, I was the fastest and best researcher. I feel so different now.

Interviewer: Have there been other times in your life when you have felt depressed like this?

Maria: Not exactly like this, but I have felt very sad before, especially when I was a child.

Interviewer: Maybe this is a good time to talk about your background. We will certainly talk more today about your depression, but it will help me understand you better to put things in context. How would you feel about filling me in on your background?

Maria: Some of it is hard to talk about but I'll try. I was born in El Salvador. I never knew who my father was and my mother said she didn't know either. My mother and I lived with her mother, my grandmother. My mother worked to support us all but we were very poor and my mother said that things just kept getting worse. When I was about 7, she went to the United States to find a better job. She never told me she was leaving; she said she didn't want to see me cry. I woke up and she was gone. My grandmother told me why my mother wasn't there.

Interviewer: What was that experience like for you?

Maria: At first, I didn't mind. I guess I thought she would be back in a few days. I really didn't expect her to be gone for so many years. It got to be pretty bad.

Interviewer: Pretty bad?

Maria: Yeah, my mother sent money every few months but we really couldn't manage. My grandmother got sick and so we moved in with my Aunt Anna. My grandmother and I lived with her and her husband and three children. They did support us but they treated me like a servant.

Interviewer: That must have been very difficult.

Maria: Well, yes and no. They did let me go to school so I didn't really mind helping out. It gave me something to do. I got to feel so lonely for my mother that it sort of took my mind off how bad I felt. But then things got worse; that's the part that's hard to talk about.

Interviewer: It's up to you whether you want to talk about that now.

Maria: I guess I should tell you everything so you can help me. There was a problem with my uncle; he started looking at me a lot, following me around, saying I was developing early and becoming so beautiful. This didn't feel right!

Interviewer: How did you handle that?

Maria: I couldn't do anything but stay away from him as much as I could. I was very shy and had no girlfriends. I had no one to talk to. I didn't want to upset my grandmother and I was afraid that if I told my aunt, she'd throw us out and then what would I do? Sometimes I couldn't leave the house because there was shooting and fighting outside and then I felt really scared. Things were very bad in El Salvador then. One day I came home from school and there were two dead bodies lying on the street. I was sad and scared all the time. I prayed a lot and wished that my mother would come back and get me. She kept saying she would but she didn't come back until I was 14.

Interviewer: You have been through some extremely difficult experiences!

Maria: Yes, but I survived. I didn't get killed and my uncle never really did anything to me. I don't know how I managed to take care of myself for so long but I did.

Interviewer: You must have many strengths.

Maria: I used to think so but now I'm not so sure. Maybe I just had too many problems. I thought things would be all right when my mother came for me, but that was terrible too.

Interviewer: What was that like for you?

Maria: When I was about 14, my grandmother died. I guess that is why my mother finally came back. She packed up my stuff and took me to the United States with her. I didn't know this but my mother was married and had another daughter. She was 5 and could speak perfect English; I hardly knew any English and she made fun of me. And I had a stepfather who didn't like me much. He would take his daughter out for ice cream and just leave me alone at home.

Interviewer: What a disappointment that must have been for you, and what a difficult change.

Maria: It was, but at least I was away from my uncle and I had opportunities in the United States.

Interviewer: Opportunities?

Maria: Yes, I decided that I would learn English and do really well at school. I had always loved school and it became a good place for me in the United States too. I would listen to the television and try to talk like the people I saw. I would even talk to my stepfather and sister as much as I could, just to practice English. One of the teachers at school helped me; she gave me books and tapes and I learned to speak English very well. I guess that kept me out of trouble. The other kids were using drugs and dating and didn't care about school but I did. When I began my last year of high school, the teacher I liked helped me get a scholarship to college. I couldn't believe it! I went to college, got a degree, and learned to be a legal assistant. It really helped me that I was bilingual and I got lots of job offers. Good thing I took the job I did or I wouldn't have met Frederick.

Interviewer: You really turned your life around, pretty much all by yourself.

Maria: Yes, I guess I do feel pretty proud if that. Of course, the teacher helped me and my mother let me live with her while I was going to college. She and my stepfather had gotten divorced by now and she liked having me there to help out with my sister and the housework.

Interviewer: I'm glad to hear you can take pride in all you accomplished, even though you did have some help. How did your relationship with your mother develop as you got older?

Maria: We get along ok, but I never really felt close to her. We had been separated for too long. I think of my grandmother as more of a mother to me. It was very hard for me when she died.

Interviewer: That was another big loss for you.

Maria: Yes, it was. But it helped to go to the United States with my mother. My mother and I probably get along better now than we ever did but I've had to change what I expect from her.

Interviewer: How so?

Maria: When my first son was born, I wanted us to be like one big family. I would ask her to visit us and I would take my son to visit her. I did that with my in-laws and they always seemed happy to see us. But it was different with my mother. Sometimes she wouldn't show up when she said she would and then if I were going to visit her, she would sometimes be too busy to spend much time with me. She had a new boyfriend and they would always have some plan or other. I try to remember that she never had a real family herself and doesn't know what it should be like. Her father and older brother were killed. At least I didn't have it that bad. Now I'll call her every week and try to see her often, but my children hardly know her. It's not like how my grandmother and I were but I have strong spiritual beliefs and I know I must maintain a relationship with my mother.

Interviewer: Tell me more about your religious and spiritual beliefs.

Maria: I was raised Catholic. Church was like school for me, a quiet place where I felt safe and special. Frederick has a very different background. His family is Protestant and they hardly ever go to church. This has been an issue for us and I've had to make some compromises, but I always have God in my heart. Frederick and his family really respect that about me.

Interviewer: That means a great deal to you.

Maria: Yes, I do have wonderful in-laws. They are always so happy to see me and the boys. All of my pregnancies have been difficult but they have always been there to help me.

Interviewer: Tell me some more about that.

Maria: I guess each pregnancy was hard in a different way. When my husband and I got married, I had been working as a legal assistant for about 5 years. I loved my work and did very well. I was making more money than I ever imagined. I had my own apartment and I would go out to dinner with two good friends I had. I could buy nice clothes and help out my mother. It was a wonderful time in my life, but I always hoped I would get married and have my own family. When Frederick and I got married, he said he earned plenty of money and I didn't need to work. I wanted to work for awhile but when I got pregnant, I left work to get ready for the baby.

Interviewer: That must have been a big change for you.

Maria: It was, but I wanted my children to have a real family and to have everything we could give them. I understand why I was depressed when my mother left and when I had to live with my aunt and uncle, but I can't understand why I get so depressed each time I get pregnant. I've heard of people who get depressed after they have a baby, but I'm more depressed during the pregnancy.

Interviewer: What sense do you make of that?

Maria: I don't really know. When I first got pregnant, I felt sad because I stopped working and seeing my girlfriends, but my husband and I decided that was the right thing to do. So why should I have been depressed?

Interviewer: I can hear that it's puzzling to you. That is something we can talk about next time. I'd like to talk just a bit more about the things that are bothering you now before we end our session. It sounds like you have had several episodes of depression; when your mother left, when you were living with your aunt and uncle, and then each time you got pregnant.

Maria: Yes, but I didn't really get so depressed when I was pregnant with my second son or even the third. It was worst with my first pregnancy and it's pretty bad now.

Interviewer: Have you even felt the opposite of depressed, sort of like you were on top of the world and couldn't stop thinking of new exciting ideas.

Maria: No, I never felt that way.

Interviewer: Did you ever take any drugs to help you with the depression?

Maria: No, I don't take any drugs unless I have the flu. I used to have a glass of wine sometimes but now I've been pregnant so much of the time, I haven't even had any wine in years.

Interviewer: Have you had any serious illnesses or hospitalizations?

Maria: Just to deliver the babies. I've been lucky that I have been pretty healthy. Maybe that's why it bothers me so much now that my back hurts. I just don't feel like myself.

Interviewer: I wonder if you are sometimes still bothered by memories of the way your uncle treated you and the frightening things you saw in El Salvador?

Maria: I was very bothered by it for many years. I used to have nightmares and couldn't stand to be alone. I felt anxious all the time and wouldn't go out when it was dark. It was pretty bad, even long after I left El Salvador. But then when I went to college, somehow it changed and gradually got better. I'll never forget all that but it doesn't haunt me the way it used to.

Interviewer: Even though those strong reactions have greatly diminished, there probably are many ways in which those experiences still affect you. I wonder what you think about that?

Maria: Yes, you're right about that. If I could do it, I'd make sure no other child ever went through what I did, not really having a mother or father while I was growing up and being exposed to all those terrible things. I want to make sure that my children have a very different life. My husband says I worry too much about them, that they have loving parents and a good home and they'll grow up just fine but that's not good enough for me. Bringing a child into the world is such a big responsibility; I have to do the best I possibly can for them.

Interviewer: It sounds like you work very hard to do all you can for your family. I wonder what effect that has on you and your marriage.

Maria: I do get tired sometimes, and frustrated with myself that I can't do more, especially now that I'm having a tough pregnancy. As for my marriage ... we decided to have a big family and my husband has to understand that the children come first. We'll have time when they are older.

Interviewer: How do you think your husband feels about that?

Maria: He works very hard too. He would like us to have more time alone but I won't leave the children with anybody but his parents and lately I haven't even been comfortable leaving the children with them. My mother-in-law fell and I don't think she should be picking up a child.

Interviewer: So you and your husband have very little time together?

Maria: Yes, but how can we do that right now, with three children and another on the way? My husband said he thought this should be our last child. I'm not sure, but if she is, in 5 years or so she'll be in school and I won't mind leaving the children with a good baby-sitter then.

Interviewer: I can hear how dedicated you are to your children. As we continue to meet together, we will talk more about your family as well as your depression. You have told me a great deal already. I wonder if I have missed anything that you want to be sure I know about today?

Maria: No, I think you covered most of the important information.

(The session now would conclude by summarizing the session, asking for her reactions to the session, and setting up an appointment for her next session.)

NATURE OF AN INTAKE REPORT

The report of an extended intake interview typically includes the following 12 topics:

- Identifying information
- Overview of the presenting problem, its symptoms, and impact on the person
- Information on the MSE
- Other problems and difficulties
- Present life situation
- Information on family of origin and present family
- Developmental history, important incidents
- Medical and treatment history
- Case conceptualization, including strengths and areas of difficulty
- Multiaxial diagnosis
- Treatment plan and other recommendations
- Conclusion and summary

REPORT OF INTAKE INTERVIEW

Client: Maria Sanchez   *Interviewer*: Anne Eastment, M.A., LPC
Birthdate: 2/3/68   *Date of interview*: 5/9/04

Identifying Information

Maria Sanchez, a 36-year-old married Latina woman, was self-referred for counseling at the New England Community Mental Health Center. Ms. Sanchez is currently pregnant. She lives with her husband and three sons, ages 3, 5, and 7, and is
a full-time homemaker. A college graduate, Ms. Sanchez had been successfully
employed as a legal assistant.

Presenting Problem

Ms. Sanchez reports depression, lasting approximately 2 months. Symptoms
include overeating, difficulty falling asleep, feelings of guilt about her perceived
inability to give her children sufficient care and attention, and feelings of being
overwhelmed. Her symptoms are compounded by what Ms. Sanchez described as a
difficult pregnancy, including back pain and excessive weight gain, and by her
reluctance to accept help with child care. Despite recurrent episodes of depression,
this is the first time Ms. Sanchez has sought counseling. Ms. Sanchez reported
a difficult childhood and adolescence including no knowledge of her father, a
lengthy separation from her mother, emotional abuse by an uncle, and multiple
traumatic experiences in El Salvador, where she spent the first 14 years of her life.

Mental Status Examination

Ms. Sanchez presented for the interview wearing a loose blouse, jeans, and sneak-
ers. She had a casual and natural style and was dressed appropriately for the
weather. She had no unusual physical characteristics but was visibly pregnant. She
stated that she was 5'6" tall and weighed 196 lb, which she perceived as overweight,
although she was in the sixth month of pregnancy. Ms. Sanchez related well to this
interviewer and seemed motivated and eager for help. She made appropriate eye
contact, except when discussing her troubling experiences in El Salvador, and manifested no unusual behaviors. Her speech was quiet but audible with little trace of
an accent. Ms. Sanchez was articulate and expressed herself clearly. She appeared
depressed and somewhat anxious, sometimes sighing deeply or wringing her
hands. No signs or reports of suicidal ideation were evident. The client's affect
varied little and was consistent with the serious topics she was discussing, although
she did smile occasionally when discussing her children.

Ms. Sanchez was in good contact with reality and manifested no difficulties in concentration, attention, or memory, even when talking about her experiences in El Salvador. Her thinking was clear and coherent and she seemed capable of insight, although her judgment sometimes seemed flawed. Ms. Sanchez is probably of at least above average intelligence; she learned English quickly upon immigrating to the United States, successfully completed college, and was employed as a legal assistant. However, she is experiencing low self-esteem and self-blame and currently feels too overwhelmed to make good use of her problem-solving abilities. She has few leisure activities and allows herself little time apart from her children. At the same time, she has many strengths; she is open and expressive, she is motivated to make some changes, she reports a strong and supportive relationship with her husband, is a mature and responsible woman who has overcome considerable adversity, and is dedicated to her children.

Other Current Problems and Difficulties

Ms. Sanchez was born in El Salvador. She never knew who her father was and lived with her mother and grandmother until age 7, when her mother left El Salvador without saying goodbye to Ms. Sanchez and went to the United States to earn money for the family. The two had almost no contact for the next 7 years. When the grandmother became ill 2 years after the mother's departure, Ms. Sanchez and her grandmother moved in with an aunt and uncle and their children. Ms. Sanchez reported being treated like a servant and experiencing emotional as well as threatened sexual abuse from the uncle.

The political unrest and violence in El Salvador compounded the situation at that time. Ms. Sanchez reported seeing dead bodies lying in the street and being terrified by violence. Ms. Sanchez apparently developed a Posttraumatic Stress Disorder at that time; symptoms included nightmares, fear of being alone, and high anxiety. These symptoms continued until age 18.

When Ms. Sanchez was 14, her grandmother died, prompting Ms. Sanchez's mother to return home and bring her daughter back to the United States. Unbeknownst to Ms. Sanchez, her mother had married and had a daughter. This was a difficult transition for Ms. Sanchez. However, she learned English rapidly, focused her attention on succeeding at school, earned a scholarship to college, completed her bachelor's degree, and found employment as a legal assistant.

Ms. Sanchez reports several coping skills: her spiritual and religious beliefs and her determination to succeed, especially via education. Nevertheless, she has experienced many episodes of depression, including when her mother left, when she lived with her aunt and uncle, her early years in the United States, her first pregnancy, and now during her fourth pregnancy.

Present Life Situation

Ms. Sanchez describes college and her subsequent years of employment as a legal assistant in very positive terms. Her husband is a lawyer in the firm where she was employed and, after dating for 2 years, the two married. Her husband is 10 years older than Ms. Sanchez and has a Protestant background. Ms. Sanchez is Catholic and reports that her religion is important to her. The couple has been married for 10 years; they have three sons, ages 7, 5, and 3. Ms. Sanchez is now 6 months pregnant and is expecting a daughter. The family live in a large home in a suburban community. Ms. Sanchez assumes full care for her children, accepting only occasional help from her in-laws and someone to clean the house. Her husband works long hours in the law firm and the two rarely have time as a couple. In addition, Ms. Sanchez has few friends or leisure activities, devoting herself entirely to care of her home and family.

Ms. Sanchez maintains contact with her mother and half-sister but reports that her mother, now divorced, is unreliable and unable to help her. The client reports positive relationships with her in-laws but states that they, too, can provide little help because of their age and health.

Family

Ms. Sanchez comes from a difficult family background. Although separation from a parent who is seeking economic improvement is not unusual in Ms. Sanchez's culture, the circumstances of her separation from her mother, including lack of preparation for the separation, minimal contact, living with an elderly grandmother, and an emotionally abusive aunt and uncle, were particularly difficult. In addition, the client was ill prepared for her return to the United States, where she was surprised by the presence of a stepfather and half-sister.

Ms. Sanchez exerts enormous effort to counteract the inadequate parenting and limited early education she received by setting high and probably unrealistic goals for her role as wife and mother. She seems to be teaching her children skills they may not be ready to master, allows herself no time for friends or leisure activities, puts her marriage second to her role as mother, and will not even make allowances for herself now that she is pregnant.

Developmental History

Important events in Ms. Sanchez's history are primarily family events, described above. Ms. Sanchez attended a neighborhood school as a child and viewed that as an escape from the aversive conditions of her early years. A shy child, her social maturity seems to have lagged behind her physical and intellectual maturity.

Family responsibilities allowed her little leisure time. Only after college did she develop some friendships.

Medical and Treatment History

Ms. Sanchez is currently 6 months pregnant; medical tests reveal she will give birth to a girl. She reports back pain and fatigue, stemming at least in part from her pregnancy. Otherwise, Ms. Sanchez is and has been in good health.

Case Conceptualization, Including Strengths and Areas of Difficulty

Ms. Sanchez has much strength. Her history reflects remarkable resilience. Through her spiritual beliefs, intelligence, determination, strong values, and support from her grandmother and a teacher, she survived adversity in both her family and her environment and became a well-educated and self-supporting young woman. She and her husband seem to have a strong marriage despite the pressure of three children.

On the other hand, the combination of Ms. Sanchez's difficult early years, her low self-esteem, her extremely high standards, and her limited support systems have contributed to her depression. Although she does not seem to be in danger, she is likely to experience even more stress during the rest of her pregnancy and after the birth of her fourth child. She has difficulty attending to her own needs and those of her husband but is driven by personal and background factors to devote all her energy to her children. This is probably compounded by anxiety stemming from her insecure and traumatic background and her lack of information on healthy parenting.

Diagnostic Impression

Although Ms. Sanchez presently seems to be taking adequate care of herself and her family, her self-esteem and social functioning are impaired. She struggles with depression, feelings of failure and self-blame, and a history of abuse and difficult family relationships. At the same time, she has much strength. She is an appropriate candidate for counseling at present. A multiaxial assessment of Ms. Sanchez follows:

Axis I.   296.32 Major Depressive Disorder, recurrent, moderate, with
            interepisode recovery
            309.81 Posttraumatic Stress Disorder, prior history
Axis II.   V71.89 No mental disorder on Axis II
Axis III.   Pregnant, reports fatigue and back pain

Axis IV.   Pregnancy, three young children
Axis V.   57

The treatment plan for this case is presented in Chapter 7.

                                                    THE BRIEF INTAKE INTERVIEW

Many mental health agencies use a brief approach to intake interviews. Such interviews typically last 30–50 minutes and culminate in a relatively short written report. This approach is particularly prevalent in agencies that are understaffed or that advocate one of the brief, solution-focused approaches to treatment, discussed in Chapter 7.

The primary goals of the brief intake process are similar to those of the extended intake process. They commonly include the following:

- Assessing and dealing with the urgency of the person's concerns
- Gathering demographic data
- Orienting the person to the policies and procedures of the agency as well as to counseling
- Understanding the presenting problem and reasons for seeking help
- Evaluating mental status
- Obtaining information on the person's current situation
- Gathering salient information on relevant history, especially previous treatment
- Conceptualizing the case in such a way as to make sense of the person's concerns
- Determining suitability for counseling and identifying issues that seem amenable to treatment
- Developing a diagnosis and treatment plan

In a brief intake interview, particular emphasis is placed on presenting concerns. The brief model assumes a less analytical approach, generally accepting the person's statement of his or her goals with only limited exploration. The interviewer typically pays far less attention to history taking and undertakes only limited exploration.

Examples of Brief Intake Interview Reports and Information Forms ————

An intake interview, whether brief, extended, or in-between, often begins with the gathering of some factual written information from the client. Sometimes this information is obtained by a receptionist or mental health aide rather than by a mental health professional. A sample of such an information sheet follows. It has been completed with data obtained from a person whose brief interview report also is presented in the following section.

Although the content areas of brief intake reports are fairly consistent, the formats used tend to vary from one agency to another. What follows are two brief intake reports, completed according to two different models. The first of these is based on an interview with a young boy named Jefferson Lawrence. The second report is based on Maria Sanchez.

INFORMATION FORM FOR JEFFERSON LAWRENCE

NAME: Jefferson Lawrence   ADDRESS: 452 Wayne Street, Fairfax,
                                                                    Virginia 22030
HOME PHONE: (703) 555-3854   WORK PHONE: (703) 555-8345 (father)
DATE OF BIRTH: 2/21/94   PLACE OF BIRTH: Hoboken, New Jersey
SEX (underline one) Male   Female   AGE: 10
RACE: African American   MARITAL STATUS: Single
EDUCATION: In the fourth grade   OCCUPATION: Student
REFERRAL SOURCE: Dr. Sareoum Kry, physician
Have you ever been seen at this Mental Health Center before? NO
Have you received prior counseling or psychiatric treatment? NO
Are you taking any medication? NO   If YES, what? _____

INTAKE REPORT ON JEFFERSON LAWRENCE

Intake Interviewer: Leslie Sok, Ph.D.   *Date*: January 11, 2004

Presenting Symptoms. Jeff, as he is called, was brought to the interview by his father. Since the beginning of school, Jeff has been behaving in unusual ways. He expresses frequent concern about contracting the illness of a disabled boy in his class. To avoid "catching his germs," Jeff has refused to sit in seats or touch objects that might have been touched by the other boy. He insists on wearing only his "lucky clothes" to school, reserving other garments for wear at home. If he has a cut or sore, he refuses to attend school because "the germs can get in."

Mental Status Examination. Jeff, a tall, slender boy, was casually and appropriately dressed. He was oriented to time, place, person, and situation. However, several unusual behaviors were noted. Jeff brought a cushion with him and sat on the cushion rather than on a chair. He insisted on wearing his long raincoat throughout the interview, stating that it protected him from germs. Jeff seemed anxious and continually scanned the room, once peering under the desk.

Despite these behaviors, his memory, concentration and attention were satisfactory and he seemed to be an intelligent and articulate boy. He readily spoke about the fears he had about germs and contagion and his apprehension about contact with the boy in his class. He also acknowledged that his behaviors were unusual, but saw them as necessary to safeguard his health.

Present Situation and Relevant History. Jeff was born in Hoboken, New Jersey, the older of two children. He currently lives with his father, who is a history teacher, his mother, who is a travel agent, and his sister, age 6, who is in the first grade. Jeff was somewhat slow to develop physically but began talking and reading very early. He was identified as gifted in the second grade. Although he sometimes socializes with other boys, Jeff prefers to play action games on the computer. He is especially interested in trains, airplanes, and ships and has done a great deal of independent reading on these subjects. About 6 months ago, Jeff's mother was diagnosed with breast cancer. Although she has an excellent prognosis, she has undergone surgery, chemotherapy, and radiation since her diagnosis. Jeff and his sister have often stayed with relatives during this time. When his mother was first diagnosed, Jeff asked many questions about the illness but lately has rarely talked about it. Jeff's father described his wife as a "very anxious person" and stated that her mother had been diagnosed with Obsessive–Compulsive Disorder (OCD).

Prior Treatment. Jeff has received no prior counseling. He is physically healthy.

Multiaxial Assessment

Axis I.   300.3 Obsessive–Compulsive Disorder, moderate
Axis II.   V71.09 No mental disorder on Axis II
Axis III.   No medical conditions reported
Axis IV.   Mother diagnosed with breast cancer, undergoing treatment; child spending considerable time with relatives; boy with disabilities in class
Axis V.   Current: 53

Jeff is experiencing an Obsessive–Compulsive Disorder (OCD), probably triggered by anxiety and stress related to his mother's diagnosis with cancer. He may well have a genetic predisposition to develop OCD. Jeff's reluctance to attend school regularly and socialize with his peers seems likely to impair his emotional and academic development. Although he is a bright boy with many strengths, this disorder warrants immediate attention because of its impact on the client and his family. Attention also should be paid to how Jeff is dealing with his mother's illness.

Overview of Treatment. Individual counseling, family counseling, and a medication evaluation are recommended. Individual counseling will afford Jeff a safe environment in which he can express his concerns about his mother's disease and its impact. Family counseling is likely to help them cope with both the mother's diagnosis and Jeff's difficulties. Behavioral interventions, incorporated into both individual and family counseling, should enable Jeff to find other ways to alleviate his anxiety, reduce his fear of germs, and gain control over his compensatory behaviors. Because medication often is useful in treatment of OCD, a referral has been made.

BRIEF INTAKE REPORT—MARIA SANCHEZ

Another example of a brief intake report is presented here, this one focusing on Maria Sanchez, whose intake interview appeared earlier in this chapter. This report can be compared with the longer report of the interview with Maria Sanchez already presented in this chapter.

Client: Maria Sanchez   *Counselor*: Anne Eastment   *Date*: 2/17/04

Presenting Symptoms and Concerns. Ms. Sanchez, a 36-year-old married Latina woman, sought counseling because of depression and the related symptoms of difficulty sleeping, overeating, guilt, hopelessness, and impaired functioning. Ms. Sanchez is pregnant with her fourth child. She described this pregnancy as difficult and reports fatigue and back pain. Although she has some family help, Maria insists on taking on nearly total responsibility for her home and children, setting apparently unrealistic standards for herself and the children.

Mental Status Examination. Ms. Sanchez is motivated toward counseling and related well to this examiner. She is oriented to reality and manifested no unusual behaviors. Her communication skills are good and she expresses herself clearly. Memory is intact. Intelligence is above average or better. Depression, as well as some anxiety, was evident although client does not present a danger. Impairment in self-esteem, judgment, and insight were noted.

Present Situation and Relevant History. Ms. Sanchez was born in El Salvador. She lived with her mother and grandmother until the mother left for the United States when the client was 7. For most of the 7-year separation from her mother, client lived with relatives who reportedly were emotionally abusive. Exposure to violence and death in her country also affected Ms. Sanchez. She made a difficult transition to the United States at age 14. Despite family conflict, she actively pursued her education, graduating from college and obtaining employment as a legal assistant. She married her husband 10 years ago and has three sons (7, 5, 3).

Prior Treatment. No significant prior medical or psychological treatment was reported.

Multiaxial Assessment

Axis I.   296.32 Major Depressive Disorder, recurrent, moderate, with interepisode recovery
309.81 Posttraumatic Stress Disorder, prior history

Axis II.   V71.09 No mental disorder on Axis II
Axis III.   Pregnant, reports fatigue and back pain
Axis IV.   Pregnancy, three young children
Axis V.   57

Case Formulation and Overview of Treatment. Ms. Sanchez experienced an extremely difficult childhood and early adolescence including separation from her only parent, emotional abuse, and traumatic experiences. Her determination and intelligence enabled her to extricate herself from her negative environment, obtain an education, maintain successful employment, and marry and have a family. However, she now seems driven to provide her children a positive and intellectually stimulating home environment at all costs. Her difficulty in meeting her high standards due to the stress of her pregnancy and the demands of three young children seems to have led to a recurrence of a Major Depressive Disorder. Ms. Sanchez probably will benefit from weekly cognitive-behavioral counseling, emphasizing interventions designed to alleviate depression and anxiety, improve self-esteem and realistic goal setting, and promote coping skills, as well as social support and leisure activities. Attention also will need to be paid to her history of abuse and trauma; she needs to understand the impact this has had on her and how, even now, it affects her self-image and judgment. Family dynamics, as well as relationships with mother and husband, also should be a focus of treatment. Individual counseling is recommended initially; however, once some progress has been made, this client seems likely to benefit from couples counseling and perhaps participation in a women's support or therapy group. A psychiatric evaluation to determine her need for medication is indicated.

MAKING THE TRANSITION FROM INTAKE TO TREATMENT

An intake interview generally culminates in the formulation of a diagnosis and a treatment plan, as it has in this report. Detailed information on diagnosis is provided in Chapter 3 and on treatment planning in Chapters 6 through 9. In some agencies, the intake interviewer has the responsibility for determining the diagnosis and treatment plan while in others this is accomplished through a case conference.

Case conferences make diagnosis and treatment planning a group process, presumably increasing accuracy because input from a number of people is obtained. The case conference can also serve as the vehicle for assigning clients to mental health therapists. A typical case conference is a regular weekly meeting, perhaps 1–2 hours in duration, of a group of mental health workers in a particular agency. Intake interviewers will describe each new client, including a brief summary of history and concerns and the interviewer's impressions of the client. The group will then collaborate to determine a viable case formulation, diagnosis, and treatment plan for each client. Then the case is assigned to an appropriate mental health professional, based on the expertise of the staff members, their interest in particular types of clients and approaches to treatment, the treatment needs of the client, and the schedules of clients and staff. Case conferences also can be used to help counselors with ongoing clients. More information on case conferences is presented in Chapter 12.

6

The Nature and Importance of Treatment Planning

The initial or intake interview (discussed in Chapter 5) and the multiaxial assessment according to the *Diagnostic and Statistical Manual of Mental Disorders* (discussed in Chapter 4) are the first two steps in effective counseling. These steps provide counselors with the information they need for step three, the development of a treatment plan.

"Treatment planning in counseling is the process of plotting out the counseling so that both counselor and client have a road map that delineates how they will proceed from their point of origin (the client's presenting concerns and underlying difficulties) to their destination, alleviating troubling and dysfunctional symptoms and patterns and establishing improved coping mechanisms and self-esteem" (Seligman, 1993, p. 288).

Treatment planning plays many important roles in the counseling process:

1. A carefully developed treatment plan, well grounded in research on treatment effectiveness, provides assurance that counseling is likely to succeed.
2. Written treatment plans enable counselors to demonstrate accountability and effectiveness. Treatment plans, along with posttreatment evaluations, can substantiate the value of counseling. They can assist counselors in obtaining funding for programs and in receiving third-party payments and can provide a sound defense in the event of a malpractice suit. In fact, "changes in behavioral health practice now require writing cost efficient and highly specific symptom-focused treatment plans based on assessment" (Pollak, Levy, & Breitholtz, 1999).
3. A treatment plan specifying goals and procedures helps counselors and clients to track progress, determine whether goals are being met, and, if not, facilitate revision of the plan.

4. Treatment plans also provide structure and direction to counseling. They help counselors and clients to develop shared and realistic expectations and promote optimism that progress will be made. Research has demonstrated a positive relationship between treatment plan compliance and success of treatment (Wiger & Solberg, 2001).

Typically, counselors develop treatment plans with input from their clients and then share either all or appropriate sections of the treatment plan with clients so that counselor and client can form a team, following the same path to success. With experience, counselors can usually prepare a treatment plan in about 30 minutes. This chapter presents a systematic and comprehensive model to facilitate that process.

SUITABILITY FOR COUNSELING

Before counselors develop a treatment plan for a particular person, they must determine whether that person is likely to benefit from counseling. In order to assess this, counselors should review intake, diagnostic, and other information on that person, paying particular attention to three areas: motivation, characteristics of the person, and nature of the problem.

Motivation

People come to counseling from various referral sources and with varying degrees of motivation. Asking people, "What led you to seek counseling now?" is a good place to begin to assess motivation. An assessment of a person's motivation generally can be made by examining the nature of the referral, the urgency and magnitude of their difficulties, and any precipitating events.

Nature of Referral

People may seek counseling on their own initiative, at the suggestion of another person, or via a professional referral or mandate. Self-referred clients usually have looked at their lives and believe that change is warranted; they have selected counseling as a way to achieve that change. Generally, people who are self-referred are motivated to participate in counseling, although they still may have unrealistic expectations and barriers to change.

People's family or friends sometimes suggest they seek counseling. People motivated by another's success are a positive example. These people have an incentive to seek counseling, although they may not understand that process. However, many people who seek counseling because of pressure from others do not have intrinsic motivation to engage in counseling. They may resent being told to seek help, resist engaging in treatment, and transfer their resentment to the counselor. While clients referred by family or friends may be excellent candidates for treatment, counselors should be sure to explore expectations and strengthen their motivation.

Motivation also varies considerably among people who are referred to counseling by another professional such as a physician, member of the clergy, lawyer, or other therapist. Involuntary clients, such as those who are court-mandated to treatment, typically have more extrinsic than intrinsic motivation and may manifest resistance to the counseling process. Treatment planning must take account of their motivation. Short-term contracts and concrete, readily attainable goals generally should be established and progress assessed at regular intervals.

Urgency and Magnitude of Difficulties

These dimensions of people's difficulties often provide valuable information on their motivation. However, urgency does not necessarily imply high motivation. For example, Bettina, diagnosed with alcohol dependence, presented for counseling upon learning that she was pregnant. She knew her alcohol use could harm the fetus, so she viewed her concern as urgent. However, Bettina had little genuine interest in changing her lifestyle or examining her attitudes and behaviors; she refused to attend AA meetings and soon discontinued counseling.

A crisis in people's lives often prompts them to enter counseling. This often leads them to be receptive to counseling but, of course, this is not a guarantee they will engage productively in counseling. It just opens the door. Whether the counselor is allowed through that door depends on the skills of the counselor and the motivation of the clients.

Counselors occasionally encounter people whose motivation is so low they cannot be engaged in the counseling process. Such people may refuse to disclose more than identifying information, may be verbally abusive toward the counselor, or may misunderstand the nature of counseling. If efforts to clarify the nature of counseling, develop rapport, and identify goals do not succeed, the counselor probably should suggest that counseling is not appropriate at present. A referral for other services can be made or, if warranted, an appointment for a follow-up visit in a few weeks or months can be scheduled. This is not a failure but, simply, an acknowledgment that counseling is not the cure for all ills.

Characteristics of the Client

Most counseling approaches are designed for people who are not severely impaired in their verbal and intelligence levels and who have a reasonable degree of organization in their lives. Such people usually keep scheduled appointments, follow through on agreed-upon tasks, and discuss their concerns.

People without those characteristics pose more of a challenge to counselors and call for particularly careful treatment planning. Support systems may be enlisted to help bring clients to scheduled appointments. Counseling sessions may be held in the person's home or in inpatient or day treatment facilities. Verbal tactics may be deemphasized while behavioral and teaching models might be used extensively. The field of counseling today is sufficiently broad to accommodate the needs of people who are not the affluent, articulate, and self-disciplined clients so often depicted in early case studies. However, people who have little intrinsic motivation toward counseling, difficulty keeping appointments, and verbal skills that are well below average may benefit more from community services or other programs.

Nature of the Problem

In order for people to benefit from counseling, they must have concerns that are amenable to treatment by counseling. Categories of common concerns include:

- Relationship and communication difficulties
- Confusion about goals and direction
- Poor or unclear self-image
- Indecision
- Troubling behaviors or habits
- Depression or anxiety
- Difficulty coping with a change, crisis, or loss

Counseling is appropriate for a wide range of concerns. However, people sometimes present with goals or concerns outside the scope of the counseling process. Examples include people who want to make someone else change, people seeking a friend or defender, people asking for help outside of the counselor's range of expertise (e.g., on financial affairs or divorce law), and people who want the counselor to force them to do something such as lose weight. Such goals are not too far afield from the counseling process. For example, people who seek friendship through counseling can be helped to improve their social skills and form better friendships outside of counseling. However, if such presenting concerns cannot be redefined through counseling, clients will need to be referred to other sources of help. Counselors should bear in mind, though, that people's presenting problems often are not what is really troubling them and considerable effort should be channeled toward clarifying their underlying concerns before determining that counseling is not warranted. Especially when working with multicultural clients, counselors should be sure their clients understand the nature and purposes of counseling and help clients deal with any discomfort or expectations that interfere with their efforts to obtain help.

Counseling as the exclusive treatment intervention also has a low probability of success with some people. Those with severe personality disorders and a history of treatment failures, people who unwaveringly externalize the source of their difficulties, people with oppositional attitudes who seek to prove the counselor to be ineffective, and people with cognitive mental disorders or psychotic disorders typically make challenging clients. Although some of these benefit from treatment, their motivation must be addressed and perhaps a medication evaluation obtained before an effective treatment plan can be developed.

Frances, Clarkin, and Perry (1984) concluded, "The findings of outcome research demonstrate psychotherapy to be, on the average, significantly more effective than no treatment" (p. 214). About 60–70% of people improve in response to counseling, and some of those who do not improve would probably have deteriorated further without help. Occasionally, however, no treatment or another treatment is the best recommendation.

MODEL FOR TREATMENT PLANNING

Few widely accepted models for treatment planning are available. However, the DO A CLIENT MAP, developed by this author (Seligman, 1990), has been adopted by many clinicians. The first letters of the 12 steps in this model serve as a mnemonic device, spelling DO A CLIENT MAP. The purpose of a treatment plan is to map out the counseling process for a given client. This format of treatment planning includes the following 12 steps:

1. Diagnosis, according to the *Diagnostic and Statistical Manual of Mental Disorders* (DSM)
2. Objectives of treatment
3. Assessments
4. Clinician
5. Location of treatment
6. Interventions
7. Emphasis
8. Number of people
9. Timing
10. Medication
11. Adjunct services
12. Prognosis

Whatever format for treatment planning is followed, counselors must make decisions regarding some or all of the 12 elements in the MAP. Consequently, mastering this format probably will enable counselors to understand and use effectively any structured format for treatment planning. The rest of this chapter describes the 12 elements of the DO A CLIENT MAP in greater detail.

DIAGNOSIS

A multiaxial assessment or diagnosis according to the *DSM* is the first step in a treatment plan. The details of the plan will then stem from the information provided in the diagnosis about a person, his or her mental disorders and conditions listed on Axis I and Axis II, medical conditions listed on Axis III, stressors listed on Axis IV, and level of functioning rated on Axis V. Chapter 3 of this book provides guidelines for making a multiaxial assessment according to the *DSM*.

OBJECTIVES OF TREATMENT

Objectives (or goals) should be developed early in a counseling relationship. These can be described as desired end points in treatment. Objectives may change and evolve as counseling progresses, with new goals replacing older ones as gains are made. Nonetheless, objectives are necessary to develop a treatment plan, assess progress, and focus the counseling process. They direct and energize clients, mobilize use of skills and knowledge, and promote effort (Locke & Latham, 2002). Particularly motivating are goals of moderate difficulty; very difficult or simple goals can easily limit progress and usually do not build feelings of competence.

Typically, objectives focus on at least one of the following areas (Wiger & Solberg, 2001):

- Improving subjective well-being
- Reducing symptoms
- Improving functioning

Johnson and Johnson (2003) provide another viewpoint on goal setting; they suggest that, in order of importance, goals might focus on protection, stabilization, motivation, direction, education, and reintegration. Objectives should reduce symptoms associated with disorders and conditions listed on Axes I and II as well as promote coping skills to address medical conditions listed on Axis III and stressors listed on Axis IV. Accomplishment of these objectives should lead to an increase in Global Assessment of Functioning rating listed on Axis V.

Most objectives are directly linked to clients' multiaxial assessment. However, counselors should think not only in terms of ameliorating problems and pathology, but also should view people from preventive and developmental perspectives, seeking to help them establish more rewarding lives and master the skills they need to cope successfully with future difficulties. Having a model of what it means to be psychologically healthy can help counselors gather information and establish objectives. Witmer and Sweeney (1992) identified five areas of optimal health and functioning. Considering people's strengths and difficulties in these five areas can facilitate determination of objectives that promote healthy development.

1. *Spirituality*—a sense of inner peace, clear values, optimism, enjoyment of life, and direction.
2. *Self-regulation*—self-worth and self-esteem; being physically fit and healthy; feeling resilient and in control of one's life; having creativity and problem-solving skills and a sense of humor; and being realistic, spontaneous, and intellectually stimulated.
3. *Work*—whether work means employment, volunteer activities, education, or leisure activities, work that provides psychological, social, and economic benefits is part of a balanced life.
4. *Friendship*—support systems and positive interpersonal relationships.
5. *Love*—a long-term relationship that is mutually intimate, cooperative, trusting, and sharing.

Establishing objectives should be a mutual process, involving both clients and counselors. Sometimes counselors believe they know what would be best for clients and what their goals should be. However, shared goals are more likely to facilitate counseling and motivate clients. Counselors should begin the goal-setting process by eliciting goals from the client, should rephrase them if necessary, and write them down. If people have difficulty articulating goals, counselors can facilitate that process by asking questions such as the following:

- What exactly are you like when you are experiencing this difficulty?
- Before you developed this problem, how did you feel and what was your life like?
- What has been the most rewarding time of your life and what made it so?
- Suppose a miracle happened overnight and, when you awoke in the morning, all these difficulties were resolved. How would you know? What would be different? (deShazer, 1991).
- If you resolved this problem, what changes would other people notice? What would you be doing that you are not doing now?

Once the client's goals have been thoroughly explored, attention can shift to any other objectives the counselor might have. Counselors have the right to suggest goals to clients and even to make them a condition of treatment. For example, a counselor might say, "I know that your primary concern is the conflict you have had with your last three supervisors. However, that conflict seems related to your use of alcohol. I don't think I can help you with your work problems unless we also try to change your use of alcohol. How would you feel about adding an objective related to reducing or eliminating your use of that substance?"

Identified objectives should be clear and measurable. Clients often express goals such as "feeling better about myself" and "getting along better with others." While such changes may well be achieved through the counseling process, these objectives are vague and hard to measure. Such objectives make development of interventions and assessment of progress very difficult. Consequently, counselors should work with clients to determine, for example, exactly how they will know they are getting along better with others. Will they have fewer fights with colleagues, have lunch with friends more often, or have a longer list of people they would invite to a party? Subjective self-report data (e.g., "I really do have more self-confidence these days") are indicators of counseling progress. However, such feelings can be ephemeral and may not be solid building blocks in the counseling process. People seem to develop the soundest self-help skills and the greatest sense of their own competence and independence if they understand what they have done to effect positive changes in their lives and what the specific indications of those changes are.

Johnson and Johnson (2003) suggest a mnemonic device to keep in mind when formulating objectives. They use the acronym SMART (specific, measurable, action oriented, realistic, and time bound) to guide goal-setting. Compare the following objectives to see the difference between a SMART goal and a goal that does not meet these criteria:

Weak Objective: I will do my best to get to work early as often as possible.

SMART Objective: On at least two days in the next work week, I will set my alarm for 6 a.m., arise immediately, follow the morning routine I planned, and arrive at work by 8 a.m.

Gintner (1995) delineated the following five-step process for establishing objectives:

1. Describe the problem as specifically as possible.
   Example: Gets to work at least 30 minutes late 4 out of 5 days a week.
2. Transform the problem into an objective by stating it as something that needs to be increased, decreased, or done differently.
   Example: Arrive at work daily by 9 a.m.
3. Make the objective measurable by stating it in terms of at least one of the following:

   a. Frequency (e.g., change the number of times a behavior is performed)
   b. Intensity (e.g., reduce score on the Beck Depression Inventory to 20 or less)
   c. Duration (e.g., spend at least 30 minutes per day in conversation with my husband)
   d. Amount (e.g., write 10 pages per day).

4. Establish criteria for achieving the objective.
   Example: Increase time spent exercising to at least 30 minutes a day, 4 days a week.

5. Identify a time frame for achieving the objective.
Example: By the end of the month …

Phrasing objectives in quantifiable terms is optimal. Some objectives are readily quantifiable and can easily be measured and tracked via client reports. Other objectives can be assessed via brief standardized inventories such as the Beck Depression Inventory, the Symptom Checklist, and others. However, sometimes quantifying objectives is difficult. In such circumstances, counselors can establish an informal rating scale for their client's use. For example, the counselor might say, "On a 1 to 10 scale, where would you say your self-esteem is now? … Where would you say it was before you became depressed? … Where would you realistically like it to be in 3 months? … In a year?" Similar is the Subjective Units of Distress Scale, another subjective ordinal scale that people can use to rate negative emotions, or the linear analog described in Chapter 4. Most people have no difficulty using these rating scales, despite their unscientific nature. They provide a useful vehicle for measuring change.

Counselors often think of objectives in terms of short-term, medium-term, and long-term goals. Approximately three to five objectives should be listed under each relevant time frame. This number of goals is not overwhelming yet affords options in terms of where clients channel their efforts. A challenging goal might be phased in incrementally over all three levels with a short-term goal being to read about nutrition and exercise and develop a plan to improve physical health; medium-term goals might reflect some changes in eating habits; and long-term goals might include a weight loss of 20 pounds, more changes in eating habits, and maintenance of an exercise routine.

Short term usually refers to objectives that can be accomplished in days or weeks; medium term, in weeks or months; and long term, in months or even years. Short-term objectives always should be developed, regardless of the anticipated duration of counseling. Short-term objectives, easily accomplished and evaluated, provide both counselors and clients a sense of progress, optimism, and reinforcement. Examples of short-term goals are obtaining college applications, writing a letter, and eating ice cream no more than twice a week.

Medium- and long-term objectives guide the overall direction of the counseling process. Examples of medium-term goals are remaining alcohol-free for 3 months, identifying and applying to four appropriate colleges, and beginning a home business. Long-term objectives are developed only if long-term counseling is anticipated or if client and counselor understand that those are goals to be pursued after the completion of counseling. Long-term goals might include completing college, obtaining a more rewarding job, and running a marathon.

The format for listing objectives (illustrated later in this chapter) also should include consecutive numbering of items. This facilitates linking objectives with interventions designed to promote their accomplishment.

ASSESSMENT

In order for counselors to establish objectives that are clear and realistic, they must have a good understanding of their clients as well as of the nature and possible causes of their difficulties. Assessment tools and procedures can provide information not otherwise available to counselors and can serve as a double-check on the counselor's own interpretation of a problem. Assessment may be done by the counselor, by another mental health professional, or by a specialist in another field. Detailed information on assessment tools is presented in Chapter 4. Physicians, neurologists, psychologists, and other professionals also can conduct assessments.

CLINICIAN

According to Glauser and Bozarth (2001, p. 142), "The variables most related to success in counseling outcome research are the client-counselor relationship and the personal and situational resources of the client." Herman (1993) agreed, stating, "… nonspecific factors such as therapist personal characteristics may be the primary determinants of successful outcome" (p. 29) and "… the quality of the therapeutic bond has a significant impact on therapy outcome" (p. 30). Evidence is accumulating that counselors' personal and professional qualities can have a profound impact on the nature and effectiveness of counseling.

Counselors who are emotionally stable, well adjusted, and optimistic and who have fulfilling lives are more likely to be effective (Sexton & Whiston, 1991). Other counselor qualities associated with a positive outcome include being friendly, likable, patient, and flexible. Effective counselors have realistic self-esteem; skill in communicating warmth, empathy, positive regard, and concern; involvement in the counseling relationship; and credibility as perceived by the client. Effective counselors typically assume a collaborative stance in relation to their clients, prepare clients for the part they will play in treatment, and encourage active client involvement, a problem-solving attitude, and a sense of appropriate responsibility for their difficulties. Effective counselors communicate genuineness, respect, and immediacy. They are interested in and committed to their profession and view their clients as capable, trustworthy, dependable, and friendly (Terry, Burden, & Pedersen, 1991). These counselors pay attention to the development of a working alliance and take time to establish mutually agreed upon objectives with their clients. Clients who anticipate positive and realistic outcomes from counseling and whose expectations are congruent with those of their counselors are more likely to achieve those outcomes (Beutler, Crago, & Arizmendi, 1986).

Part of treatment planning is identifying a suitable counselor for a client. Many variables should be considered when matching counselor and client, in addition to the characteristics mentioned above. Experience and training in treating people with problems and symptoms like those of the client are important counselor variables.

A related but perhaps more difficult issue is that of the counselor's comfort. Even if counselors have relevant expertise, they may have emotional reactions to certain clients or concerns. Although counselors must maintain a strong measure of objectivity and generally refrain from imposing their own values on clients, counselors inevitably have feelings toward their clients and their behaviors. These reactions often are strongly colored by the counselors' own backgrounds and experiences. When these reactions bear little relation to the reality of the clients' behaviors but are more a reflection of the counselors' inner experiences, the reactions are termed countertransference. An example is a counselor who was severely punished for lateness as a child who became angry with a client for being 10 minutes late. Other counselor reactions may be more grounded in objective reality. For example, many counselors would feel angry and upset when a client described sexually abusing his 6-year-old daughter.

Neither countertransference reactions nor other emotional reactions to clients are, in themselves, problems or grounds for referral. However, counselors should pay attention to and understand their own feelings. Strong emotional reactions to clients, especially of a countertransference nature, perhaps should prompt counselors to seek supervision or counseling for themselves. Especially if more than a few counseling sessions have taken place, counselors should avoid referring a client due to their own emotional reactions since the client might perceive that as a rejection. Only in extreme circumstances should a referral be made because the counselor's reactions to a person prevent the development of a positive counseling relationship.

Counselors occasionally are aware in advance that they are likely to be emotionally uncomfortable working with a particular client. An example might be the counselor who does not want to counsel people considering abortions because he is morally opposed to abortion or the woman who has been raped and fears that her anger will get in the way of counseling a person who has been convicted of rape. In such cases, the counselors' supervisors can be made aware of those constraints so that clients with these issues can be channeled to other counselors. However, counselors in mental health agencies may have little opportunity to choose their clients. In general, counselors should try to deal with their biases and work through negative reactions so that they can counsel a broad range of clients.

Although research suggests that general qualities of the counselor, discussed above, are more important than demographic variables, the impact of counselor demographic variables also should be considered during treatment planning. Age, gender, and ethnic background of the counselor are probably the most important of these, although others, such as the counselor's marital status, whether he or she is a parent, and religious preference also can have an impact on the counseling process.

Few clear answers are available as to how and even whether clients and counselors should be matched demographically. However, particular notice should be taken of:

1. Great disparities between counselor and client—a 65-year-old client, adjusting to retirement, may have difficulty accepting help from a 25-year-old novice counselor.
2. Great similarities between counselor and client—a client who is struggling with the pressures of becoming a single parent may overidentify with or become envious of a counselor who also is a single parent.
3. Strong feelings on the part of the client toward particular groups—a client who has always assumed a passive role in relation to women may have difficulty engaging in a productive counseling relationship with a female counselor, for example.

Of course, these are only hypothetical examples. Very different reactions may ensue. The 65-year-old retiree may find that the youthful counselor sharpens his awareness of the breadth of his life experiences, leading to increased self-confidence. The single parent may benefit from the empathy and support he receives from the counselor in similar circumstances. The client who has had difficulty relating to women may learn new ways to interact through a female counselor. Predicting the impact of demographic variables on the counselor–client relationship is difficult. However, counselors still should attend to such variables, drawing on their insight and skills, as well as client preferences, to handle the impact of such variables on that relationship.

LOCATION

Identifying the type of counseling agency or practice best able to help a particular person is another important step in treatment planning. Whether treatment should be provided in a standard or intensive outpatient setting, at a partial or day hospital setting, at a group home or residential setting, or in an inpatient hospital facility can be determined by examining the following variables:

- Nature, severity, progression, and duration of symptoms
- Threat client presents to self or others
- Type and effectiveness of previous treatments
- Support systems and living situation
- Preferences of client and significant others
- Likelihood of client keeping outpatient appointments
- Insurance coverage and financial resources
- Overall objective of treatment (e.g., symptom removal, rehabilitation, maintenance)

Counselors should pay particular attention to the level of supervision and the frequency of treatment needed by the person. People should be seen for counseling in the least restrictive environment that can provide them the safety and services they need. Although most clients are appropriate for treatment in outpatient settings, people who present a danger to themselves or others, who have a serious mental disorder accompanied by severe impairment, or who are unable to perform activities of daily living and keep themselves safe require more intensive treatment.

In addition to identifying the appropriate level of care for a client, a treatment plan also should specify the particular type of agency (e.g., rehabilitation counseling center, substance abuse treatment program, agency providing counseling to children and their families). Determining location of treatment may be unnecessary if the client already has sought out an appropriate counseling facility. However, if this has not happened, a referral may be indicated.

INTERVENTIONS

The interventions section is really the heart of the treatment plan. Here clinicians specify exactly what they will do to accomplish the objectives that have been determined. The interventions section of a treatment plan has two parts. First, clinicians indicate the theoretical framework that will guide their work with a particular person. Ten theoretical models of counseling (psychodynamic, Adlerian, person-centered, cognitive, behavioral, reality, solution-based brief therapy, constructivist, multimodal, and developmental) are discussed in detail in Chapter 7. Others are briefly reviewed. Although some clients and concerns call for a relatively pure theoretical approach, counseling is more likely to involve an eclectic or integrated approach. If so, the treatment plan should specify the nature of that approach. For example, the counselor might plan to begin with a person-centered approach to build rapport and strengthen self-esteem, then shift to a cognitive-behavioral approach to mobilize the person and reduce dysfunctional thinking, and finally shift to a psychodynamic approach to promote understanding of underlying concerns in order to build coping mechanisms and prevent a recurrence.

In the second part of the interventions section, counselors list the specific strategies they will use, such as *in vivo* desensitization, imagery, discussion of earliest memories, or modification of distorted cognitions, to accomplish their objectives. Each intervention should link to one or more objectives and all objectives should be addressed by one or more interventions. In this way, counselors can be sure they have created a treatment plan that is carefully structured yet comprehensive enough to target all identified objectives. Information on strategies associated with the major theoretical approaches to counseling is reviewed in Chapter 7.

Considerable research through the 1980s and 1990s focused on differential therapeutics, seeking to determine which models of counseling are most effective and under what circumstances. Particularly relevant is research conducted under the auspices of the American Psychological Association (APA). In 1993, a task force report by Division 12 of APA established criteria for identifying empirically supported psychotherapies. Three years later, this task force (Chambless et al., 1998) published a list of treatments that met the criteria for being well established or probably efficacious in treating specific disorders and conditions. For example, cognitive therapy was found effective in treatment of depression, and dialectical behavioral therapy proved effective in treatment of Borderline Personality Disorder.

Although research on treatment effectiveness does not yet support the validity of a prescriptive approach, in which specific interventions are indicated for treating each mental disorder, research such as the report by Chambless et al. does provide some guidelines as to what is likely to be effective and what is not (Seligman, 1998).

The following section organizes most of the mental disorders and conditions described in the *DSM* into seven broad categories, listed roughly in order of prognosis, along with treatment recommendations for each category.

1. *Problems of Adjustment and Life Circumstance*—This section includes the Adjustment Disorders (mental disorders) and the Conditions (not mental disorders). Conditions include such concerns as Partner Relational Problem, Bereavement, Occupational Problem, and Phase of Life Problem listed in the *DSM*. These difficulties are very common; approximately 10% of adults and 32% of adolescents will experience an Adjustment Disorder (Maxmen & Ward, 1995). People described as having a Condition or Adjustment Disorder typically have difficulty coping with a specific stressor (e.g., divorce, relocation, death of a loved one, job loss) or a life circumstance (e.g., retirement, career dissatisfaction, a chronic illness). They need help in gaining a clear and realistic perspective on their situation, perhaps via reading and information gathering; the opportunity to explore and express their feelings; emotional support; and identification and mobilization of coping skills. Problems in this category typically respond well to short-term counseling that follows a crisis intervention model. Support groups, including people facing similar stressors, are also helpful; they can provide understanding, empathy, suggestions, and useful role models as well as reassurance that the client is not alone. Successful treatment of Conditions and Adjustment Disorders often promotes both symptom reduction and sustained personal growth.

2. *Behavioral Disorders*—Included in this category are disorders characterized by problems in habits, behaviors, or impulses such as Substance Use Disorders, Sexual Dysfunctions, Paraphilias, Conduct and Oppositional Defiant Disorders, Attention-Deficit/Hyperactivity Disorders, Eating Disorders, Sleep Disorders, and Impulse-Control Disorders such as Pyromania and Kleptomania.

People with these disorders typically manifest a cycle of dysfunction in which they experience a buildup of tension, along with a craving for or pressure toward some harmful activity. When the tension is eventually released through the activity, then a quiescent or regretful period may follow until the tension starts to build again, continuing the cycle.

Treatment of these disorders is usually primarily behavioral in nature, using such techniques as goal setting, contracting, stress reduction, and response prevention. Peer support groups, such as Rational Recovery or Overeaters Anonymous, as well as group counseling are important additions to treatment; the role models offered by group members can promote development of coping skills and provide reinforcement. Family counseling and education are other important treatment ingredients. Some of these disorders, such as Attention-Deficit/Hyperactivity Disorder, Eating Disorders and Sleep Disorders, often benefit from medication as well as counseling. Although most people with behavioral disorders respond positively to treatment, relapse prevention must be part of treatment. In addition, many people with behavioral disorders often have underlying Mood or Anxiety Disorders that also need attention.

3. *Mood Disorders*—Included in this group are Major Depressive Disorder, Dysthymic Disorder, Bipolar I and II Disorders, Cyclothymic Disorder, and Depressive Disorder NOS. Major Depressive Disorder probably is the disorder most often treated in both inpatient and outpatient mental health settings. Depression, a feature of most of the disorders in this section, has been shown to respond well to both cognitive-behavioral therapy and interpersonal psychotherapy, a form of brief psychodynamic psychotherapy. Psychotropic medication is usually combined with counseling in the treatment of Bipolar I and II Disorders and Major Depressive Disorder and also may be used for the other Mood Disorders. Interventions that encourage physical activity, experiences that provide pleasure and promote feelings of competence, and self-help opportunities between sessions are especially useful in alleviating depression. Suicidal ideation often accompanies depression and must be addressed. Relapse prevention also is a component of treatment because of the high rate of Mood Disorder recurrence.

4. *Anxiety Disorders*—Anxiety Disorders are characterized by a combination of worry, fear, and apprehension along with physical manifestations of anxiety such as avoidance, withdrawal, fatigue, and muscle tension. In a 1-year period, approximately 12.6% of the population will experience an Anxiety Disorder (Maxmen & Ward, 1995). This category includes such disorders as Phobias (Specific, Social, and Agoraphobia), Panic Disorder, Obsessive–Compulsive Disorder, Acute Stress Disorder, Posttraumatic Stress Disorder, Generalized Anxiety Disorder, and Separation Anxiety Disorder. These disorders usually respond well to cognitive-behavioral interventions, particularly when treatment includes relaxation, systematic desensitization with exposure to the feared stimulus, and other anxiety

management strategies. Supportive interventions and psychoeducation can empower people to deal effectively with their fears. Disorders triggered by a traumatic experience typically benefit from group counseling with people who have undergone similar experiences, while Obsessive–Compulsive Disorder usually requires medication in addition to counseling.

5. *Disorders that Combine Physical and Psychological Complaints*—Included in this category are the Somatoform Disorders, the Factitious Disorders, and a broad range of Mental Disorders Due to a General Medical Condition. Counselors should work collaboratively with physicians in the treatment of these disorders. The physicians must determine whether a medical condition is present and what treatment it requires. Typically, people with these mental disorders focus on their physical complaints and neglect other areas of their lives. The body often becomes their vehicle for self-expression. Counseling can help these people to increase socialization and activity levels and to become more aware of and able to verbalize their feelings. Secondary gains of the physical complaints need to be identified and possibly reduced. Techniques such as relaxation and pain management also can be useful. A combination of person-centered/supportive counseling and cognitive-behavioral counseling usually is indicated for these disorders. Some exploration of a client's history may also be useful in clarifying messages about how the person is supposed to act and how he or she obtained attention and nurturing as a child. People with disorders in this group, particularly Factitious Disorder, often are difficult to engage in treatment; gradually forming a positive treatment alliance is essential.

6. *Personality Disorders*—These deeply ingrained and long-standing disorders may cause less impairment than some of the Mood, Anxiety, and Somatoform Disorders but typically are more challenging to treat. Personality Disorders are very common and are present in approximately 15% of the general population and 30–50% of clinical populations (Gunderson, 1988). Treatment of Personality Disorders can be lengthy, often at least several years in duration. At the same time, people with Personality Disorders typically want rapid assistance with their difficulties and usually do not have a great deal of insight or intrinsic motivation to make changes. In light of this conflict, treatment of these disorders tends to be most successful when it has two phases. In phase one, active, directive, and structured approaches such as cognitive and behavioral counseling predominate, addressing the person's presenting concerns. Once progress has been made, and if the person is willing to engage in long-term treatment (often not the case for these clients), psychodynamic interventions can be combined with the cognitive-behavioral ones to help the person address long-standing concerns and patterns as well as underlying problems. Specific interventions vary, depending on which Personality Disorder is diagnosed. For example, people with Schizoid Personality Disorders usually need help with assertiveness, communication, and socialization while people with Histrionic Personality Disorders benefit from help in developing insight, making sound decisions, and managing their emotions.

7. *Cognitive, Psychotic, and Dissociative Disorders*—People with these disorders typically have difficulty maintaining a clear sense of reality. They may have memory loss, confusion and disorientation, or delusions and hallucinations. The primary treatment for people with Cognitive or Psychotic Disorders usually is medication, and psychiatrists typically oversee their treatment. However, behavioral counseling that promotes adjustment and maximizes functioning also can be very helpful, as can supportive interventions to encourage and calm clients. Family counseling usually is needed, either in addition to or instead of individual counseling for people whose symptoms put them in danger and prevent them from successfully caring for themselves. Dissociative Disorders vary considerably, as does their treatment; people with Depersonalization Disorders may need only some help in reducing anxiety while people with Dissociative Identity Disorders typically need long-term psychodynamic psychotherapy.

EMPHASIS

Once counselors have determined the theoretical model, and perhaps also the interventions they will use in treating a particular person, they should determine how that approach will be adapted to the particular needs and personality of that client. For example, cognitive behavioral counseling may well be helpful to a fragile, elderly woman experiencing severe depression, but that treatment approach may need to be tempered by considerable empathy, support, and positive regard; focus, at least initially, will probably be on the present. Cognitive behavioral counseling also might be the treatment of choice for an adolescent female who has many personal resources but who was abandoned by her father at an early age and has begun using harmful drugs at the urging of her boyfriend. Her treatment is likely to be structured to use caring confrontation and to address the connection between her early loss of her father and her present unhealthy relationship with her boyfriend. Counselors may consider the following dimensions in deciding how to individualize their counseling and what aspects of an approach to emphasize:

1. *Level of Directiveness and Structure*—People who respond best to a counseling approach that is active, structured, and directive usually are those who are uncomfortable with verbal interaction or self-disclosure, who have limited motivation and insight, and who have concerns that are urgent and behavioral in nature. On the other hand, people who are self-motivated, insightful, and functioning fairly well but who are prone to self-doubts and low self-esteem often respond better to approaches that rely more on clients to give direction.

2. *Level of Confrontation*—Confrontation may sound like a threatening process, but it simply entails calling people's attention to discrepancies. An example of a gentle confrontation is, "I'm confused by what you said. Earlier, you talked

about how tight finances were and how you were trying to save money to buy a house; now you've told me that you are planning a costly wedding. Help me understand how all this information fits together." In general, people who are both resistant to counseling and fairly resilient are candidates for confrontation and structure while people who are fragile or in poor contact with reality benefit from considerable support.

3. *Level of Exploration*—Exploratory counseling encourages people to look beyond their presenting concerns and may focus on the antecedents of those concerns, earlier difficulties, dysfunctional and recurrent patterns, and family dynamics. While presenting concerns certainly are not ignored, efforts are made to understand them from a holistic or lifelong perspective. This process may entail loosening some defenses, raising clients' anxiety levels, and opening up concerns that had been suppressed, denied, or avoided. People suitable for an exploratory emphasis in counseling have the emotional resources necessary to take a close look at their developmental concerns and life patterns. Ideally, they should have an interest in personal growth and time and motivation for counseling that goes beyond their presenting concerns. People who do not fit this profile may benefit more from counseling that strengthens their existing defenses and maintains a present-oriented focus.

All of the dimensions related to Emphasis are on a continuum; counselors should think not in terms of whether they should have a confrontational or supportive style but, rather, where on the continuum ranging from very confrontational to very supportive they should focus their counseling with a particular person. Counselors also should keep in mind that use of these variables often shifts during counseling. A person in crisis may require supportive counseling but, once the crisis is resolved, that person may benefit from more structured counseling to address self-destructive behaviors.

NUMBER OF PEOPLE

Another aspect of treatment planning is determining how many people and which people will be involved in the counseling process. Three broad categories are considered in answering this question: individual counseling, group counseling, or family counseling.

Individual Counseling

Individual counseling is the most common form of treatment. Almost any concern that is amenable to counseling can be treated through individual counseling.

Sometimes individual counseling is used because it seems more likely to help the person than group or family counseling. For example, the client might be extremely shy and anxious, very angry and hostile, in poor contact with reality, or coping with an urgent crisis. People such as these are at least initially more likely to benefit from individual counseling.

Individual counseling also may be the method of choice for pragmatic reasons. An appropriate group may not be available or the client's family may refuse to attend counseling. In such cases, counselors can bring elements of group or family counseling into one-to-one counseling. Strategies such as role-playing or the empty-chair technique help people deal with family or other interpersonal issues in individual counseling. Counselors also can view clients through a family dynamics perspective even though family members are not present. Homework assignments, focusing on client interaction with others, can further broaden the scope of individual counseling.

Group Counseling

Group counseling, like individual counseling, can be employed for both therapeutic and pragmatic reasons. Some counseling agencies rely heavily on group counseling in order to provide services to more clients than they could through individual counseling. However, group counseling should not be thought of as simply a more efficient approach to counseling.

Group counseling is well suited for some concerns and contraindicated for others. Many people with interpersonal difficulties benefit from group counseling. However, participation in a counseling group does require at least a minimal level of confidence and communication skills. Group counseling also can be more stressful and anxiety producing than individual counseling, at least until the group has developed a supportive and cohesive environment. Consequently, people who have severe depression or anxiety, have very weak interpersonal skills, or are in crisis probably should not participate in group counseling until their symptoms have been somewhat reduced. However, for reasonably well-functioning people who need improvement in communication skills and who are confident enough to benefit from peer feedback, group counseling can be effective in improving clients' social skills and helping them become more aware of how others react to them.

Counseling groups also enable people to feel less alone and can help them learn from the insights and efforts of others in similar situations. Counseling groups can be supportive, especially to fragile or emotionally damaged clients. Homogeneous groups are particularly helpful to people in marital or career transitions, people who have been abused, and people with life-threatening illnesses, to cite just a few. Disorders involving problem behaviors (e.g., Substance Use Disorders, Eating Disorders, and Intermittent Explosive Disorder), as well as disorders that develop in response to a trauma (Acute Stress Disorder, Posttraumatic Stress Disorder) also typically benefit from group counseling. Chapter 9 presents additional information on group counseling.

Even when group counseling is not the primary mode of treatment, it can be a valuable source of additional help for some people. Such people might be in individual and group counseling concurrently or might be referred to counseling or support groups after progressing in individual counseling. Alternatively, group counseling might be recommended for one aspect of a person's concerns, such as social anxiety, while individual or family counseling is used for other aspects, such as a history of abuse. Of course, treatment planning will need to be pragmatic as well as therapeutic, considering the client's time and resources as well as the services of the agency.

Family Counseling

Family counseling has been growing in importance as a mode of treatment and is discussed further in Chapter 8. Some counselors believe that nearly all difficulties stem from family dynamics and prefer to see an entire family together for counseling whenever possible. Other counselors use family counseling more selectively. When planning the treatment, counselors should consider the client's diagnosis, relevance of the person's family background and current family patterns to the presenting problems, the willingness of the client to involve family members, and the reported motivation of family members to attend sessions. Family counseling should be included in the treatment of most children and adolescents, and usually should be part of the treatment of people with Substance Use Disorders and Psychotic and Cognitive Disorders to help families cope more effectively with those disorders. If family counseling is warranted, counselors then should consider who should be present (e.g., partner, children, siblings, parents, grandparents). Type of family counseling also must be determined.

Family counseling, like group counseling, can be combined with other modes of treatment. For example, a person is seen for a few sessions of individual counseling, followed by some joint sessions with a partner or parent, and then continues individual treatment once the counselor has gathered information on family dynamics and helped improve family interaction and communication. Although family counseling may be the most effective mode of treatment in some cases, changes can be made in a family by working with an individual, especially if a counselor can assume a family dynamics perspective regardless of who is present at the counseling session.

TIMING

Many decisions enter into planning the timing of the counseling process. Counselors must decide the length of the counseling sessions, their spacing and frequency, their approximate number, and whether counseling will be time-limited. Pacing and sequencing of the counseling process also should be considered as part of timing. Timing is determined by the interaction of several factors: the motivation of the client, the diagnosis, the objectives, and any constraints such as the person's financial circumstances or limitations of their insurance coverage.

Length of Sessions

Most counseling sessions are 45–50 minutes in length. However, sometimes reasons exist for deviating from that time frame. Children and people with significant cognitive or intellectual deficits may feel more comfortable with shorter sessions; families sometimes need longer sessions so that everyone has an opportunity to participate fully.

Frequency of Counseling

Generally, people are seen for counseling once a week. However, here, too, another pattern might be more helpful. People who are in crisis, who present a danger to themselves or others, or who have severe and incapacitating symptoms often are seen more frequently. On the other hand, people who have made good progress and are approaching termination of counseling may shift to bimonthly or monthly sessions as a way to gradually complete counseling. Intermittent treatment sometimes is used for people with chronic concerns to help them maintain their stability and monitor their functioning. Counselors can be flexible in the frequency of the counseling they provide a client, adapting the schedule to the client's needs.

Duration of Counseling

Crisis intervention, the briefest form of counseling, is designed for fairly healthy people with immediate concerns often accompanied by considerable distress and dysfunction. Examples might include a man whose wife was killed in an accident, leaving him feeling overwhelmed by his loss, and a woman who has been diagnosed with cancer with an excellent prognosis.

Short-term counseling, approximately 8–20 sessions in duration, often is indicated when an otherwise well-functioning person presents a relatively circumscribed concern. The widowed man described above, for example, might become a candidate for short-term counseling once he has dealt with his crisis; short-term counseling might help him to grieve the death of his wife, clarify his role as a single parent, resume a social life as a single person, and redefine his future goals.

Short-term counseling also may be indicated for a person with limited motivation who has multiple long-standing problems. An example is a 52-year-old woman who presents with concerns about her mother. The woman sought counseling to help her decide whether to place her mother in a nursing home and to better cope with her guilt and anger toward her disinterested siblings. During counseling, the woman stated that she was experiencing marital strain and had been feeling sadness and lack of direction since her youngest child entered college. However, she was not motivated to look at these issues at present, but only wanted help with her concerns about her mother. (The client returned for career and marital counseling a year later.)

Medium-term counseling, defined roughly as longer than 20 sessions but shorter than 50 sessions, often is needed for people with two or more coexisting mental disorders or with long-standing or severe symptoms. However, counselors should bear in mind that considerable progress during counseling typically occurs by the eighth session. Kopta, Lueger, Sanders, and Howard (1999) reported that 50% of clients have resumed normal functioning by the sixteenth session; 75% by the fifty-eighth session.

Long-term counseling has become uncommon in most clinical settings. Counselors should be cautious about recommending long-term counseling. It can tax a person's finances and schedule, may lead to undesirable dependency on the counselor, and fail to yield benefits that are significantly greater than short- or medium-term counseling. However, long-term treatment of some disorders such as the Personality Disorders or Dissociative Identity Disorders almost always is indicated. Counselors should be sure that long-term counseling really is the best treatment for the client. According to Frances, Clarking & Perry (1984, p. 170), "Most studies fail to demonstrate a significant advantage of longer treatment."

Clients sometimes ask how long counseling will take. The experienced counselor probably can estimate approximately how long it usually takes to deal effectively with the sorts of concerns the person presents. Questions about duration typically reflect apprehension about counseling, and this should be explored. If the question reflects a reluctance to make a significant commitment of time and energy, the counselor might suggest that the person agree to a predetermined number of sessions, after which the counseling is reevaluated. Time-limited counseling can focus and intensify the process and can contribute to treatment effectiveness. Flexibility and change are needed in determining duration. Counselors might find that crisis intervention can evolve into medium-term counseling, while unmotivated clients may halt plans for long-term treatment.

Pacing and Sequencing

Treatment plans should take account of people's readiness for change and be paced accordingly. A gentle, gradual approach to counseling might be used with an anxious person with few support systems, while a more rapid approach might be adopted with a well-functioning person in a situational crisis. The sequence of treatment elements is another consideration, closely linked to pacing of treatment. A fragile client may first be seen in individual counseling and then, when confidence has grown, be placed in a counseling group to improve social skills. A more resilient client might be able to tolerate concurrent career and family counseling. Pacing and sequencing, then, also should be considered as part of timing.

MEDICATION

Medication sometimes is prescribed to people in counseling to help them overcome debilitating anxiety, prolonged and severe depression, mood swings, attention deficits, psychosis, and other symptoms. Although counselors are not qualified to prescribe medication, the following reasons indicate why counselors should be knowledgeable about the types and effects of medications that are commonly used to treat mental disorders:

• Clients may already be taking prescribed medication. Knowledge of that medication, its purpose, and side effects can provide counselors important information about the person's condition. It also can give counselors an idea of how the person functioned before taking medication and what the person might be like without it.

• By knowing what medication can and cannot do for people, counselors can decide when to refer a person to a psychiatrist for a medication evaluation.

• Counselors typically see clients more frequently than a collaborating psychiatrist who prescribes medication for those clients. Consequently, counselors are in a better position to monitor treatment compliance as well as the effectiveness of the medication and to suggest another visit to the psychiatrist if the medication does not seem to be helping.

• Similarly, counselors are likely to learn quickly of a change in a client's medical condition, such as a pregnancy or the diagnosis of a physical illness. Such information should prompt a strong recommendation from the counselor that the client taking medication should contact the psychiatrist immediately.

• In addition, clients may not be as open with a psychiatrist, seen for brief monthly visits, as they are with a counselor whom they see weekly. For example, a person who is abusing alcohol may not disclose that to a psychiatrist, but may share this information with the counselor. Some drugs can be fatal if combined with alcohol. The well-informed counselor can remind the client of any dangers associated with the medication being taken and can ensure that the psychiatrist has full information on the person's condition.

• Medication brings many benefits but also can cause a wide range of sometimes serious and occasionally lethal side effects. Common side effects (in alphabetical order) include anxiety, appetite changes, bowel changes, breast enlargement, breathing difficulty, cardiovascular changes (heart rate, blood pressure), confusion, depression, dizziness, drowsiness, facial grimaces, faintness, gastrointestinal upset, hair loss, headaches, impaired coordination, jaundice, light sensitivity, memory impairment, menstrual irregularities, mouth dryness, muscle spasms and tremors, nausea, nightmares, pains, panic, perspiration, rashes, restlessness, ringing in ears, sexual difficulties, sleep disturbance, slurred speech, tingling sensations, tongue changes, urinary difficulties, visual abnormalities, weakness, and weight change. Side effects vary in nature and severity, but all medications have side effects.

When clients are taking medication, counselors may have difficulty determining whether symptoms are caused by emotional factors or are side effects of the medication. Side effects also can be confusing and upsetting to clients. Some side effects, such as hair loss, sexual dysfunction, and weight change, can have an adverse impact on people's self-images and their interpersonal relationships, while others, such as confusion, panic attacks, and pain, can be frightening and dangerous. Counselors should know the potential side effects of common medications and should consult with physicians, with the client's permission, when worrisome side effects occur.

A brief overview of the major categories of psychotropic medications is presented here. Additional information can be obtained from the *Physicians Desk Reference*, available at nearly every medical facility in the United States. Briefer references, such as *The Pill Book*, *The Complete Pill Guide*, and *The PDR Pocket Guide to Prescription Drugs*, can also be useful and convenient references.

The following are the major categories of medication commonly used to treat mental disorders and their symptoms:

1. *Benzodiazepines and Anxiolytic Medications*—These medications are prescribed to reduce anxiety, panic attacks, and insomnia; facilitate withdrawal from drugs or alcohol; enhance the effect of antipsychotic medication; and serve as muscle relaxants. Included in this category are Ativan (lorazepam), BuSpar (buspirone), Halcion (triazolam), Klonopin (clonazepam), Librium (chlordiazepoxide), Restoril (temazepam), Serax (oxazepam), Valium (diazepam), Xanax (alprazolam), and others. Occasional or temporary use of these drugs can help reduce severe and debilitating symptoms. However, these drugs have addictive properties and can be lethal when combined with alcohol. More judicious use is being made of these medications, but they are still frequently prescribed.

2. *Mood Stabilizers/Anticonvulsants*—These medications are used to stabilize and regulate moods. They are especially helpful to people diagnosed with

Bipolar Disorders and to people who tend to be impulsive and aggressive. Frequently used medications included in this category include Depakote (divalproex), Clozaril (clozapine), Lamictal (lamotrigine), Lithobid and Eskalith (lithium carbonate), Neurontin (gabapentin), Tegretol (carbamazepine), and Trileptal (oxcarbazepine). Forms of lithium carbonate are the best known of these; they help control manic episodes and reduce the severity of depressive episodes in people with Bipolar I and II Disorders. Lithium (as well as many of the other medications in this category) also can be effective in ameliorating the symptoms of Cyclothymic Disorder, recurrent Major Depressive Disorder, and Schizoaffective Disorder. Although 80–90% of people with Bipolar Disorders show significant improvement in response to lithium, they may need to take the drug for many years and have regular blood tests because the medication can upset electrolyte balance.

3. *Tricyclic Antidepressants*—These well-established medications are particularly useful for people experiencing Major Depressive Disorders (especially those accompanied by melancholia), Dysthymic Disorder, and Panic Disorders but also are used to treat Enuresis, Posttraumatic Stress Disorder, and a variety of other disorders. Examples of medications in this category include Anafranil (clomipramine), Elavil (amitriptyline), Pamelor (nortriptyline), Tofranil (imipramine), and Vivactil (protriptyline). Anafranil also has been found effective in treating Obsessive–Compulsive Disorder and Trichotillomania. The onset of the effect of these drugs typically requires 10–14 days. About 4–6 weeks may be needed for the full impact of the drug to be felt, so rapid improvement should not be anticipated. Weight gain and other side effects are associated with this category of medication. An overdose of tricyclic antidepressants can be fatal, so they should be prescribed cautiously for people experiencing confusion or suicidal ideation.

4. *Monoamine Oxidase Inhibitors* (MAOIs)—A second category of antidepressant medication, MAOIs, includes Nardil (phenelzine) and Parnate (tranylcypromine). They, too, require several weeks to take effect and are used in the treatment of such symptoms as depression, panic attacks, anxiety, phobias, obsessional thinking, hypochondriasis, and depersonalization. MAOIs are particularly effective in the treatment of depression accompanied by one or more of the above symptoms. The ingestion of foods containing tyramine (e.g., ripened cheese, beer, wine, and yeast) or use of nasal decongestants in combination with these drugs can cause an adverse reaction.

5. *Serotonin Selective Reuptake Inhibitors* (SSRIs)—This group of antidepressant medications is newer than the above two groups and is more often used despite some controversy surrounding their impact. Examples of these medications are Celexa (citalopram), Effexor (venlafaxine), Lexapro (escitalopram), Luvox (fluvoxamine), Paxil (paroxetine), Prozac (fluoxetine), and Zoloft (sertraline). These antidepressants generally have fewer side effects than earlier medications and are effective in treatment of depression and associated disorders such as Eating

Disorders, Obsessive–Compulsive Disorder, Panic Disorder, Social Anxiety Disorders, Somatoform Disorders, and Sleep Disorders.

6. *Other Antidepressant Medications*—Medications such as Remeron (mirtazipine), Serzone (nefazodone), and Wellbutrin (buproprion) do not fit into the above three categories but also are used in treatment of depression. In addition, Wellbutrin is used for Attention-Deficit/Hyperactivity Disorder and smoking cessation.

7. *Antipsychotic Medication*—These medications are used primarily to reduce psychotic symptoms and to prevent relapse of Schizophrenia and other Psychotic Disorders. Some have other important uses. Haldol, for example, is used to treat Tourette's Disorder. Several of these drugs can ameliorate the symptoms of Pervasive Developmental Disorders and Cognitive Disorders. This category includes older medications such as Haldol (haloperidol), Mellaril (thioridazine), and Thorazine (chlorpromazine), which are not widely used today. More likely to be used are the newer antipsychotic medications, including Clozaril (clozapine), Risperdal (risperidone), Seroquel (quetiapine fumarate), and Zyprexa (olanzapine), which have fewer side effects and usually are more effective. Long-term use of some of these medications can lead to Tardive Dyskinesia, characterized by such symptoms as facial grimacing and tongue protrusion.

8. *Barbiturates*—These drugs, including Amytal (amobarbital), Nembutal (pentobarbital), and Seconal (secobarbital), produce prompt and sustained sedation. They often are used to relax people prior to surgery and are effective in reducing insomnia and anxiety. However, use of these drugs is limited because they are highly addictive, have many side effects, and can be lethal if an overdose is taken. They also can cause drowsiness and may interfere with driving.

9. *Central Nervous System Stimulants*—Medications in this category are particularly useful in the treatment of Attention-Deficit/Hyperactivity Disorders. They also may be used to treat excessive fatigue and sleepiness, as in Narcolepsy. Medications in this category include Adderall (amphetamine), Cylert (pemoline), Dexedrine (dextroamphetamine), and Ritalin or Concerta (methylphenidate).

10. *Other Medical Treatments*—Methadone, Naltrexone, and Buprenorphine are used to help people who have been dependent on narcotics. Naltrexone may also be helpful to people who are diagnosed with alcohol dependence. Antabuse (disulfiram) is another medication that has been used as part of the treatment of alcohol abuse or dependence.

Although not a form of medication, electroconvulsive therapy (ECT) also is sometimes recommended and can be helpful when medication and counseling have been unsuccessful. ECT has received much negative publicity, and some counselors are surprised to learn that it is still used. In fact, approximately 100,000 people each year receive ECT (Smith, 2001). ECT works quickly and is at least as effective as antidepressant medication in relieving acute depressions, especially those characterized by melancholia. However, ECT can cause temporary or permanent memory impairment, is more costly and less convenient than medication, and often results in only temporary improvement. Consequently, ECT should almost always be accompanied by other treatments and generally is used only after other treatment approaches have failed.

Deciding Whether to Refer for Medication

In 1994, 9% of prescriptions were for psychotropic medication (Ingersoll, 2000). A blend of counseling and medication is often superior to either alone. Counselors and their clients should not construe a need for medication as an indication that counseling has failed. Rather, medication is one more tool that counselors can use to enhance treatment effectiveness.

Counselors should not specify particular medications in their plans but should leave that decision to the psychiatrists. The treatment plans should indicate only whether or not a referral for a medication evaluation is needed. That decision will be based primarily on the nature and severity of a person's symptoms. If a medication evaluation is indicated, counselors should refer the person to a psychiatrist with whom they have a collaborative relationship and should obtain written permission from the client to confer with the psychiatrist.

The following indicates likelihood of needing a medication referral for most of the mental disorders. This can help counselors decide whether to include such a referral in a treatment plan:

- *Always*—Bipolar I and II Disorders, Cognitive Mental Disorders, Mental Disorder Due to a Medical Condition, Pervasive Developmental Disorder, Psychotic Disorders, Tourette's Disorder.
- *Almost Always*—Major Depressive Disorder, Obsessive–Compulsive Disorder, Substance-Induced Disorders.
- *Usually*—Attention-Deficit/Hyperactivity Disorder, Eating Disorders, Cyclothymic Disorder, Panic Disorders, Sexual Disorders, Sleep Disorders.
- *Sometimes*—Anxiety Disorders, Conduct Disorders, Dissociative Disorders, Dysthymic Disorder, Factitious Disorders, Impulse-Control Disorders, Mental Retardation, Personality Disorders, Substance Use Disorders.
- *Rarely*—Adjustment Disorders, Learning Disorders, Oppositional Defiant Disorder, Other Conditions that are not mental disorders.

Of course, people with disorders such as Factitious and Somatoform Disorders probably will already have ongoing contact with physicians. Even if psychotropic medication is not indicated, counselors should confer with these physicians, with the client's permission.

ADJUNCT SERVICES

Most clients benefit from adjunct services: sources of help, support, and information that are outside of the counseling relationship. These can enhance and contribute to the effectiveness of counseling and accelerate progress toward goals.

Recommended adjunct services and ways of providing them can be determined during the course of treatment planning as well as throughout counseling. When deciding whether to recommend adjunct services, counselors should consider the following five questions:

1. *When* should the adjunct services be obtained? For example, should they begin immediately or after the person's mood is somewhat improved?

2. *What adjunct services* should be recommended? Typically, the counselor suggests not only the type of adjunct services that are needed but also sources for these services. Many clients benefit from adjunct services that promote physical activity and increase their contact with other people.

3. *What connection* will be maintained between the counselor and the provider of the adjunct services? Will the counselor simply give the client the name of an agency or service provider without follow-up? Will the counselor follow up at a distance by occasionally inquiring about the person's involvement with and reactions to the adjunct services? Or will the counselor contact the providers of adjunct services so that they can work as partners in implementing the client's treatment plan? People who are fearful, confused, resistant, or in poor control of their impulses typically require considerable support in their efforts to obtain adjunct services. A close connection between a counselor and the provider of adjunct services also is indicated if the services are closely related to the counseling process (e.g., career counseling, assertiveness training) rather than representing other disciplines (e.g., tutoring, speech therapy, exercise class).

4. *Who* will oversee the treatment plan? One of the pitfalls of a multifaceted treatment plan is the lack of clarity surrounding the question of who will oversee, coordinate, and take responsibility for the implementation of that treatment plan. Designation of the primary counselor or case manager should be clear.

5. *What will be the sequence* of the adjunct services? Sometimes several adjunct services are recommended as part of a treatment plan. Treatment plans should specify whether the services are sequential (e.g., communication skills training should precede a person's involvement in a social organization), concurrent (e.g., exercise class and a weight control program), or determined by client preference and availability of services.

The needs of the client, the philosophy of counseling and style of the counselor, and the treatment setting all determine the choice and appropriate use of adjunct services. The following is a list of some frequently used adjunct services that might become part of a treatment plan.

- *Skill Development*—Tutoring, study skills, assertiveness training, parenting, job-seeking skills, communication skills, academic courses.
- *Focused Counseling*—Career counseling, art therapy, biofeedback, sex therapy.
- *Personal Growth*—Values clarification, relationship enhancement, image enhancement.
- *Support Groups*—Twelve-step programs such as Alcoholics Anonymous and Overeaters Anonymous, support groups for people with severe illnesses or disabilities, men's or women's support groups, Tough Love.
- *Alternate Care or Living Arrangements*—Halfway houses, group homes, low-income housing, day treatment centers, foster homes, shelters for the homeless, homemaking services, facilities providing nursing care or rehabilitation.
- *Professional Services*—Gynecologists, urologists, and other specialized physicians; legal assistance; financial planning; accounting; divorce mediation; acupuncture; employment agencies.
- *Other Health-Related Services*—Weight-control programs, exercise classes, physical rehabilitation, meditation.
- *Organizations for Socialization and Leisure Activities*—Social clubs, organized sports activities, special interest groups (e.g., bridge clubs, gardening clubs), cultural societies or groups, religious or spiritual organizations, nature-oriented activities (e.g., Sierra Club, hiking or biking groups), Parents Without Partners, professional associations.
- *Governmental Services*—Aid to dependent children, food stamps, Social Security, unemployment compensation, subsidized housing.

Knowledge of the communities in which counselors work and the typical needs and resources of people in those communities should enable counselors to identify and select appropriate adjunct services for their clients. Adjunct services can greatly enhance treatment.

PROGNOSIS

Prognosis is the last piece of the treatment plan. It indicates the likelihood of accomplishing the objectives in the treatment plan according to the methods identified in that plan. Prognosis is determined primarily by two important factors:

- The usual prognosis for the mental disorders with which the client has been diagnosed
- The particular client and that person's motivation, personal characteristics, and supports.

In general, a good prognosis is associated with disorders that begin late, that have a precipitant, that are of short duration, and that receive rapid treatment. A good prognosis also is more likely for clients who are in distress, are motivated to seek help, have only one mental disorder, have good premorbid functioning, take appropriate responsibility for their concerns, and have strong support systems. Adjustment Disorders, Depressive Disorders, and Anxiety Disorders typically have a positive prognosis while the outlook for helping people with Personality Disorders, Schizophrenia, Eating Disorders, Substance Dependence, and Factitious Disorders is not as positive. Approximately 65% of clients make positive changes as a result of counseling (Altekruse & Sexton, 1995). Usually these changes are enduring. However, 6–7% of clients deteriorate during counseling (Sexton & Whiston, 1991).

Terminology used to describe prognosis includes excellent, very good, good, fair, poor, and guarded. For people with multiple diagnoses, the prognosis may differ for each of the disorders. Counselors should strive to develop a treatment plan that has an optimistic prognosis. This involves establishing realistic objectives as well as interventions that have proven their value.

Chapters 7–9 provide additional information on theories and techniques of individual, family, and group counseling to facilitate treatment planning. Sample treatment plans are included in each of those chapters for counselors to use as models for their treatment planning.

Theories and Strategies of Individual Counseling

Counseling is effective! Study after study has arrived at conclusions similar to that of Sexton and Whiston (1991, p. 345): "… while some clients do improve on their own, in comparison, those in counseling improved more and at a faster rate … ."

However, researchers are still trying to determine why counseling works, when it works, and how to improve the process. This area of inquiry was launched by the 1980 study of Smith, Glass, and Miller. Using meta-analysis to summarize the results of 475 controlled outcome studies, they concluded that psychotherapy was effective and that the 2-year relapse rate was small. However, when Smith, Glass, and Miller tried to draw more specific conclusions about effectiveness, their findings were limited. They did discover that cognitive, cognitive-behavioral, and behavioral interventions were highly effective in treating a broad range of disorders. The psychodynamic approaches also demonstrated effectiveness. However, the less well-researched humanistic and developmental approaches did not receive the same support.

Research since 1980 has sought to provide more definitive information on treatment effectiveness. However, that endeavor is a challenging one for several reasons. The outcome of counseling depends not only on the treatment that is provided but also on existing factors in the client, the counselor, and the setting, and on their interaction during the therapeutic process. In addition, over 400 separate schools of psychotherapy have been identified (Lazarus & Beutler, 1993).

This complex situation makes it unlikely that one theoretical model will emerge as superior. Nevertheless, counseling should not be a haphazard process. Treatment effectiveness seems to depend on five dimensions:

- Common factors in effective counseling approaches
- Common factors in effective counselors

- The personal and situational resources of the client
- A sound match of treatment to client and diagnosis
- The therapeutic alliance

Prochaska and Norcross (1994) viewed the following *factors as characteristic of most approaches to counseling*: feedback, education, corrective emotional experiences, stimulus control, self- and social liberation, counterconditioning, reevaluation, and contingency management. Nearly all counseling approaches also provide information on human functioning, on how problems arise, on interventions, and on desired outcome (Hershenson, 1993). Most counseling approaches follow a common pattern of treatment: (1) problem exploration; (2) problem definition; (3) identification of alternatives; (4) planning; (5) action and commitment to change; and (6) assessment and feedback. Most approaches to counseling, then, have an underlying similarity.

Research also has identified *common factors of effective clinicians*. These include having strong interpersonal skills, realistic self-confidence, rewarding lives, self-efficacy, an orientation toward growth, sensitivity to others, emotional stability, and optimism.

Client variables associated with a positive treatment outcome include recognition of a need for personal change, motivation to make positive changes, optimistic expectations for treatment, being realistic and willing to engage in problem solving, intelligence, financial and emotional support, and psychological-mindedness. The ability to form positive interpersonal relationships is especially important, particularly in the development of a sound therapeutic alliance.

Client–counselor alliances form early in treatment and have an enduring impact. Mutuality and collaboration, the client's identification with and admiration of the counselor, and shared warmth and respect characterize *positive therapeutic alliances*.

Current research on empirically supported interventions, as well as a large body of both data-based and theoretical information on treatment effectiveness, facilitates selection of an appropriate treatment approach for a given client and diagnosis. The challenge for counselors is not to find the one perfect approach to all counseling, but to develop a sound treatment plan for each client that matches interventions to client, disorder, and clinician skills. According to Sexton (1995, p. 57), "It is ... the skillfulness of the counselor that is the most significant factor .... A skilled counselor who skillfully applies techniques that focus clients on their presenting concerns, and who uses various techniques matched with clients' presenting concerns, will be effective regardless of their theoretical perspective."

Reflecting this conclusion, increasing numbers of counselors are gravitating toward eclectic and integrated treatment models discussed later in this chapter. McWhirter and McWhirter (1991, p. 74) provided a useful definition of eclecticism: "Eclecticism means to select methods or doctrines from various sources or systems." It is not "… an indiscriminate and arbitrary collection of scraps and pieces" but rather draws concepts and interventions from identified sources and integrates them via the style and personality of the counselor. Current emphasis on integrated, rather than eclectic models, also mandates that so-called eclectic approaches have a theoretical coherence and consistency.

Altekruse (1995) reported that 40.2% of mental health counselors surveyed described their theoretical orientation as eclectic. Specific orientations reported by the counselors included Cognitive-Behavioral and Rational Emotive Therapy, 17.4%; Humanistic/Existential/Person-Centered, 11.7%; Adlerian, 6%; Psychoanalytic, 5.7%; Developmental, 4.3%; Reality Therapy, 3.2%; Transactional Analysis, 2.5%; Gestalt, 1.4%; and other, 7.5%.

Whether counselors identify themselves as eclectic or affiliate with a specific approach to counseling, counselors now need knowledge of and facility with a broad range of approaches and interventions. Although research has not (and probably never will) provide recipes for the treatment of each disorder and client, most counseling approaches work better with certain types of people or concerns than they do with others. This chapter considers the major approaches to individual counseling in relation to diagnosis and treatment planning. (Group and family counseling are considered in later chapters.) This book assumes that readers already possess some familiarity with important theories of counseling. Although a review of the essential ingredients of these approaches is provided, the intent of this book is not to teach theories of counseling. Neither is it the intent to encourage counselors to become chameleon-like and adopt a different counseling approach for every person they see. Most counselors develop their own counseling styles, which they are understandably unwilling or unable to modify radically. However, counselors can shift their styles within broad parameters, can borrow from a variety of counseling approaches such as those described in this chapter, and can develop ways of relating to and helping each person that is uniquely suited to that person's needs.

PSYCHODYNAMIC PSYCHOTHERAPY

Psychodynamic psychotherapy is derived from psychoanalysis and was developed by Sigmund Freud. Although psychoanalysis has waned in popularity, psychodynamic psychotherapy has received increasing attention and support. Traditional versions of this approach include Object Relations Theory, as well as the work of Harry Stack Sullivan, Karen Horney, Anna Freud, and others. Modern psychodynamic psychotherapy is reflected in the work of Heinz Kohut, Peter Sifneos, Gerald Klerman, David Malan, Habib Davanloo, Hans Strupp, and others who adapted psychoanalysis to modern counseling, leading to the development of brief psychodynamic psychotherapy (BPT) and interpersonal psychotherapy.

Description of Approach

Careful selection of suitable clients is key in BPT, which is relatively brief (usually no more than 6 months) and encourages an active and challenging stance on the part of the clinician. BPT typically seeks to ameliorate a recurrent focal concern or dysfunctional pattern—often problems in relationships—and helps people handle similar concerns more effectively in the future. Dysfunctional patterns in the person's past are explored in order to understand their impact on present functioning. Underlying emotions are uncovered and processed. Some attention is paid to transference, dreams and fantasies, defense mechanisms, and the unconscious, but far less than would be done in conventional psychoanalysis.

Techniques associated with psychodynamic psychotherapy include:

- Support and empathy
- Identification of repeated dysfunctional patterns
- Identification of a focal, usually interpersonal, concern
- Questioning, exploration, and active probing
- Linking of past to present concerns
- Interpretation, designed to promote insight and awareness, reduce repression, modify defenses
- Analysis of transference, early memories, dreams, and fantasies
- Challenge and confrontation
- Direct advice
- Working through
- Teaching improved coping skills

Application to Clients

BPT can be effective in treating depression, anxiety, and situational disorders reflecting repeated patterns, while long-term psychodynamic approaches are useful with more deeply ingrained disorders, once any initial crisis has passed. The following disorders and conditions are likely to respond well to treatment via a psychodynamic approach:

- Mood Disorders—including Major Depressive Disorder, Dysthymic Disorder
- Anxiety Disorders—including Generalized Anxiety, Posttraumatic Stress Disorder
- Somatoform Disorders
- Most Personality Disorders
- Some Conditions—including grief reactions, relational problems

—————————————————— INDIVIDUAL PSYCHOLOGY/ADLERIAN COUNSELING

Alfred Adler, once a colleague of Freud's, developed an approach now known as Individual Psychology or Adlerian counseling. In the past 20 years, a resurgence of interest in this approach has developed, especially for counseling children.

————————————————————————— Description of Approach

Adler's approach has a strong philosophical base that focuses on clients' perceptions of the world (phenomenological) and is holistic and humanistic. Like Freud, Adler emphasized the importance of the early childhood years. Adler believed that children have strong feelings of inferiority that they strive to overcome throughout their lives by seeking achievement, mastery, pleasure, and social acceptance. These needs, as well as whether and how they are met during the early years, lead people to develop enduring lifestyles and goals that form early in their development. Adlerian counseling, then, tends to focus on children and on the parent–child interaction because Adler believed that the seeds for rewarding adult development were sown in childhood. More recent theorists, such as Rudolph Dreikurs, Raymond Corsini, Donald Dinkmeyer, Len Sperry, Jon Carlson, and others, have elaborated and updated Adler's theory so that the approach now is used widely not only with children and their families, but also in adult personal counseling, career counseling, and marital counseling.

Adlerian counseling, also known as Individual Psychology, is characterized by:

- Emphasis on early childhood development and its impact on present attitudes and behavior
- Attention to early feelings of inferiority, the family constellation, and birth order
- Holistic examination of person and environment
- Development of rewarding and socially responsible goals and modes of achieving them
- Establishment of an improved lifestyle

Adlerian counseling encourages use of the following techniques:

- Establishment of a collaborative and positive therapeutic alliance
- Interpretation, via hunches or intuitive guesses, to promote insight and awareness of patterns
- Empowerment and encouragement; focusing on efforts rather than accomplishments
- Acting as if one can accomplish something positive
- Analysis of family constellations and birth order
- Use of early recollections as a source of information on interpersonal and other patterns

- Lifestyle analysis
- Analysis of dreams
- Immediacy and focus on present behaviors
- Development of emotional control
- Avoiding the tar baby (avoiding repetitive pitfalls)
- Spitting in the client's soup (dispelling illusions and promoting awareness of reality)
- Use of natural and logical consequences
- Development of social interest
- Advice and task assignments between sessions

The Adlerian model differs from many newer counseling approaches in that it emphasizes the importance of early childhood development and seeks to foster insight and understanding. Usually it is less symptom-focused and more oriented toward improving people's overall ability to deal with life in a rewarding and socially responsible way. It is a broad-based approach to helping people that can be used by teachers and parents as well as by counselors.

Application to Clients

Although it is an analytical approach, Adlerian counseling assumes a fairly directive role. Consequently, this model does not require a client who is highly motivated or communicative. However, the approach does seem best suited to people who are neither severely disturbed nor confronting an urgent problem or issue. Individual Psychology seems most appropriate for people who are experiencing long-standing emotional difficulties and who are having difficulty developing self-confidence, mobilizing themselves, and finding a rewarding direction. People for whom this model seems likely to be helpful might be experiencing the following:

- Disorders of Childhood and Adolescence—including Conduct Disorder (especially if mild), Oppositional Defiant Disorder, Separation Anxiety Disorder
- Mild-to-moderate, long-standing depression or anxiety such as a Dysthymic Disorder, Generalized Anxiety Disorder, or Social Phobia
- Some Conditions—including Identity Problem, Childhood or Adolescent Antisocial Behavior, Parent–Child Relational Problem, other relational problems, and Occupational Problem

PERSON-CENTERED COUNSELING

Person-centered counseling, formerly known as client-centered counseling and nondirective counseling, is a treatment approach developed by Carl Rogers in the

1940s. It has continued to evolve, becoming more flexible and advocating a more active role for counselors. Person-centered counseling has provided the basis for many more recent counseling approaches. The growing appreciation for the importance of the client–counselor relationship has affirmed the importance of Rogers's ideas.

Description of Approach

The overriding principle of person-centered counseling is the idea that if the counselor can provide clients with a genuine relationship in which they feel understood, accepted, and valued, their self-esteem will blossom and they will increasingly be able to draw on their own resources to help themselves. This humanistic approach views each person as unique and able to strive toward self-actualization and achievement of his or her full potential. The person-centered model is characterized by the following qualities:

- Present-oriented
- Advocates a holistic view of people as well as a belief in the human potential
- Phenomenological (emphasizes the person's experience, perceptions, agenda, and goals)
- Promotes a strong therapeutic alliance in which the counselor communicates empathy, acceptance, genuineness, and congruence
- Focuses primarily on lifelong development, self-esteem, self-awareness, healthy functioning, and self-actualization, although specific problems also are considered
- Emphasizes feelings and emotions
- Encourages concreteness and specificity as well as exploration

Person-centered counselors, who generally pay little attention to the past and rarely use advice giving and confrontation, are very different from psychodynamic or Adlerian therapists. Person-centered counseling makes little use of structured techniques and interventions, preferring to let clients take the lead in the treatment process. Grant (1990, p. 78) refers to the stance of the person-centered counselor as "principled nondirectiveness" or providing "therapeutic conditions in the belief that they are expressions of respect and with the hope that the client will make use of them." The interpersonal skills of the counselor and the creation of a psychological environment that encourages self-actualization are the most important treatment strategies. Others include:

- Immediacy
- Empathy and reflection of feeling
- Acceptance and positive regard, support and encouragement
- Genuineness, modeling, rapport building

- Exploration, including use of clarification, paraphrase, open questions
- Goal setting

Application to Clients

Some elements of the person-centered model, such as empathy, concreteness, and a focus on the present, are included in many approaches to counseling. Others, such as the emphases on emotions, self-actualization, and the counselor–client relationship, characterize some approaches but not others. Aspects of the person-centered model can be integrated into many approaches to counseling without making full use of this model. However, the person-centered model is particularly well suited for some clients. The concerns presented by such people include primarily mild *DSM* disorders and conditions including:

- Adjustment Disorders
- Other Conditions that may be a Focus of Clinical Attention, particularly Phase of Life Problem, Occupational Problem, Bereavement, Identity Problems, Religious or Spiritual Problems, and Acculturation Problems

Such people usually can accept the responsibility for their own growth that is inherent in the person-centered model, have resources they can draw on, and are interested in change via a collaborative treatment process. They can tolerate the sometimes leisurely pace of the person-centered model and can make changes in emotions, perceptions, and self-concept leading to changes in behavior, thinking, and relationships. People who experience successful treatment via person-centered counseling typically develop a greater sense of well-being and the ability and courage to take responsibility for their lives.

Because this model is a supportive and positive one, it can also be used with people who are not high-functioning, such as those with Psychotic or Cognitive Disorders. Although medical treatment usually will be the primary approach to helping these people, many can benefit from a supportive, affirming, and nondemanding counseling relationship that helps them maximize their functioning, promotes their self-esteem, and enhances their adjustment.

GESTALT COUNSELING

Like person-centered counseling, Gestalt counseling, developed by Fritz Perls and Laura Perls, has had a powerful impact on the field of counseling, particularly during the 1970s. Gestalt therapy, too, emphasizes the importance of the whole person and of promoting self-actualization. Although its use has declined, Gestalt counseling has become an established approach in the field.

Description of Approach

Gestalt therapists help people access neglected aspects of themselves, bring closure to unfinished experiences, develop a greater sense of responsibility, and become more aware of their potential. Counselors using this approach typically assume a directive role in which they may frustrate, interpret, lead, and interact with clients. The focus is primarily on present experiences. Counselors' attention to the whole picture leads them to attend to mind, body, and spirit; emotions, behavior, and cognitions; verbal and nonverbal communication; and person and environment. By attending to these, Gestalt counselors promote awareness, wholeness, integration, and balance.

Gestalt counseling uses a broad range of techniques including the following:

- Focus on the here and now (rather than the past) and on what and how (rather than on why)
- Encouragement of responsibility for the self via I statements
- Exploration of dreams and fantasies
- Giving voice and action to physical sensations, nonverbal cues, and emotions
- Exaggeration of emotions and movements to clarify the message
- Role play using an empty chair to simulate dialog with another person or part of the self
- Topdog/underdog (reflecting dominant and submissive parts of the personality)
- Confrontation
- Homework
- In group therapy, use of the hot seat (person receives feedback from the group) and making the rounds (group member says something to each member of the group)

Application to Clients

Because of its confrontational nature and its emphasis on making the unconscious conscious, the Gestalt approach generally is not appropriate for people who are severely disturbed, in a crisis, or poorly motivated to change. The model appears most useful for people who intellectualize, have trouble clarifying their feelings, feel immobilized, and cut themselves off from aspects of themselves (e.g., the person who neglects relationships and overemphasizes work). Gestalt counseling also might be useful with people presenting psychosomatic or other physical symptoms that are linked to emotional difficulties. Such people may benefit from help in attending to and making better use of the bodily messages that they are receiving and sending. People for whom Gestalt Therapy seem useful might present with the following disorders and conditions:

- Mood Disorders—including Dysthymic Disorder, Cyclothymic Disorder

- Generalized Anxiety Disorder
- Somatoform Disorders
- Factitious Disorders
- Adjustment Disorders, especially of long-standing
- Mild Personality Disorders or Traits—including Avoidant, Dependent, Narcissistic, Histrionic, and Obsessive–Compulsive Personality Disorders and Traits
- Conditions—including Psychological Factors Affecting Medical Condition, Identity Problem, Phase of Life Problem, Relational Problem, Occupational Problem.

For more severe disorders, the Gestalt approach generally should be used only if client motivation and emotional strength are adequate, and if the approach is tempered by other approaches. The Gestalt approach seems well suited to many of the problems resulting from the pressures of modern life. It is a rich model with a broad repertoire of techniques, many of which can be used to enhance or expand on other models of counseling.

RATIONAL EMOTIVE BEHAVIOR THERAPY

Albert Ellis developed rational emotive behavior therapy (REBT), previously known as Rational-Emotive Therapy, in the 1950s. Ellis became disillusioned with the psychoanalytic model and sought a more effective counseling approach. The seeds of Ellis's psychoanalytic training are evident, however; he viewed emotional difficulties as stemming from a pattern of childhood development that leads people to care too much about what others think of them and behave in ways that will win them favor. People with these attitudes tend to be outer- rather than inner-directed, have little confidence in their own skills and attributes, and have beliefs that Ellis termed irrational. These beliefs, such as the thought that they must be fully competent and achieving in all areas to be viewed as worthwhile, are characteristic of people who awfulize, as Ellis put it. They overgeneralize, focus on should's and must's, think in extremes, feel disaster lurking around every bend, and believe they have little control over their lives. Behavioral and emotional difficulties grow out of these dysfunctional thoughts.

REBT has evolved over the years. It has become more humanistic, preventive, growth promoting, and flexible, paying attention to emotions and behaviors as well as to thoughts. In addition, Ellis and Dryden (1997) have delineated two tiers of REBT; general REBT targets immediate concerns while elegant or preferential REBT seeks to effect deep, enduring changes.

Description of Approach

Ellis's model views the onset of difficulties and their resolution according to six steps:

- A, an *activating* event occurs and is identified and described
- B, *beliefs* emerge about the event, leading to rational or irrational thoughts
- C, the thoughts and beliefs lead to *consequences* that can be harmful or helpful
- D, client and counselor *dispute* irrational and harmful beliefs
- E, interventions promote *effective* rational beliefs and philosophies
- F, new *feelings* and behaviors emerge that are more helpful to the client.

REBT is characterized by many strategies including the following:

- Emphasis on the present, though past and future both receive attention
- Focus on thoughts as the key to changing both emotions and behavior
- Counselor assumes a directive and instructional role; rapport is necessary but not sufficient
- Encouragement of client responsibility and acceptance of oneself as fallible
- Use of ABCDEF model (presented above)
- Modification of dysfunctional thoughts via disputing, Socratic questioning, persuasion
- Reduction of ideas to absurdity, other uses of humor
- Shame-attacking exercises
- Role playing (often a dialog between rational and irrational thoughts)
- Imagining the worst and promoting tolerance and ability to cope with it
- Use of contracts and homework assignments to promote action
- Skill training, including problem solving, decision-making, assertiveness
- Promoting will power and determination

Application to Clients

REBT's emphasis on cognitive analysis and restructuring seems best suited for people who have strengths in verbal fluency, intellectual ability, contact with reality, motivation to change, and self-discipline. REBT is particularly appropriate for people who are affected by dysfunctional emotions and behaviors stemming from extreme, perfectionistic, and distorted cognitions. Such people might be experiencing the following disorders:

- Mood Disorders—including Major Depressive Disorder, Dysthymic Disorder
- Anxiety Disorders—especially Generalized Anxiety Disorder

- Mild-to-Moderate Impulse-Control Disorders
- Adjustment Disorders
- Mild-to-Moderate Personality Disorders and Personality Traits

For more severe disorders, such as Bipolar Disorders, medication or other treatment modalities often are combined with REBT to accelerate progress.

Both REBT and Reality Therapy (discussed later in this chapter) are characterized by their developers as serving a broad spectrum of the population. Both can be used by teachers as well as by counselors and offer ways of helping troubled people, as well as those who are functioning satisfactorily, to think, feel, and act in healthier and happier ways. These modes of treatment certainly are not ideal for all people, but they do have wide application.

COGNITIVE THERAPY

Cognitive Therapy, related to REBT, was developed by Aaron Beck and his colleagues in the 1960s and 1970s. Cognitive therapy assumes that emotions and behavior are influenced by underlying assumptions or cognitions derived from previous experiences. This is a directive, structured approach that identifies and corrects distorted cognitions.

Description of Approach

Cognitive Therapy differs from REBT in the approach used to effect change in thinking (Beck, 1995). Cognitive therapy is a structured approach that begins each session by establishing an agenda. Then, presenting concerns are identified and associated emotions, actions, and thoughts are explored, assessed, modified if necessary, and then reassessed. Cognitive therapy consists of specific learning experiences designed to teach people to:

- Recognize links among cognition, affect, and behavior
- Identify, monitor, and record negative automatic thoughts
- Reality test dysfunctional thoughts
- Replace dysfunctional thoughts with more accurate and helpful ones
- Identify and change underlying core beliefs leading to biased and distorted cognitions

Cognitive therapy makes extensive use of strategies to promote change. Among these are:

- Diaries of events, emotions, actions, and cognitions
- Hypothesis testing, using exaggeration, reattribution, and other strategies to assess and modify cognitions

- Systematic assessment of alternatives
- Labeling the distortion
- Cognitive and covert modeling
- Diversions, distractions, and thought-stopping
- Self-talk and affirmations
- Activity scheduling and rating activities for mastery and pleasure
- Graded task assignments
- Assessment of mood via the Beck Depression and Anxiety Inventories and other tools
- Stress inoculation
- Cognitive rehearsal and role-playing

Application to Clients

Cognitive interventions usually are combined with behavioral interventions (discussed next) for a particularly powerful treatment plan. Research has given considerable support to the effectiveness of cognitive therapy in the treatment of depression, anxiety, substance use, and eating problems (Chambless et al., 1998). Either alone or in combination with behavioral strategies, cognitive therapy often is helpful to people experiencing:

- Mood Disorders—especially Major Depressive Disorder
- Anxiety Disorders—including Panic Disorder, Social Phobia, Obsessive–Compulsive Disorder, Posttraumatic Stress Disorder, Generalized Anxiety Disorder
- Eating Disorders—especially those involving binge eating
- Somatoform Disorders and chronic pain
- Some Substance Use Disorders
- Adjustment Disorders
- Some Personality Disorders

Cognitive Therapy is a sophisticated and complex approach that has received considerable attention and support in recent years. The apparent usefulness of the model, especially with people who are depressed, suicidal, or anxious, makes it an approach with which all counselors should be familiar. It is one of the forerunners of a group of time-limited, directive, cognitive-behavioral, and strategic approaches that are establishing new directions for counseling.

BEHAVIOR THERAPY

Originating with the work of B. F. Skinner in the late 1930s and 1940s, the behavioral model of counseling has become an essential tool. Whether or not clinicians emphasize behavior therapy in their work, this approach offers a wealth of ideas and treatment strategies that can be productively integrated into most other treatment approaches.

Description of Approach

Behavioral counselors generally believe that personality is shaped by environmental reinforcers. If undesirable traits and behaviors have been learned through modeling, conditioning, and reinforcement, then behavior therapy can teach and reinforce positive behaviors while eliminating maladaptive ones. Behavior therapy is characterized by the following dimensions:

- Generally present oriented, though it pays attention to how problems developed
- Problem/symptom focused
- Counselor primarily responsible for agenda of sessions, but work is collaborative
- Concreteness and specificity encouraged
- New learning, leading to behavioral change, is the primary goal
- Considerable use of information giving, inventories, homework assignments, other techniques
- Exploration of interface between person and environment
- Focused on goals, using contracts, plans, and regular evaluation of progress

The behavioral model has been criticized for neglecting people's inner needs. However, this reflects a misunderstanding. Most behaviorists now view the counselor–client relationship as important. Counselors communicate empathy and acceptance and time is taken for accurate listening, development of rapport and a collaborative counselor–client relationship, as well as understanding people's symptoms in light of their history and context. Nevertheless, the ultimate goal of behavioral therapy is symptom removal and behavioral change; the counseling relationship is viewed as an important condition for change rather than the cause of change.

- Behavior therapy follows a fairly predictable pattern: identify the problem behavior, establish a baseline, develop goals and a behavior change contract, implement change strategies, establish rewards and/or consequences, assess progress, change goals and strategies if needed, solidify and extend gains, and maintain progress. The following additional techniques also are associated with Behavioral Counseling.
- Natural consequences and aversion therapy (e.g., time out, negative imagery, Antabuse).
- Incompatible alternatives.

- Reinforcement schedules, token economies.
- Cueing, anchoring.
- Behavioral rehearsal.
- Satiation, flooding.
- *In vivo* or imaginal systematic desensitization.
- Relaxation strategies.
- Role-playing and modeling by self or other.
- Acting as if one is someone who is admired.
- Activity schedules.
- Assertiveness and other skill training.

Application to Clients

People for whom behavior therapy is likely to be effective present disorders of behavior or habit control. Behavior therapy can be particularly useful with children or adults who lack the motivation or verbal facility for extensive self-exploration. Treatment typically is short term and time-limited in nature and so may appeal to people who do not have the interest, patience, or resources to engage in prolonged counseling and who are seeking circumscribed and measurable changes. Behavior therapy is likely to be useful to people with disorders such as the following:

- Disorders of Children and Adolescents—including Attention-Deficit/Hyperactivity Disorder, Conduct Disorder, Oppositional Defiant Disorder, Pica, Elimination Disorders (Encopresis, Enuresis), Separation Anxiety Disorder
- Anxiety Disorders—including Phobias (Specific Phobia, Social Phobia, Agoraphobia), other Anxiety Disorders (including Panic Disorder and Obsessive–Compulsive Disorder)
- Sexual Disorders—including Sexual Dysfunctions and Paraphilias
- Eating Disorders, especially those involving overeating
- Some Sleep Disorders—including Insomnia and Circadian Rhythm Sleep Disorder
- Trichotillomania
- Some Personality Disorders, including Borderline Personality Disorder (treated via Dialectical Behavior Therapy) and Avoidant Personality Disorder

Behavior therapy also can be helpful in modifying the behaviors of people with other Personality Disorders, Cognitive Disorders, Psychotic Disorders, Anorexia Nervosa, Mood Disorders, and Adjustment Disorders, although behavioral counseling probably will need to be combined with other approaches in their treatment. Behavior change strategies often accelerate client growth and change even when another model of treatment is primary. For example, a person with low self-esteem and strong feelings of insecurity may require the pace and support of a person-centered counselor but may benefit considerably from the inclusion of assertiveness training and communication skills in the treatment plan.

REALITY THERAPY/CHOICE THERAPY

William Glasser first wrote about Reality Therapy in the 1960s. Since that time, reality therapy, also known as choice therapy, has evolved and gained popularity. It has been adopted by many substance use treatment programs and correctional facilities, and also is used in many schools because of its emphasis on prevention and responsibility.

Description of Approach

Reality therapists generally believe that people who behave responsibly, seeking to fulfill their needs in a socially acceptable manner and in a way that attends to the real world, are most likely to develop what Glasser called a success identity. Reality therapy suggests that all people are born with five basic needs: Survival, belonging, power/achievement, fun/enjoyment, and freedom/independence (Glasser, 1998). The relative strengths of these needs are reflected in people's personalities. According to reality therapy, all behavior is purposeful and is directed at satisfying these needs. Procedures involved in reality therapy are reflected by the acronym WDEP, signifying exploration of WANTS, reviewing DIRECTION and DOING, EVALUATING actions and attitudes, and PLANNING effective action.

Reality Therapy can be characterized by the following dimensions:

- Present and future oriented, remedial as well as preventive
- Emphasis on importance of counselor–client rapport and involvement
- Focus on behavior, not emotion; emphasis on what and how, not why
- Encouragement of client self-evaluation, goal setting, planning, and contracting
- Elimination of punishment and excuses; people learn through natural consequences
- Never giving up; if one approach doesn't work, try another.

Reality therapy uses many of the strategies of behavioral therapy as well as some borrowed from cognitive therapy. Additional strategies associated with reality therapy include:

- Caring confrontation
- Encouragement to establish positive "addictions" such as exercise or meditation

- Use of verbs and "ing" words (e.g., angering) to suggest control over emotions

Many similarities exist between behavior therapy and reality therapy. However, reality therapists place particular emphasis on the establishment of a warm, understanding counseling relationship. Reality therapists also are concerned with clients' self-esteem and environment. Reality therapy seeks to help people give and receive love, and perceive themselves as valuable members of society.

Application to Clients

Glasser developed his approach while working with adolescent girls exhibiting delinquent behavior. Reality therapy is effective with people like these who have difficulty meeting their own needs, tend to violate the rights of others, behave irresponsibly, and disregard social norms. Such people might have the following *DSM* disorders and conditions:

- Conduct Disorder
- Oppositional Defiant Disorder
- Substance Use Disorders
- Disorders of Impulse Control including Pathological Gambling, Pyromania, Intermittent Explosive Disorder, and Kleptomania
- Some Personality Disorders, especially Antisocial Personality Disorder
- Adult, Adolescent, or Childhood Antisocial Behavior

People with disorders such as these tend to be reluctant to engage in treatment and have difficulties that manifest themselves behaviorally. Reality therapy often is effective in helping people with this combination of characteristics. This approach also can be a useful part of a treatment program for people in crisis, people who are depressed or angry, and people with Somatoform Disorders.

SOLUTION-FOCUSED BRIEF THERAPY

Solution-focused or solution-based brief therapy has become an important treatment approach in recent years. Emphasizing behavior change, this approach has much in common with reality therapy. Both emphasize the present and the future, help people identify and achieve their wants and goals, stress the importance of planning, and build on successes. Current leaders in this approach include Steve de Shazer, Bill O'Hanlon, and Michele Weiner-Davis.

Description of Approach

Solution-focused brief therapy is a phenomenological approach; it takes the position that unrewarding and harmful behaviors stem from distorted or self-destructive worldviews. Counselors advocating this treatment model believe that small changes shift people's worldview, enabling them to expect and make positive changes. This will have a ripple effect, leading to more and greater changes. Little time is devoted to the origins, causes, or purposes of concerns; rather, this is an active approach that quickly encourages positive movement and action. Counselors take an optimistic view of clients, giving them a message that they have the strengths and resources they need to resolve their difficulties. Stages in treatment include identifying a complaint that is solvable, setting goals, creating an intervention, suggesting strategic tasks that will promote change, highlighting positive changes, consolidating gains, and completion of treatment.

Use of creative strategies is a hallmark of this approach. Some of the important strategies associated with solution-focused brief therapy are:

- Gearing treatment and tasks to a person's worldview and readiness for change
- 1–10 scale to assess complaints, symptoms, and progress
- Changing repetitive, nonproductive sequences of behavior
- Miracle question (discussed further in Chapter 8)
- Reframing
- Promoting use of positive behavior already occurring and expanding upon positive exceptions
- Developing new and more helpful behaviors
- Use of practical and specific goals and solutions
- Strategic tasks designed to empower as well as nurture new skills
- Compliments and encouragement
- Using suggestion and solution-based language to create an expectancy of change (e.g., "If you weren't using that time to argue with your partner, what might you be doing instead?")
- Use of indirect strategies such as stories and metaphors
- Videotalk (describing concerns in action terms).

Application to Clients

Largely because it is such a new approach, research, especially on the enduring impact of solution-focused brief therapy, is limited. However, existing research as well as extensive case studies suggest that this treatment approach is sufficiently flexible to be used, either alone or in combination, with a broad range of clients and complaints. The following diagnoses and problems seem likely to be helped by this approach:

- Anxiety Disorders
- Mild-to-Moderate Depressive Disorders
- Mild-to-Moderate Personality Disorders
- Somatoform Disorders
- Impulse-Control Disorders
- Substance Use Disorders
- Sexual, physical, and emotional abuse.

ECLECTIC AND INTEGRATED MODELS OF COUNSELING

A trend toward eclecticism in counseling has been gaining ground since the 1940s. Although most counselors seem to have a preferred theoretical orientation that forms the basis of their work, most counselors are flexible, drawing from many treatment approaches and exhibiting an extensive repertoire of interventions. Since the early 1990s, the field has witnessed a particular effort to develop integrated models of counseling that are effective, although most counselors today who do not adhere to a specific theoretical model are probably better described as technical or systematic eclectics, borrowing from several theoretical models, rather than true theoretical integrationists (Prochaska & Norcross, 1994).

Multimodal Behavior Therapy

The first well-known eclectic treatment model is Multimodal Behavior Therapy. Arnold Lazarus developed this present-oriented approach to counseling, which integrates and expands on many of the approaches discussed in this chapter. Lazarus's model enables counselors to take a systematic and comprehensive look at a person, determine areas of strength and weakness, and develop a treatment plan designed to have a multifaceted impact. Multimodal therapists view counseling as a holistic learning process and believe that change in one aspect of a person will affect and be encouraged by change in other aspects of that person. This approach advocates a sevenfold model, represented by the acronym BASIC I.D., for assessing the person and planning the treatment. Assessment of these seven areas leads to the development of a Structural Profile to guide the counseling process. The seven categories in this model follow, along with selected strategies associated with each element in the model.

1. B/Behavior (observable habits and activities)—contracts, teaching new coping skills, reinforcement, consequences, extinction, conditioning

2. A/Affect (feelings and emotions)—recognizing, modifying, and expressing feelings; abreaction
3. S/Sensation (physical concerns, sensory responses)—relaxation, pleasuring
4. I/Imagery (images, dreams, and fantasies)—visual imagery, changing self-image
5. C/Cognition (beliefs, thoughts, plans, philosophies)—cognitive restructuring, education
6. I/Interpersonal relations (relationships with others)—modeling, social skills training
7. D/Drugs, biology (biological functioning)—improving nutrition and exercise, changing use of harmful substances

The behavioral origins of the multimodal approach are evident. However, this approach goes beyond behaviorism in breadth and flexibility. Even if people present difficulties in only one or two of the seven areas, the BASIC I.D. framework enables counselors to ensure not only that obvious problems receive attention, but that all important areas of functioning are explored. This model also helps counselors define and build on people's strengths.

Multimodal counseling has a contribution to make to almost every sort of client concern. However, some types of people, difficulties, and circumstances lend themselves particularly well to this sort of an approach. This model seems best for a client who is reasonably well motivated, in satisfactory contact with reality, and capable of planning, organizing, and self-monitoring. People who present a range of diverse concerns (e.g., depression, eating problems, and poor social skills) might be especially responsive to the multimodal model, which can help them develop a systematic approach to their concerns and reduce feelings of being overwhelmed and discouraged, common in multiproblem clients.

Developmental Counseling and Therapy

A treatment approach with a carefully crafted and integrated structure is Developmental Counseling and Therapy (DCT) for individuals and its companion, Systemic Cognitive-Developmental Therapy (SCDT) for families (Rigazio-DiGilio, Ivey, Ivey, & Simek-Morgan, 1997). Formulated by Allen Ivey, Sandra Rigazio-DiGilio, and associates, DCT/SCDT is a developmental approach that redefines pathology as blocks or delays that need to be alleviated to free people for further growth. This holistic model considers mind, body, and context, matching treatment to a person's developmental orientation.

Although research is needed to demonstrate the effectiveness of this theoretical model, it reflects multicultural and postmodern perspectives, may apply to a broad range of people and disorders, and provides useful guidelines for treatment planning and selection of interventions. DCT/SCDT postulates the existence of the following four cognitive-developmental orientations, based on the developmental stage theory of Piaget:

1. *Sensorimotor*—People in this stage are present oriented. They typically rely on their senses and are not introspective. They tend to be reactive and easily overwhelmed. Counseling focuses on eliciting their experiences and understanding.

2. *Concrete-Operational*—People in this stage can describe and plan, following a linear model of causality. They have difficulty with empathy, generalization, and change. Counselors can work with these people best if they focus on facts, sequential descriptions, and perceptions of events.

3. *Formal Operational*—These people are analytical, can see their place in their environment, and can see patterns and multiple perspectives. However, they sometimes emphasize reflection at the cost of action and have trouble changing basic assumptions. They need to focus on present experience of roles, relationships, and patterns of thoughts, feelings, and behaviors.

4. *Dialectic/Systemic Operational*—Although people in this group also may focus too much on thinking, they have a capacity for integration, for challenging their own assumptions, and for understanding context and complexity. They need help in reviewing their assumptions and alternatives, changing patterns, and integrating aspects of their lives.

Thinking-Feeling-Acting Model

The Thinking-Feeling-Acting (TFA) model, developed by Mueller, Dupuy, and Hutchins (1994), is another holistic model that seeks to match interventions to clients. Using the Hutchins Behavior Inventory, counselors adopting this model identify a person's strengths and limitations in three areas: thinking, feeling, and acting. Strategies are then adapted to both the person's primary orientation and to areas that need development.

Adaptive Counseling and Therapy/Readiness Model

The Adaptive Counseling and Therapy/Readiness Model (ACT) also matches therapist approach to clients' needs (Nance & Myers, 1991). Treatment approaches are described in terms of two dimensions: support and direction. The model describes four counseling orientations based on these dimensions. Approaches that are low in directiveness and high in support are basically supportive approaches; those high in directiveness as well as support emphasize teaching; those low in support and high in directiveness focus on telling; while those low in both emphasize delegating. This approach, like TFA and DCT/SCDT, shows promise but needs further study.

Stages-of-Change Models

Stage models link interventions to both the stage of a person's readiness for change and the progression of their treatment. An influential example of this sort of model is the *transtheoretical model* developed by Prochaska and others (Prochaska & Norcross, 1999, p. 495). This approach suggests that "change unfolds over a series of five stages: precontemplation, contemplation, preparation, action, and maintenance."

OTHER MODELS OF TREATMENT

Other theoretical models, not as well established as those discussed earlier in this chapter, also have made a contribution to the counseling profession. The following are worthy of mention.

Existential Therapy

Developed by May, Yalom, Frankl, Binswanger, Bugental, and others, the Existential model addresses such troubling aspects of the human condition as loneliness, guilt, meaninglessness, loss, and death. Existentialism is less a treatment model and more a phenomenological and humanistic philosophy that seeks to help people know and express themselves fully. Using such techniques as life review and paradoxical intervention, this model helps people to move toward self-actualization and relatedness with others, create meaning in their lives, make rewarding choices, and develop responsibility and self-confidence. Existential therapy seems best suited for use with fairly healthy people experiencing mild depression, anxiety, or situational difficulties, who need a sense of purpose and direction in their lives.

Transpersonal Counseling

Transpersonal counseling, derived primarily from eastern traditions and beliefs, also has a strong philosophical emphasis. Focusing on spirituality and transcendence of the material world, this approach can provide a powerful antidote to our hurried and stressful lives. Transpersonal counseling seeks to raise people's awareness of the interrelatedness of all beings, our purpose and place in the universe, and our potential for higher levels of awareness. This approach encourages use of intuition, spiritual development, meditation, and other practices designed to promote inner peace and enlightenment. Adherence to structured religious beliefs and practices may or may not be part of the sort of growth that is valued by transpersonal counselors.

Postmodern, Constructivist, and Multicultural Approaches to Counseling

A series of approaches have been developed, beginning in the 1990s and gaining importance in the 21st century, that emphasize an epistemological viewpoint encompassing multiple perspectives of reality. Their advocates believe that knowledge is not an objective representation but, rather, is a creation of thought and language that grows out of social interactions and cultural backgrounds (D'Andrea, 2000; Guterman, 1994). They emphasize change and process rather than content and suggest that each person has a unique perspective and life experience as well as an individual logic and wisdom. They believe that clients and counselors should cocreate definitions of problems and directions for change, with the therapeutic relationship being an integral element in the change process. These approaches emphasize culture and society as well as the individual, strengths and development, and prevention and education. Language, metaphors stories, and dialog are important ingredients in these approaches. Important examples of postmodern approaches to treatment include narrative therapy and feminist therapy.

Narrative Therapy

Narrative therapy has its roots in Australia in the work of Michael White and David Epson. Narrative theorists believe that people's self-images, their worldviews, and the way they lead their lives stem largely from internalized stories learned from their family, cultural group, and society. The goal of this approach is to help people tell and explore their stories, deconstruct them, and then revise them. New stories can lead to new perceptions that, in turn, can lead to improved functioning and healthier development. Sharing written documents and revised stories with others helps clients make the new stories a part of their lives.

This approach seems likely to be helpful to underserved and disenfranchised groups such as the poor, people with disabilities, the elderly, and people from some ethnic and cultural groups. Changing their stories can help people such as these reclaim their rightful place in society and embrace positive messages about themselves.

Constructivist Therapy

Constructivist therapy is another phenomenological approach that takes an optimistic view of people. Emphasizing background as well as social context, this approach helps people make meaning of their lives so that they see new possibilities and live in more creative and rewarding ways. Language is important in this approach to both clarify and change meaning.

Feminist Therapy

Feminist therapy is designed to address not only the common concerns that people present in treatment but also to help women overcome negative societal messages regarding sex role, gender stereotypes, physical beauty, and other aspects of their lives. Sands (1998, p. 44) described three basic principles inherent in feminist counseling:

1. The Personal is Political: counselors must work for social change.
2. Egalitarian Relationships: counseling should be a collaborative process.
3. Valuing the Female Perspective: counseling should help women value their gender-related strengths including cooperation, intuition, relationships, and interdependence.

Motivational Interviewing

Motivational interviewing, another new and promising treatment approach, was developed by Miller and Rollnick. According to Miller (1999, p. 2), "Motivational interviewing is a directive, client-centered counseling style for eliciting behavior change by helping clients to explore and resolve ambivalence." Working collaboratively with clients, therapists using motivational interviewing reduce barriers to change via strategies such as open-ended questions, affirmations, reflective listening, and summarization. "Change talk" helps reluctant clients to recognize and express their problems, become hopeful that change is possible, and make a commitment to change. Originally intended to promote relapse prevention in people who misused drugs and alcohol, this approach has useful suggestions for promoting motivation and change in all clients.

Power and Energy Therapies

Power and energy therapies reflect another innovative way to help people. Included in this group are eye movement desensitization and reprocessing (EMDR), thought field therapy (TFT), neuro-linguistic programming (NLP), traumatic incident reduction (TIR) and others. Underlying most of these approaches is the belief that traumatic experiences are captured and held within the body. Posttraumatic Stress Disorder and other painful emotions can be alleviated by interrupting the physical responses associated with those emotions (Gallo, 2002). Bilateral stimulation via eye movements, tones, or pulses (EMDR); tapping (TFT); and other techniques are part of these approaches. The best known and best researched of these, EMDR, has received considerable support as a treatment for Posttraumatic Stress Disorder and other anxiety-related concerns.

Additional Models

Several hundred other approaches to counseling are available, including Jungian analytical psychology, transactional analysis, and a broad range of expressive therapies (e.g., art therapy, play therapy, poetry therapy). Approaches to counseling are constantly being developed and modified. This chapter is not intended to provide a comprehensive discussion of all models of counseling. Rather, its purpose is to help readers appreciate the broad range of counseling approaches and make appropriate use of treatment systems and strategies.

Even though most counselors have preferred modes of counseling, they often borrow from other approaches to counseling. The best treatment often can be provided by counselors who are knowledgeable and flexible enough to select ingredients from several theories in helping their clients. Counselors should be able to elaborate on and justify their approach, selecting interventions that have proven their effectiveness in addressing particular problems or disorders and systematically tailoring their counseling approach to each client.

SAMPLE TREATMENT PLANS

This section will present three abbreviated counseling cases along with treatment plans that have been developed to suit the particular needs of these clients. These examples are designed to illustrate the application of principles discussed in this chapter as well as in Chapters 3–6.

Case 1—Maria Sanchez

The first treatment plan, following the format of the DO A CLIENT MAP, focuses on Maria Sanchez, the 36-year-old Latina woman whose intake interview was presented in Chapter 5. Review that intake interview and the report that follows it before reading this treatment plan.

Diagnosis

Axis I.   296.32 Major Depressive Disorder, recurrent, moderate, with interepisode recovery
309.81 Posttraumatic Stress Disorder, prior history
Axis II.   V71.09 No mental disorder on Axis II
Axis III.   Pregnant, reports fatigue and back pain
Axis IV.   Pregnancy, three young children
Axis V.   57.

Objectives

Short-Term Objectives

1. Maria will manifest a reduction in depression as evidenced by a drop in her score on the Beck Depression Inventory (BDI) of at least 3 points.
2. Maria will begin a relaxation program of her choosing.
3. Maria will gain some insight into the nature of her depression as evidenced by being able to verbalize at least three possible reasons for her sad mood.
4. Maria will show improvement in her enjoyment of her role as mother as evidenced by her identifying at least one rewarding activity that she does with her children each week.

Medium-Term Objectives

5. Maria's mood will be in the normal range as evidenced by her score on the BDI.
6. Maria will report that she continues her relaxation program and has carved out at least 2 hours per week for leisure activities by herself or with other adults.
7. Maria will be able to describe fully her difficult childhood and adolescence and explain the connection between her experiences in El Salvador and her present concerns.
8. Maria will continue to report increased enjoyment in her role as mother and will have developed a rewarding vision and plan for her life after her fourth child is born.

Assessments

Beck Depression Inventory, Life History Questionnaire.

Clinician

Maria will probably work best with a female counselor who is her age or older. A counselor who is knowledgeable about multicultural issues and about Posttraumatic Stress Disorder is recommended. That counselor should demonstrate support and caring as well as recognition of Maria's strengths and also needs to understand and honor the choices Maria has made, even though they seem overwhelming for her now. However, the counselor also needs to gently help Maria modify these choices so that she has a sense of control over her life.

Location

Maria is not in danger and seems likely to keep scheduled appointments. Consequently, she should be treated in an outpatient setting, perhaps a counseling program for women, a private practice, a community mental health center, or an agency focused on helping people with Hispanic and Latino backgrounds.

Interventions

The overriding theoretical framework for counseling this client will be cognitive therapy. Psychodynamic, behavioral, and feminist elements also will be integrated into the treatment.

Specific Interventions

- Identification, assessment, and modification of cognitive distortions (Objectives 1, 4, 5, 8)
- Life review, helping Maria recognize the impact of her cultural background on her wants and self-image and process the sexual and emotional abuse she experienced (3, 7)
- Teaching simple relaxation techniques such as deep breathing and stretching (2, 6)
- Planning activities that provide pleasure and mastery (1, 4, 5, 8)
- Affirmations (1, 4, 5, 8)

Additional interventions can be added to treatment, based on Maria's response to counseling.

Numbers

Maria's counseling will initially be one-to-one. Once she has made progress, become less depressed, and improved her self-esteem, joint sessions with her husband should be useful.

Timing

Maria will be seen for weekly counseling with sessions lasting 45 minutes. She will probably need about 6 months of treatment. Pacing can be moderate, since Maria has many strengths despite her current depression and is not in immediate danger.

Medication

People with Major Depressive Disorders usually benefit from antidepressant medication. However, Maria is pregnant and does not want to take medication as long as she is pregnant. If her mood has not improved significantly in approximately 2 months, she will be encouraged to consult with a psychiatrist to see whether she can safely take any medication.

Adjunct Services

Maria needs to build up a support system. At the same time, she is already busy and probably has little time for friends or group meetings. Exploration of online support groups for pregnant women or women with young children, play groups and gyms with child care where she can have contact with other parents while still caring for her children, and similar social and support opportunities might help her find a source of support that does not place further demands on her time. Eventually, Maria does need to develop leisure activities, but probably not until after she gives birth.

Prognosis

Major Depressive Disorder generally has a positive prognosis. In addition, Maria is a resourceful woman with much strength. This combination suggests a very good prognosis. However, Major Depressive Disorder does have a high likelihood of relapse. Treatment will have to pay particular attention to relapse prevention.

Case 2—Marty Leone

Marty Leone, a 14-year-old Caucasian male, was recently arrested for shoplifting. This is only one of a long series of illegal and aggressive acts, including violence against younger children, stealing from school and family, and truancy, that began at least 6 years ago. Marty has always been a poor student. Although his inventoried intelligence is in the average range, he has never gotten a grade better than a C and was required to repeat fourth grade. Marty does have some friends and reportedly enjoys basketball and other sports but has never gotten involved with sports at school. Marty's mother described him as having a temperament like his father. Marty's father is currently in prison following a conviction for breaking and entering. Marty is in good health except for a broken arm, suffered in a fall from a fence on which he was climbing.

Diagnosis

Axis I.	312.81 Conduct Disorder, childhood-onset type, severe
Axis II.	V71.09 No diagnosis on Axis II
Axis III.	Client reports broken arm resulting from a fall
Axis IV.	Recent arrest for shoplifting, academic difficulties, father on probation
Axis V.	53.

Objectives

Short-Term Objectives

1. Marty will reduce illegal and aggressive behavior as evidenced by self-report and reports from mother and teacher.
2. Marty will learn ways to manage anger better as evidenced by fewer conflicts with peers, family, and authority and self-reports of using anger management strategies.
3. Marty will attend school daily with no unexcused absences as evidenced by attendance records.
4. Marty will articulate the consequences associated with his behaviors and begin to identify other ways to meet his needs as evidenced by his discussions with the counselor.

Medium-Term Objectives

5. Marty will engage in no illegal and aggressive behavior as evidenced by self-report and reports from his mother and teachers.
6. Marty will continue to have no unexcused absences from school and will improve his grades at school by at least one letter grade.
7. Marty will engage in two positive social interactions per day with peers, family, and teachers as evidenced by self-report and reports from his mother and teachers.
8. Marty will identify negative, destructive thoughts and behaviors and replace them with constructive, positive cognitions and behaviors as evidenced by self-report.
9. Marty will identify and become involved in one rewarding extracurricular activity.

Assessment

Achenbach's Child Behavior Checklist (parent and teacher versions), as well as the Connors Teacher Rating Scale, will be used to obtain information on Marty's behavioral difficulties and to determine whether he has comorbid disorders such as Attention-Deficit/Hyperactivity Disorder. The Beck Depression Inventory also will be used to assess mood level. A drug and alcohol screening will determine whether Marty is misusing substances.

Clinician

Marty will probably work best with a male counselor who can serve as a positive role. That counselor should have experience in dealing with adolescents with Conduct Disorders who are reluctant clients. A counselor who is firm and understanding, patient and calm, but who can set limits and is comfortable with a structured counseling approach seems best.

Location

Initially, treatment will be at a family counseling agency that is experienced in helping acting-out adolescents and collaborating with family and school to promote treatment goals. If Marty's behavior worsens or does not improve soon, he probably should be treated in an intensive day treatment or similar program.

Interventions

The overriding theoretical framework for Marty's treatment will be reality therapy, incorporating a variety of cognitive and behavioral strategies.

Strategies

- Establishment of rapport and a collaborative therapeutic alliance (all)
- Assessment of the relative strength of Marty's five basic needs as well as his progress in meeting those needs (1, 4, 5, 7)
- Identification and modification of distorted cognitions (1, 2, 4, 5, 8)
- Use of WDEP model (exploration of wants, reviewing direction and doing, evaluating actions and attitudes, planning effective action) (all)
- Caring confrontation (all)
- Skill development, focused on study skills and interpersonal skills (1, 2, 3, 6, 7, 8)
- Encouragement of involvement in a positive activity, preferably one that is physically active and involves peer interaction (2, 7, 9)
- Self-esteem building (all)
- Planning and making written commitments to responsible behavior (all)
- Anger management and impulse control training (1, 2, 5, 7, 8)
- Use of rewards and natural consequences (all)

Numbers

The primary vehicle for counseling Marty will be individual counseling. However, some sessions also will be held with his mother and with Marty and his mother together. Marty also would benefit from concurrent group therapy with other adolescents engaged in antisocial activities and manifesting poor academic performance.

Timing

Marty will initially be seen twice a week (once in individual therapy and once in group therapy). Additional family therapy sessions will be scheduled as needed. Sessions will be 50 minutes in length. Marty's intensive treatment seems likely to last for 3–6 months. Sessions will then be reduced to once a week and eventually to every other week but will last for at least 1 year. Pacing will be moderate to rapid; Marty needs to make changes quickly because he presents a danger to others.

Medication

Unless Marty is found to have an additional underlying disorder such as a Dysthymic Disorder or Attention-Deficit/Hyperactivity Disorder, medication is not indicated at present. However, if he does not respond well to counseling, medication should be considered to help stabilize his moods and reduce impulsivity.

Adjunct Services

Marty will be referred to a psychoeducational group to help develop his social and academic skills. In addition, he will be encouraged to engage in a physically active extracurricular activity with other young people.

Prognosis

The prognosis for alleviating Marty's Conduct Disorder is probably fair to good. Negative prognostic factors include the diagnosis itself, the length of time Marty has manifested symptoms of this disorder, and Marty's father's criminal behavior and incarceration. However, Marty's mother, as well as his teachers and school counselor, are committed to helping him change. In addition, he is of at least average intelligence and is physically healthy.

SAMPLE CASES

Readers are encouraged to develop their skills by completing treatment plans, following the DO A CLIENT MAP, for the following five cases:

1. Dee, aged 10, has always been very shy and has not enjoyed parties and group gatherings. About 6 months ago, while she was at a party, a bunch of balloons burst right behind her. Since then, she has refused to attend any parties and cries when her parents insist that she attend school when parties are planned. On several occasions when balloons were brought into the classroom, she developed extremely high anxiety and had to leave the room. She even became anxious

when watching parades on television that featured balloons. Other than these difficulties, Dee does well at school, seems to have good relationships with family and teachers, and is well behaved. Dee has asthma but is otherwise healthy.

2. Evan, a 25-year-old man, sought counseling at the suggestion of his father. Evan reported that his father thought there was something wrong with his son because he didn't have a girlfriend. In fact, Evan had never had a date and had no interest in close relationships. He had graduated from college and was successfully employed as a computer programmer; he had a computer at home and rarely went into the office, preferring to work by himself. He raised purebred dogs and devoted a great deal of time and energy to his pets. Although he did not enjoy showing them, he did sell them and enjoyed photographing them. He stated that although he did not feel very close to his family, he was in contact with them and had dinner with them once a month. Evan described his life as stable and satisfactory and reported no particular difficulties other than his current conflict with his father. Evan was in good health.

3. Nancy, a 29-year-old woman, presented herself for counseling seeking help in deciding how to handle an unplanned pregnancy. She had become pregnant on her first date with a man she had met at a bar. She subsequently informed him of her pregnancy, but he expressed no interest in continuing their relationship and advised her to have an abortion as soon as possible. Nancy was upset, confused, sad, and angry but still managed to perform her work and denied suicidal ideation. Nancy also reported mild depression since the death of her mother 3 years ago. Nancy has severe eczema, especially during the summer, but is otherwise healthy.

Nancy currently lives alone. She reported feeling very lonely and isolated. Although she wanted to have close relationships, her shy and unassertive manner made it difficult for her to develop such relationships. She did have two close women friends with whom she enjoyed spending time, but she generally waited for them to call her rather than initiating contact with them. This has been her pattern since at least early adolescence.

4. Until about 6 months ago, Peter, age 13, had been well behaved and cooperative at home, an above-average student at school, and active in his church youth group and with his soccer team. Rather abruptly, his behavior changed. He became emotionally unpredictable, sometimes acting as he usually did but at other times becoming angry or withdrawn. He associated with a new group of friends who generally did poorly in school and often received detention. Peter's parents, both busy professionals, had assumed he was just going through a difficult stage, but now they, as well as Peter's teachers, are concerned. His parents noticed that many household substances, including nail polish remover, paint thinner, and cleaning fluid, have disappeared. Peter was born with scoliosis but thus far no treatment has been required.

5. The client, a 47-year-old man who insisted on being called Gauguin, was brought to counseling by his wife. She reported that throughout most of their 10-year marriage, her husband had been very stable except for two periods when he seemed quite depressed for 3 or 4 months. Now she was seeing a new side of him. The client reported that he had recently realized he was destined to be a famous painter like the original Gauguin. He was making plans to sell the family home so they could move to the South Seas, where he was sure he would be inspired to paint his masterpieces. He had painted as a hobby for many years but had never spoken of aspirations like these. The client's wife reported that he seemed to be sleeping little, had become much more talkative, and was neglecting his responsibilities in their home mail order business in order to spend time painting furiously or attending private art exhibitions to which he had not been invited. The client smokes heavily and has emphysema.

Diagnosis and Treatment Planning for Families

Family counseling has been rapidly growing in use and influence for over 75 years. Research indicates that couples and family counseling is at least as effective as other forms of counseling in the treatment of many concerns. Diamond, Serrano, Dickey, and Sonis (1996) found that, on average, people treated with family-based treatments improved more than 67% of families treated with alternative approaches or who received no treatment. Family counseling theory offers a variety of approaches that are useful in diagnosis and treatment of individuals, couples, and families. It also provides a framework for understanding people in a family context.

This chapter provides counselors with information on analyzing and diagnosing family difficulties and a review of the major approaches to family counseling so that counselors can make family counseling part of their treatment plans. The chapter assumes that readers have some prior knowledge of family counseling or that they will acquire further learning in this area if they intend to practice family counseling.

Family counseling began to gain acceptance in the 1920s and 1930s. The child guidance movement, drawing heavily on the work of Alfred Adler and Rudolph Dreikurs, promoted awareness of the impact of the family on children's development. Mothers usually were interviewed when their children were brought in for treatment. Family-life education programs were initiated to prevent family difficulties. The 1930s saw the beginning of marriage counseling.

Stress and conflict in families escalated during the 1940s as a result of World War II. This further increased clinicians' awareness of the importance of family treatment, as did Bowlby's work on attachment theory and Fromm-Reichmann's research on so-called schizophrenogenic mothers (women who were domineering, rejecting, and insecure). During that same decade, the precursor of the American Association for Marriage and Family Therapy was founded, providing a professional organization for family therapists.

Several researchers gave great impetus to the development of family counseling in the 1950s. Murray Bowen on the East Coast, and the Palo Alto group (Jay Haley, Gregory Bateson, John Weakland, Don Jackson, and others) at the Mental Research Institute on the West Coast, explored family stability and communication and the family context of people with schizophrenia. Bowen focused on the process of intergenerational transmission, while Bateson and his colleagues emphasized the importance of the double-bind, a form of communication in which incompatible messages are transmitted simultaneously. For example, a parent might verbally encourage affection but then act cold and unresponsive when the child becomes affectionate. Theodore Lidz's writing reminded clinicians that attention should be paid to the impact of the father and the marital relationship as well as to the mother.

In the next decade, Virginia Satir's *Conjoint Family Therapy* (1967) focused attention on the development of healthy families and on the importance of family communication and the family unit. Satir also promoted training of family therapists. Nathan Ackerman founded the first family therapy journal, *Family Process.*

Salvador Minuchin contributed significantly to the family counseling movement during the 1970s by focusing attention on family structure and ways in which it could be modified to improve family functioning. Outcome studies on the effectiveness of family therapy were initiated during those years, along with new approaches to and increased use of family counseling. Certification and licensure of family therapists began during the 1970s.

Approaches to family counseling emerging in the 1980s generally advocated a brief, directive, and problem-focused approach to treatment, exemplified by strategic family therapy (Madanes, 1981). This decade witnessed development of many assessment tools for families, as well as models of self-help for families (e.g., marriage enrichment, parent effectiveness). Clinicians became more aware of the importance of individual and family differences and special needs.

By the 1990s, family therapy was well established. The American Counseling Association added a division for family counseling, the International Association of Marriage and Family Counselors (IAMFC), which published the first issue of its journal in 1993. Many family counselors advocated integrated treatment models encompassing aspects of brief, structural, strategic, and systemic family therapy. Innovators in family therapy during this decade focused on epistemology, which is the process of knowing and describing social construction of reality. This led to new models of family counseling that emphasized understanding a family's view of their lives and the impact of the therapist–family interaction on those perceptions.

Paralleling the development of individual counseling, family counseling during the early years of the 21st century emphasized multiculturalism and attention to social issues. Understanding of family dynamics has become circular rather than linear, focusing on feedback loops and multiple perspectives. Research has supported the effectiveness of family counseling with a broad range of problems and client groups including, but certainly not limited to, treatment of Schizophrenia (Diamond et al., 1996), Mood Disorders (Sexton & Alexander, 2002), Anxiety Disorders, Conduct Disorders, Eating Disorders, Attention-Deficit/Hyperactivity Disorder, Sexual Dysfunctions (Millner & Ullery, 2002), Substance Use Disorders (Meyers, Apodocia, Flicker, & Slesnick, 2002), and domestic violence. Family counseling is especially important in the treatment of people who are cultural minorities or socially disenfranchised, such as those living in poverty (Brown, 2002) and people who are gay, lesbian, bisexual, or transgendered (Janson & Steigerwald, 2002). In people such as these, emotional and behavioral difficulties are commonly linked to the social systems in which they exist, particularly the family.

According to Sexton and Alexander (2002, p. 238), family-based interventions are growing in importance and prevalence, primarily for three reasons:

1. Many problems in individuals can be successfully treated via family interventions.
2. Many qualitative and quantitative studies "provide convincing support for the efficacy of family interventions."
3. A growing number of treatment protocols have demonstrated success in treating families with a broad range of problems, geographic locales, ethnic and cultural background.

This provides only a cursory overview of the development of family counseling. However, it does offer readers a context in which to consider current approaches and methods of treatment.

ASSESSMENT OF FAMILY FUNCTIONING

No taxonomy comparable to the *Diagnostic and Statistical Manual of Mental Disorders* (*DSM*) exists for the diagnosis and assessment of family functioning. However, the following categories for understanding families have been drawn from the literature and provides a comprehensive framework for analyzing families and a structure for conducting a sort of family mental status examination.

These assessment categories, as well as the theories of family counseling considered later in this chapter, are illustrated with reference to the Wood family. This African American family consists of John Wood, age 49; his son, John Jr., age 19, from John's first marriage; John's present wife, Olivia, age 35; her son, Nathan, age 8, from her first marriage; and Keesha, age 2, the daughter of John and Olivia.

John is a successful businessman who owns a printing company. His first wife was killed in an automobile accident approximately 6 years ago.

Olivia had been married briefly to Nathan's father Neil but was divorced before Nathan's birth. Olivia attributed the divorce to her first husband's misuse of alcohol and his infidelity. She and Nathan have had no contact with Neil since the divorce. Olivia reported that Neil is currently incarcerated. Prior to her marriage to John 4 years ago, Olivia supported herself and Nathan by working as a waitress while establishing a career as an artist. She has had some success as a fabric painter, selling many of her designs.

John Jr. is a freshman in college, living with John and Olivia. He is majoring in business and works in his father's printing company during summer vacations.

Nathan is in the third grade. He has been diagnosed as having Attention-Deficit/Hyperactivity Disorder, Predominantly Hyperactive-Impulsive Type, and a Learning Disorder in Reading. A Developmental Coordination Problem also is suspected. Although he is affectionate and reasonably well behaved, Nathan is a boisterous and awkward child who has had little social and academic success. Attention from his mother as well as special help at school enabled him to pass each grade, but he seems to be falling further behind his class each year.

Keesha thus far has been a delight to the family, a healthy and happy child. Her father dotes on her, and Nathan is strongly attached to Keesha.

Presenting Problem

Family counseling, like individual counseling, usually begins with an exploration of the problem that led the family to seek help, along with discussion of the kinds of changes the family would like. With families, as with individuals, presenting concerns may not represent the fundamental issues troubling the family. Satir (1967) observed that families often seek help for a child with a behavioral problem. Satir dubbed this child the Identified Patient (IP) and found that the IP often was the healthiest family member, acting out to obtain help for the family. The attribution of a family concern to a particular person can make understanding the family's difficulties a challenging task. This task can be further complicated if family members have divergent views of family problems.

When Olivia and John Wood presented for counseling, they did indeed have different ideas about their family problems, with each one attributing those problems to different family members. Both agreed that they had been arguing increasingly and that the comfortable and loving family environment they had hoped for had not materialized. John blamed these problems on Nathan, stating that Nathan's noisy, acting-out behavior destroyed the peace he valued in his home. According to John, Olivia spent so much time with Nathan and Keesha, and with her art work, that she had little time left for him. Olivia, on the other hand, attributed the difficulties to John Jr. She believed that he was misusing alcohol and spending too much time with friends rather than his studies. She also complained that John ignored these problems. She resented his giving John Jr. money for car payments and social activities rather than paying for a private school for Nathan.

Transgenerational Family History

Bowen (1974) believed that families should be viewed from a longitudinal perspective. This promotes understanding of what he called the intergenerational or transgenerational transmission process in which patterns and traits are passed on from one generation to the next. Bowen used a genogram (diagram of generations) to facilitate understanding of this process. A partial genogram of the Wood family is provided (Figure 8.1). In a genogram, females are represented by circles; males, by squares. An X indicates a deceased family member. Siblings are listed in order of birth, from left to right. The husband's family is on the left; the wife's, on the right.

John and Olivia come from different family backgrounds. John's family was traditional and middle class. His father established the business that John now owns. His mother was a homemaker, involved with church and family. Values of stability, family unity, and financial success were important in the family.

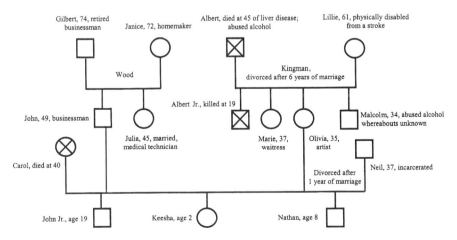

Figure 8.1. Genogram of the Wood family.

Olivia, on the other hand, came from a more chaotic family. Her mother had been the mainstay of the family, even during the years when Olivia's parents were married. Her father Albert misused alcohol, worked sporadically as a construction worker, and often stayed away from home for several days at a time. Olivia had little contact with her father from the time of her parents' divorce, when she was 5 years old, until his death.

Detailed information on John and Olivia's siblings is not included in this abbreviated genogram but would be included in a full genogram. Olivia's older brother was accidentally shot and killed at age 19 during a conflict between gangs. Her sister Marie has been divorced twice and supports herself and her three children by working as a waitress. Her brother Malcolm, who began abusing alcohol at about age 10, has not had contact with the family in nearly 15 years. John's only sibling Julia is married, has two children, and works as a medical technician.

Although more exploration is needed to determine the full nature of the transgenerational transmission process in these families, the following patterns are evident:

- Substance abuse (Albert, Malcolm, Neil).
- Gender roles are consistent within families but diverge between families; men are in charge in the Wood family while Olivia's family has strong, nurturing women and unreliable men.
- Children and the role of parenting were valued in both families.

Other patterns of importance that might affect the present family:

- Both John and Olivia reportedly were the favorite children in their families, with both having strong ties to their mothers.
- Both John and Olivia have had to cope with the loss of loved ones. John continues to grieve the death of Carol, his first wife, and sometimes compares Olivia unfavorably to Carol.

Other patterns are likely to emerge with further exploration.

Family Life Cycle

Carter and McGoldrick (1999) found that families, like individuals, go through relatively predictable developmental stages. They concluded that viewing families' symptoms and functioning over time, in relation to normal developmental stages, can promote understanding and healthy development. Carter and McGoldrick identified six stages in the family life cycle, listed below, along with some of the challenges typically associated with each stage.

1. Leaving home: single young adults.

    a. Separating from family of origin and achieving independence and responsibility.
    b. Establishing and engaging in a career, formulating financial and personal goals.
    c. Developing intimate peer relationships.

2. Marriage: the new couple and family.

    a. Forming and making a commitment to a new family system.
    b. Maintaining both separateness and intimacy.
    c. Redefining relationships with parents and friends; defining in-law relationships.

3. The family with young children.

    a. Making space for children while maintaining the spouse relationship.
    b. Establishing comfortable and compatible styles of parenting.
    c. Coping with role changes, new demands on time and finances, new responsibilities.
    d. Realigning relationships to include parenting and grandparenting roles.

4. The family with adolescents.

    a. Increasing boundary flexibility to accommodate adolescents' need for separation as well as the needs of aging parents.
    b. Coping with midlife changes in marriage, career, values.

5. Launching children and moving on.

    a. Handling financial and emotional changes associated with children in college and parents needing help.
    b. Reinvesting in and redefining the marriage.
    c. Changing roles—establishing adult relationships with grown children, dealing with disabilities and death of the older generation, becoming grandparents.

6. The family in later life.

    a. Maintaining functioning of self and couple in light of sexual, physical, role changes.
    b. Coping with aging, illness, and death.
    c. Establishing grandparenting (and maybe great-grandparenting) roles.

In general, families have the most difficulty dealing with events the first time they happen (e.g., birth of the first child), events that are unanticipated and unwanted (e.g., miscarriage, sudden job loss), and events that occur at ages that differ from the norm (e.g., the birth of a child to a couple in midlife). The process of children leaving home also can be a particularly difficult transition. Of course, each family has unique reactions to events and patterns of development.

The family life cycle can best be understood in its temporal context. Patterns such as the usual marriage age, the typical number of children, the acceptability of divorce, and gender roles are in constant flux and have an impact on how people negotiate the family life cycle. For example, half of all marriages are now expected to end in divorce, half of these within the first 7 years of the marriage; more than half of the people in the United States have been part of a stepfamily (Goldenberg & Goldenberg, 2002). The percentage of employed mothers rose from 50% in 1980 to 65% in 1996; 58% of women have completed college. The Wood family reflects many of these trends.

The family life cycle of the Wood family is complicated. Before John and Olivia married, both were single parents, John with an adolescent and Olivia with a young child. When they married, they entered the second stage, the new couple, but they also had to cope with their former stages. John became the parent of two young children at an age when most of his peers were launching their children and Olivia become the mother of an almost-launched adolescent with whom she had little opportunity to establish a relationship. Parenting responsibilities made it difficult for the couple to carry into their marriage the romance and closeness of their courtship and both felt disappointed.

The age difference between John and Olivia and the patterns of their age groups also are important. John grew up viewing women in traditional roles; that perspective had characterized his first marriage and those of most men his age. Olivia, on the other hand, matured at a time when women had more independence and opportunities. John assumed that Olivia would give up her career when they married, but Olivia had looked forward to the increased time she would have to develop her artistic skills because of the financial stability of her second marriage.

Family Structure

Many factors determine the structure of a family including:

- Composition of the family (e.g., parents, children, other relatives)
- Birth order, gender, and ages of children and other family members
- Patterns of alliance, conflict, and avoidance; similarity and difference
- Formal and informal boundaries, hierarchy and power structure
- Patterns in the families of origin

In a healthy family structure, the parents have a strong positive connection and are in charge of the family. Siblings also have a strong subsystem, particularly including

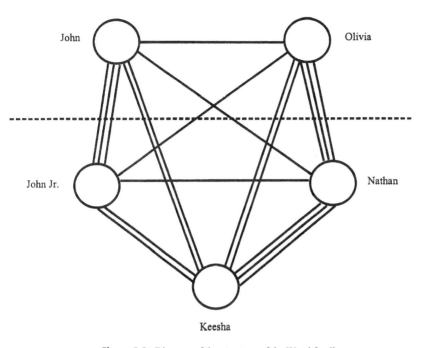

Figure 8.2. Diagram of the structure of the Wood family.

alliances being between same-gender siblings and between same-gender parent–child dyads. Patterns associated with family difficulties include each parent being closest to a child of the opposite gender, rather than to his or her partner, and the children holding the greatest power in the family.

The structure of the Wood family is diagrammed in Figure 8.2. Triple lines reflect a very strong connection; double lines, a moderate connection; and single lines, a weak connection. John and Olivia have a weak connection to each other. Both feel closest to their first child and distant from their stepchild. Nathan has not been able to bond well with either John or John Jr. and remains closest to the females in the family. Keesha is the only recipient of everyone's affection. Although the parents are in charge of this family, the boundary between the parents and the children is permeable; sometimes the children take on too much power.

Birth order provides additional information on family structure. The configuration of John Jr. and Keesha replicates John's family of origin (older brother, younger sister) and is familiar and comfortable to him. His parents held high expectations for him as the oldest child and only boy and he has transmitted those expectations to John Jr. Olivia viewed her older brother, Albert Jr., as a problem and as one reason for her parents' divorce. She has projected this negative image of older brothers and adolescent boys onto John Jr., although she does relate well to Nathan and Keesha. As often happens with middle children, Olivia followed an unconventional and artistic path, one that was accepted in her family, where personal qualities were emphasized over conventional achievement. This has helped her to understand Nathan's special needs.

Communication and Interaction Styles

Many frameworks describing family communication are available. Satir (1983) developed one of the most useful. She postulated the existence of five modes of communication:

1. Placator—views self negatively and almost always agrees with others.
2. Blamer—the self dominates, and other people and the context of situations are ignored.
3. Computer or Super-reasonable—context matters, intellectualizing is pervasive, people and their feelings are ignored.
4. Distractor or Irrelevant—communications generally ignore both people and context.
5. Congruent communicator—takes account of the self, of others, and of the context.

While people do shift styles, depending on the context, most have a preferred style of communicating. For example, John typically uses Blamer and Super-reasonable styles. Olivia, too, often assumes a Blamer style, although she sometimes is a Placator, especially in relation to issues around Nathan. Nathan himself is a Distractor, while John Jr. leans toward the Super-reasonable style but can use Placator, Blamer, and Distractor modes to avoid his father's anger.

Communication styles also may be described as visual, auditory, or kinesthetic. For Olivia, the visual mode is the most important one; her attention to her appearance and her home reflects her caring for John. However, John emphasizes a kinesthetic mode and finds Olivia distant.

Triangulation is a frequent pattern of communication in dysfunctional families, typically involving parents communicating to each other via a child. Although that pattern is not present in the Wood family, Keesha could evolve into the conduit for communication between her parents.

Family Rules, Roles, and Values

All families have rules that are stated, as well as norms, values, and expectations that may not be clearly stated. Rules such as curfews and assignment of chores typically are very specific. Norms and values tend to be less clear than rules and might include such messages as, "The children are expected to do well in school and to go to college," or "Don't talk about a family member's alcohol use." John placed great emphasis on education and consequently viewed John Jr. as successful and Nathan as a disappointment because of their different academic experiences. Olivia was brought up in a family that was damaged by uncontrolled and unacknowledged alcohol use and saw the harm that it could do; she is now trying to set limits on John Jr.'s alcohol use but is encountering resistance from her husband.

All family members also have roles determined by their official status in the family (e.g., father, youngest child) and by the needs of the family and the functioning of each person. John viewed his father as the head of his family of origin and himself as head of his current family. However, Olivia's mother had been in charge of her family and, as a single parent, Olivia took charge of her household. She was not used to yielding power to a man and envisioned her marriage with John as a partnership. Before Olivia's second marriage, one of Nathan's roles was giving a focus and purpose to his mother's life. Now that role was less important to Olivia, but Nathan still struggled to maintain his role as center of his mother's life. As in the Wood family, rules and roles are important sources of information about family functioning.

Ethnic, Cultural, Spiritual, and Socioeconomic Background

Ethnic, cultural, spiritual, and socioeconomic patterns play a significant role in determining family functioning. Although assessment of background presents risks of stereotyping and overgeneralizing, a cautious exploration can provide understanding of family dynamics.

Although both John and Olivia are African American, their socioeconomic backgrounds differ. John's father came from a poor family but used his business skills to create a comfortable life for his family. His emphasis on financial success was transmitted to John. John disapproves of Olivia's family of origin and believes that Olivia should be grateful that he rescued her and Nathan from financial instability. Olivia's background reflects patterns sometimes associated with African Americans, including strong women, artistic accomplishment, and a nontraditional family structure. She disapproves of John's traditional attitudes and wants him to acquire some of her energy and flexibility. Similar ethnic backgrounds but different cultural ones have led to discrepant values between John and Olivia.

John and Olivia both come from Protestant backgrounds and both have strong religious beliefs. However, here too similarities and differences coexist. Olivia describes herself as more spiritual than religious and has never attended church on a regular basis. In John's family of origin, however, active involvement in the church was the norm. Each modeled a different way of expressing their beliefs to their children and held different expectations for their children's religious education and involvement.

Differentiation of Self

Bowen (1974) postulated a differentiation of self scale, with scores ranging from a low of 0 to a high of 100. He used this scale as a measure of how individuated and separated people are from their families. Those at the low end (0–25) of the scale tend to have enmeshed and symbiotic relationships with their families and are self-centered and dominated by emotion. People who fall above the midpoint on the scale typically are more inner-directed, rational, secure, and respectful of others, and have fairly well-defined opinions, beliefs, and values. Although people within a family can differ considerably in their degree of differentiation, some families promote differentiation while others inhibit it. People tend to choose spouses and raise children with levels of differentiation comparable to their own. Bowen saw differentiation of self as a key ingredient in family health; one of the primary goals of his approach is to increase client differentiation.

Levels of differentiation in the Wood family fall in the middle range (25–75), with Olivia probably the most differentiated. This family is not what Bowen called an undifferentiated family ego mass; however, family members do feel pressure to conform to family and societal values rather than to develop their own value system.

Significant Physical and Mental Conditions

When someone in a family has a significant illness, disorder, or disability, it inevitably has an impact on that person's family. The impact can take many forms. In some families, the affected family member becomes the focus of the family's energy, either bonding the family or detracting from other family relationships. The affected family member may be viewed as a source of shame and embarrassment or as a source of pride. A severe or long-standing disability in a family also affects how that family interacts with the outside world. In some families, the disability causes the family to withdraw and exclude outsiders, who may intrude on the family grief or exacerbate their shame. In other families, the disability becomes a conduit for communication as family members expand their outside contacts in an effort to find treatment, information, and support. The ways in which families handle illness and disability provide information on the nature and level of their coping abilities and their attitudes toward family cohesiveness and community involvement.

Nathan's Learning Disorder and his Attention-Deficit Disorder propelled Olivia to become actively involved with his school system in an effort to obtain help for him. Her younger brother had presented similar symptoms and so Olivia was familiar with boys who demand a great deal of attention. John, however, was unfamiliar with symptoms like Nathan's and was embarrassed by his constant talking and fidgeting. John found himself avoiding family activities and preferred time alone with Olivia. Their differing attitudes toward Nathan became another source of conflict.

External Sources of Stress and Support

External sources of stress and support can have a strong impact on a family's homeostasis. Some families have a large support system, perhaps including extended family, work colleagues, neighbors, and fellow members of religious or leisure organizations. Such families typically are more able to handle stress and change than isolated nuclear families. Helping families to build support systems is an important counseling strategy.

Families have to cope with stress, as well as support, from outside sources. For example, the company where a family member is employed may close, a child may be mistreated by schoolmates, fire may destroy family possessions, or the stock market might decline.

Extended families and friends provide both stress and support to the Wood family. John's parents live in a retirement community nearby and are involved with John Jr. and Keesha, although they have difficulty with Nathan. Olivia's mother is disabled, and Olivia provides her both financial and practical help. Olivia belongs to a group of independent artists and has formed some friendships in that group; John is well respected in his church and community. Involvement in shared babysitting in their neighborhood enabled Olivia to get acquainted with nearby families. John Jr. has many friends at college and in the neighborhood. Although Nathan has few peer supports, he does have good relationships with his teachers.

Dynamics of Symptom Maintenance

Symptoms of dysfunction usually serve a purpose in a family and are almost always intertwined with the overall family dynamics. Understanding the role of a symptom can help to effect its change or elimination. Behavioral sequences, leading to the manifestation of a symptom, provide one clue to comprehending the function of the symptom. An examination of the family structure and the needs of individual members provide other clues.

Neither John Jr. nor Nathan was happy with their parents' marriage. Both had enjoyed being the center of attention and were having difficulty yielding that position. The current intensity of Nathan's symptoms, in particular, seemed to reflect his need to regain the attention and special role he had before the marriage. For John and Olivia, too, symptoms brought benefits. Both were proud of their roles as single parents; compromising the values and attitudes they held before the marriage conflicted with their self-images and therefore was resisted.

Strengths

Although the focus of analysis thus far has been on problems, the Wood family had many strengths, as do most families. Olivia and John are dedicated parents and responsible, intelligent adults. Their marriage resulted from a courtship of over a year, during which they became good friends as well as lovers. They enjoy each other's company and want to build a life together. These and other strengths enabled them to address their concerns.

Special Circumstances

In addition to exploring the 12 preceding aspects of families, counselors also should take account of any special concerns or circumstances that are present. These might include such experiences as illness, death, divorce, adoption, occupational stressors, poverty, and abuse. Remarried families, like the Wood family, typically cope with complex, conflicting, and ambiguous new roles and relationships; divided loyalties; and feelings of mistrust, guilt, and anxiety (Carter & McGoldrick, 1999). Factors such as these should be considered in understanding of family.

STRUCTURED ASSESSMENT OF COUPLES AND FAMILIES

Although interviews are the primary vehicle for gathering information on families, many inventories and nonstandardized approaches to assessment are available for use with families. These can help counselors gain insight into families and also promote increased self-awareness and mutual understanding within families.

Many inventories have been developed to assess a couple's satisfaction and adjustment. The following inventories have shown evidence of reliability and validity:

1. *Dyadic Adjustment Scale* (DAS) (Prouty, Markowski, & Barnes, 2000)—Measures quality of marital adjustment, affection, marital satisfaction.
2. *Locke-Wallace Marital Adjustment Test* (MAT) (Locke & Wallace, 1959)—Assesses marital happiness and other areas of marital adjustment.
3. *Marital Satisfaction Inventory* (MSI-R) (Snyder, 1997)—Assesses 12 aspects of marital satisfaction such as problem solving, communication, parenting.
4. *Personal Assessment of Intimacy in Relationship* (PAIR) (Olson & Schaefer, 2000)—Measures five types of intimacy.
5. *RELATionship Evaluation* (RELATE) (Busby, Holman, & Tamiguchi, 2001)—Measures quality of marital adjustment, including similarity of personality, values.

6. *Waring Intimacy Questionnaire* (WIQ) (Waring & Reddon, 1983)—Measures eight aspects of intimacy in relationships.

Although developed primarily for individuals, the Myers-Briggs Type Inventory (MBTI), published by Consulting Psychologists Press, is also useful in assessing a couple relationship. A computerized scoring of a couple's MBTI scores yields information on probable strengths and issues created by the combination of their personality types. For example, a couple in which both partners are characterized by introversion are likely to be very comfortable sharing quiet time but may have difficulty maintaining relationships with family and friends.

Also useful in the assessment of family functioning are inventories focused on the children or on the entire family. Examples are the Family Adaptability and Cohesion Evaluation Scales (FACES) (Olson, 1986), the Parent–Adolescent Communication Scale, the Family Satisfaction Scale, the Family Environment Scale, and Children's Report of Parent Behavior Inventory (Amerikaner, Monks, Wolfe, & Thomas, 1994).

In addition, a wide range of specific inventories are available for use with families; they provide assessment of such dimensions as dual-career relationships, conflict resolution skills, parenting styles, concerns of children and adolescents, sibling relationships, and family beliefs.

Many nonstandardized approaches to assessment also are available for use with families. These provide information and can be used as vehicles for discussion to promote family awareness. One is the *genogram*, discussed earlier and described particularly well by McGoldrick and Gerson (1988). Another is the *ecomap*, designed to provide a picture of the organizational patterns and relationships in a family. *Incomplete sentences* also yield family information and promote discussion. Family members complete a series of sentences individually and in writing (e.g., What I value about my family is..., The biggest problem we face is...). Responses are then shared and discussed. Another useful tool is the *family sculpture*; family members arrange themselves to create a physical representation of the family. This can be adapted to family needs by asking a particular person to create the sculpture, asking for a sculpture of the ideal family, or sculpting the family at a specific time. Discussion of the sculpture while people are still in position is particularly powerful.

TREATMENT PLANNING FOR FAMILIES

Once an assessment has been made of a family, the counselor is ready to formulate a treatment plan. Chapter 6 reviewed the DO A CLIENT MAP format for treatment plans for individuals. With minor variations (indicated below), this format can facilitate treatment planning for a family. Because the dimensions of the MAP were explored in depth in Chapter 6, they are presented briefly here, with emphasis on application to family counseling and to the Wood family.

Diagnosis—Use of the *DSM* in assessment of individuals within a family is strongly recommended. That process can shed light on family problems and patterns of interaction. For example, in the Wood family, Nathan was diagnosed with a Learning Disorder and an Attention-Deficit/Hyperactivity Disorder; these disorders have an impact on his functioning at school, his role in the family, his interactions with his mother, and his difficulties with his stepfather. John Jr. may be diagnosed with Alcohol Abuse once further information is obtained. Although neither Olivia nor John have mental disorders, John may have Obsessive–Compulsive Personality Traits, while Olivia may have Histrionic Personality Traits, reflecting very different personal styles.

Objectives—Family members and counselors should collaborate to determine appropriate objectives. For the Wood family, some of the specific objectives include the couple's having positive time together and making joint decisions regarding family roles, finances, and expectations for the children; behavioral changes in Nathan and John Jr.; and changes in patterns of subsystems and alliances.

Assessment—The primary approaches to family assessment include interviews, as well as inventories and nonstandardized procedures discussed previously. Outside sources also can provide useful information. For example, people presenting with Sexual Dysfunction usually are referred for a medical evaluation.

An important purpose for assessment of families is determining their suitability for treatment. Counselors need to decide whether the family can make a commitment to and benefit from counseling or whether the process is likely to be sabotaged by the destructive participation or absence of one or more family members. The Wood family seems suitable for counseling; both Olivia and John are motivated to improve their family relationships and neither is severely impaired. Nathan and John Jr. also have a profound impact on family dynamics and should participate in some of the family counseling sessions. Keesha probably is too young for counseling, but observing family interactions with her for a session might be informative.

Clinician—In determining who will provide counseling to a family, consideration should be given to the possible importance of such counselor variables as age, gender, family status, ethnicity, cultural background, and experience. No particular variables seem essential in a counselor for the Woods. However, they might respond best to a counselor in midlife who has experience in addressing issues of remarried families, parenting, and communication.

Location—Family counseling usually takes place in outpatient settings, although it can be combined with individual and group counseling for people in hospitals or day treatment programs.

Interventions—Determining interventions for families, as for individuals, involves identifying a theoretical orientation along with appropriate strategies that address the objectives. These choices are guided by many factors, including the motivation of the family, the nature of their difficulties, and the composition of the family. Further information on theories of family counseling and their application to the Wood family is provided later in this chapter.

Emphasis—Theories of family counseling, like those of individual counseling, need to be adapted to particular clients. Counselors should determine whether a family is unstable and has few strengths and insights, requiring a great deal of support, or whether the family is cohesive and motivated to examine past influences and underlying dynamics. The Woods are a relatively healthy, verbal, and expressive family. At the same time, they tend to blame their children for their difficulties and, as a whole family, are unlikely to welcome long-term, exploratory counseling. They would probably benefit most from counseling that is structured and problem-focused, but that also builds communication, parenting, and other family skills.

Numbers—Counselors need to determine whether to see an entire nuclear family, a couple, a subsystem (e.g., parent–child, siblings), or a nuclear family plus extended family such as grandparents. In addition, individual sessions with one or more family members might be indicated. Families also may be seen with other families or couples in group therapy. Sessions with the Wood family probably will include Olivia, John, Nathan, and John Jr. in most sessions, but couples sessions, sibling sessions, and parent–child sessions also might be held.

Timing—Family counseling sessions, like those of individuals, usually are held once a week, although each session sometimes is longer than 50 minutes to allow time for all family members to speak and interact. Contracting for a specified number of sessions is often used with families as a way to address varying levels of motivation within a family. Most models of family therapy are relatively brief, but some, like Bowen's Transgenerational Family Therapy, tend to be lengthy. The Woods probably would respond best to counseling that is short or medium in duration, with weekly sessions of at least 60 minutes.

Medication—If family members have emotional difficulties that may benefit from psychotropic medication, a referral may be indicated. Nathan already receives medication for his Attention-Deficit/Hyperactivity Disorder. The Wood family presents no other need for medication.

Adjunct Services—Families, like individuals, benefit from resources that give them support and information, increase their socialization and activity levels, and provide them rewarding and pleasurable experiences. Al-Anon groups might provide John and Olivia with information on alcohol abuse, and participation in Alcoholics Anonymous might help John Jr. More shared family activities, such as outings to the beach and family hikes that provide time together in rewarding ways, can increase the cohesiveness in this family.

Prognosis—This predicts the likelihood of the family's achieving their objectives according to the treatment plan that has been developed. In light of their motivation and emotional health, the prognosis for the Wood family is very good.

THEORIES OF FAMILY COUNSELING

Many approaches to family counseling are available. Reviewed here are some of the most important ones. Research does not definitively indicate that some family counseling approaches are better than others (Sexton & Alexander, 2002). As with individual counseling, treatment effectiveness depends on the therapeutic alliance and on the treatment plan. However, guidelines help readers understand the kinds of families, problems, and situations for which each approach is particularly useful.

Transgenerational/Systems Family Therapy

The roots of transgenerational or systems family therapy are in Freudian psychoanalytic thought. Developed by such theorists as Murray Bowen, James Framo, and Ivan Boszormenyi-Nagy, this model of long-term family counseling seeks to understand the present family by looking at previous generations from whom some of the patterns, roles, behaviors, and attitudes of the present family have been acquired. Murray Bowen probably is the best-known proponent of this approach. Bowen, who died in 1990, initially focused his work on families that had a person diagnosed with Schizophrenia. Bowen continued his work at the Georgetown Family Center in Washington, D.C., which he founded and which continues to teach his approach.

Bowen viewed the family as an interconnected system. He believed that people within that system did not function independently and that change in one person would affect the system, just as change in the system would have an impact on all family members. In addition to these feedback loops, Bowen looked at family efforts to maintain homeostasis as well as family interactions and reactions around a problem.

The following concepts are integral to Bowen's theory of family counseling:

- *Differentiation of self*—The extent to which people can think, feel, and act for themselves, assessed on a 1–100 scale. Bowen advocated a balance between togetherness and independence.

- *Transgenerational* (or intergenerational or multigenerational) transmission process.
- *Birth order* and *sibling position* as influences on alliances and roles.
- *Family triangles* as important units of analysis.
- *Nuclear family emotional system*—The focus and intensity of emotion in the family, especially the anxiety projected from one family member to another; the nature of the marital relationship; and the functioning of individual family members.
- *Family projection process*—One person projects uncomfortable or unacceptable feelings onto other family members (e.g., parents blaming a child for the family's difficulties).
- *Emotional cutoff*—A family member, often a young adult, establishes physical and emotional distance from the family in order to achieve some independence. This often characterizes the efforts of people who are poorly differentiated to separate themselves from enmeshed families.
- *Nodal events*—These are particular crises or happenings that shape a family.
- *Family secrets*—Secrets such as infidelity, abortions, and substance use are common in families and can be at the heart of family dysfunction.
- *Influence of history, context, and society*—Bowen believed these have a great influence.

In working with families, Bowen assumed the role of coach or consultant. His style and that of most of his followers tend to be cognitive and unemotional, leading people on a slowly paced journey toward gathering information, understanding their nuclear family and families of origin, and differentiating themselves via genograms, family interviews, relationship experiments, and exploration. Bowen sought to increase intimacy, objectivity, and understanding; improve communication; and decrease emotional reactivity, anxiety, and fusion in families.

Because he believed that an individual could have an impact on a system and vice versa, Bowen worked with individuals, couples, families, and multifamily groups. His approach, then, can be useful whether or not an entire family is present for counseling. In its purest form, transgenerational family therapy seems suitable for only a select group of people—those who are not in an immediate crisis and who have the time, energy, finances, and inclination to undertake a lengthy and analytical exploration of their families. A modified version of this approach, however, provides both a way of conceptualizing family functioning and many useful techniques with broad application. A genogram, for example, can promote understanding in families in which the intergenerational transmission process has had a major influence on current functioning.

The Wood family might not be willing to engage in an extended examination of their family background and so might not be good candidates for Bowen's approach. However, genograms, the impact of birth order, and differentiation might become part of their counseling.

Experiential/Humanistic/Communications Approach

Virginia Satir, who developed conjoint family therapy, is the best-known proponent of this approach to family counseling. (Other proponents include Carl Whitaker and the Duhls.) This approach emphasizes communication and self-esteem and is influenced by humanistic, experiential, existential, and phenomenological thought. Satir sought to shift the focus of the counseling from the IP to the family, especially to the couple, and to help the family reestablish intimacy, caring, cohesiveness, and congruent communication (Satir, 1983; Satir, Banmen, Gerber, & Gomori, 1991).

The following concepts are important in this model:

- The partner relationship is integral to the health and functioning of the whole family.
- Obtaining a family life chronology, beginning with the partners' families of origin and focusing on the development of the partner relationship, is important in reestablishing positive feelings.
- Low self-esteem in family members is a frequent cause of difficulties; counseling should promote individual self-esteem, maturation, responsibility, and healthy differentiation.
- Clear, open, and congruent communication is essential to healthy family functioning.
- Differing styles of communication or perception (e.g., visual versus kinesthetic) can lead to misunderstanding and conflict and need to be addressed.
- Process usually is more important than content; counseling should seek to improve family communication rather than focus on symptoms that are messages of hurt or blocks.
- Family rules, norms, and secrets exert a powerful influence on family dynamics.
- Constructive problem-solving and the ability to deal effectively with change are important ingredients in healthy families.

Satir's holistic approach, with its echoes of Carl Rogers, is probably familiar to most counselors. Satir viewed herself as a role model and resource person, communicating caring and acceptance, teaching families new ways to interact, and supporting their efforts to change and grow. Her focus was largely on the present, and she emphasized strength rather than pathology. Exercises and techniques such as analysis of communication styles, use of family sculptures, family reconstruction, parts parties (helping people value multiple aspects of themselves), awareness enhancement, meditation, touch, and reframing are important ingredients in this model.

Satir's model encourages involvement of the entire nuclear family in the counseling process, even though counselors may not meet with all family members in all sessions. Her model is particularly suitable for families with a weak partner relationship, a lack of support and nurturance, and confusing, incongruent, and limited communication. Satir's communications approach seems best suited for people who are not in crisis and who have at least a moderate degree of motivation and verbal ability. Of course, nearly all families seeking counseling have some difficulty with communication. Consequently, Satir's approach, like Bowen's, has much to offer almost all families seeking counseling.

In many ways, the communications model is well suited to treatment of the Wood family. Nathan and probably John Jr. are viewed as IPs; however, the family difficulties stem primarily from the interaction of John and Olivia, who no longer have the unity and closeness that led them to marry. They are drifting apart and becoming overinvolved with their biological children. Family members communicate in limited and ambiguous ways and little open dialog is present. Nathan, as well as Olivia and John, has low self-esteem. This family is motivated to seek help and seems capable of learning to communicate clearly and directly. Satir's model also provides a mix of supportiveness and directiveness, likely to benefit this family.

Structural Family Therapy

Salvador Minuchin is viewed as the primary developer of structural family therapy. Minuchin had a long association with the Philadelphia Child Guidance Center, which provides training and counseling in this model. Minuchin advocated taking an active and involved approach to family counseling, almost becoming a part of the family system himself, in order to unbalance and change the family structure and views of the world (Minuchin & Fishman, 1981; Minuchin, Lee, & Simon, 1996).

The following concepts are important in structural family therapy:

- *Family structure*—This includes patterns of transaction, styles of communication, coalitions, and boundaries. In healthy families, boundaries are clear yet flexible. They provide well-defined lines of responsibility and authority and facilitate independence while protecting the family. Parents are allies and are in charge of the system but are free to act childlike at times. Children have secure and clear roles, yet can occasionally assume some parental functions.

- *Subsystems*—Subsystems are essential to carrying out family functioning. These include the partner subsystem, sibling subsystems, and various combinations of parent–child subsystems (e.g., the female family members). Subsystems should be flexible and respond effectively to the situation at hand.
- *Adaptation to stress*—The manner in which families handle and adapt to stress provides information on the family structure and sources of both strength and weakness. Minuchin paid particular attention to culturally or environmentally related stressors.

Minuchin used a broad range of techniques such as accommodation, challenging assumptions, enactment, reframing, unbalancing, diagrams, and metaphors to join the family, evaluate their functioning, and then solve the problems and restructure the family, perhaps by escalating stress or using a family member as a sort of co-counselor. Structural family therapy is an active and creative approach that often is effective in overcoming resistance; it may engage even difficult families in the therapeutic process. It also is a valuable approach to helping families with boundary issues, weak parental subsystems, excluded or enmeshed family members, and related concerns. This approach often is combined with strategic interventions, discussed later.

Olivia and John are reasonably effective parents, but do not have a strong spouse subsystem. Boundaries between parents and children are sometimes inadequate, and the mother–son (Nathan) and father–son (John Jr.) subsystems are enmeshed. Although a structural approach to helping this family might be effective, the family structure was not severely dysfunctional. Attention to structural issues, therefore, might best be accomplished in the context of another approach such as the communications model.

Cognitive Behavioral Family Counseling

Cognitive therapy, behavioral counseling, and their combination have been growing in importance in family therapy since the 1980s. Many families present with behavioral concerns, such as children's misbehavior, poor communication skills, and imbalances in household responsibilities. Consequently, they often are receptive to treatment with a behavioral focus. The addition of cognitive interventions focuses attention on underlying assumptions and can deepen and empower the treatment process (Epstein, Schlesinger, & Dryden, 1988).

Behavioral family counseling, an active, directive, and symptom-focused approach, views symptoms as learned responses. It helps people unlearn harmful behaviors and learn new and more positive ones. Similar to behavioral counseling with individuals, behavioral family counseling is based on social learning theory and is particularly useful for dealing with couples or parent–child issues where a behavioral change is desired. Richard Stuart (1980) is a leading proponent of this model. Behavioral counseling typically begins with an assessment of the current family situation, the nature and level of the undesirable behavior, and its secondary gains. Inventories and checklists facilitate assessment. Next, a contract might be developed, with both partners or parents and children agreeing to make specific behavioral changes. Rewards or consequences are then specified. A range of behavioral techniques (e.g., role-playing, rehearsal, reinforcement, time out, token economies, contingency contracting, negotiation, conflict management, anger management, sex therapy) can be used to facilitate change. Structured efforts to improve relationships also play an essential role in this model. For example, couples might set aside time each day to talk or they might plan Caring Days, when they engage in behaviors their partner has identified as reflecting love, such as a massage, preparing a special meal, or an evening out. Family meetings provide a forum for sharing concerns. Follow-up sessions evaluate progress and, if necessary, modify the contract or the treatment.

Counselors using a behavioral model usually view themselves as educators, coaches, and experts, although they also emphasize rapport. They design behavioral change programs, write up contracts, and regularly assess progress. They also teach and model important skills such as problem-solving, parenting, communication, and decision-making.

The behavioral model is most likely to be effective when family concerns are fairly specific and circumscribed and when the underlying relationships are basically sound. For example, this approach can help parents develop techniques for managing their children's behavior and can help couples find a comfortable way to share household chores. Often, however, counseling that begins in a behavioral mode will unearth structural or communication difficulties. The combination of cognitive and behavioral counseling can address these underlying concerns. Cognitive family counseling stems primarily from the work of Aaron Beck and Albert Ellis. Advocates of this approach believe that negative behaviors commonly stem from underlying core beliefs. Identifying and changing those beliefs, as described in Chapter 7, and helping family members identify and understand similarities and discrepancies in their beliefs can accelerate behavioral change.

Both cognitive and behavioral interventions are likely to help the Wood family. For example, Nathan's behavior might be improved through behavioral counseling. John and Olivia could be helped to establish clear behavioral guidelines for Nathan, with rewards if they are followed and possibly consequences if they are violated. As a child who is eager to please, this could help Nathan learn to change his behavior. This approach also might help Olivia and John negotiate financial and household responsibilities.

Cognitive interventions can help the Woods to address structural and communications problems. Olivia and John have different beliefs about appropriate roles for husbands and wives. John takes a more traditional perspective and assumed Olivia would want to fit in with his lifestyle when they married. Although Olivia places great value on her family, she also values her independence and creativity. John interprets this as a sign that Olivia does not really love him and is not committed to their family. Helping the couple examine and discuss their assumptions about marriage, parenting, and gender roles is essential to helping them understand each other and their differences and find ways for those differences to enhance rather than detract from the marriage.

Adlerian Family Counseling

Adlerian counseling or Individual Psychology originally focused primarily on parent–child interactions and the healthy development of the children. However, its scope has broadened to encompass a range of family and individual concerns.

The following ideas are important to this theory and are discussed further in Chapter 7:

- Feelings of inferiority, stemming from childhood, often are related to family difficulties, as people try to overcome those feelings and reach their ideal selves.
- Birth order is important in determining family roles and relationships.
- Pampered or neglected children and children with physical or intellectual disabilities are particularly likely to present problems.
- Natural consequences, encouragement, respect, and realistic expectations help children and families to develop in positive ways.
- Family conferences and a democratic family structure contribute to the development of strong and healthy family constellations.
- Families should be considered in their social context.

Although Adlerian counselors sometimes focus their work on the couple relationship, they most often work with parents and children, together and individually. Teachers also might be included in sessions. Adlerian counselors tend to be directive, interpretive, and present oriented. Their work combines supportive and educational approaches. A focus on encouragement and health rather than on pathology makes this approach useful with a broad range of families.

Dinkmeyer and Carlson (1984) adapted this model for use with couples. They defined marital happiness as a combination of self-esteem, social interest, and a sense of humor. Using an analysis of the partners' life styles, their work promotes marital happiness and enrichment by emphasizing strengths, facilitating understanding, and building responsibility and social interest.

Aspects of the Adlerian approach can help to conceptualize and treat the difficulties of the Wood family. The family council could stimulate and improve family communication and might promote family cohesiveness. Viewing Nathan as a child with feelings of inferiority who is striving for power in self-destructive and socially unacceptable ways can lead to the development of effective approaches to helping him. Marital enrichment might be very useful to John and Olivia. In addition, discussion of the impact of birth order might promote understanding of family roles. However, the Adlerian model does not directly address the communication concerns of the Wood family and so probably is not the best method for helping them.

Strategic Family Therapy

Strategic family therapy, developed by Jay Haley and Cloe Madanes, draws heavily on the work of Milton Erickson. This theory views symptoms as a metaphor for family difficulties and advocates an active approach to removing the symptom while simultaneously improving the overall family functioning (Haley, 1987). Principles important in this theory include:

- Family structure and hierarchy are important; parents must be clearly in charge of the family.
- Transitions often precipitate family dysfunction. The departure of the children from the home is a particularly stressful transition.
- The counselor is responsible for finding ways to alleviate symptoms and help the family. If one approach doesn't work quickly, another approach should be tried until goals are accomplished.
- The counseling focuses on actions; thoughts, feelings, and insights are secondary.

Strategic family therapy is a directive, carefully planned, action-oriented approach, which puts the counselor in charge. A wide range of techniques is used. Paradoxical interventions, involving a reversal of the person's perceptions or expectations, are especially important. For example, a couple seeking help because of constant fighting might be told to schedule arguments. These interventions jostle the family's dysfunctional patterns and reduce the power of the symptom, often leading to modification in family dynamics and reduction of symptoms. The family then is likely to be receptive to learning new skills and behaviors. Other important techniques in this approach include directives, reframing, redistributing symptoms, rituals, and enactment. This approach is particularly effective with families that are resistant or passive, limited in their verbal or analytical abilities, experiencing stressful transitions and crises, and controlled by children or in-laws rather than parents.

Used with the Wood family, a strategic approach might reduce Nathan's symptoms and improve family functioning. The counselor might reframe Nathan's symptoms, telling the family that Nathan is acting out because he does not know how a young man is supposed to act. John and John Jr. could then be encouraged to model appropriate behavior for Nathan. Their attention and acceptance might give Nathan more comfort in the family and reduce his enmeshment with his mother. Other interventions could strengthen the partner relationship and promote shared parenting. However, enhancing this directive approach with a focus on the development of communication skills and understanding of the challenges of blended families could make counseling even more effective.

Solution-Focused Brief Family Therapy

Strategic family therapy has declined in use over the past 20 years but can be viewed as a precursor of the widely used solution-focused brief family therapy developed by Steve deShazer, Michele Weiner-Davis, Insoo Kim Berg, William O'Hanlon, and others. This approach is a brief, problem-focused model (Miller, Hubble, & Duncan, 1996). It assumes that people want to change; emphasizes strengths, resources, and solutions as well as past successes; and helps people use those to make small but rapid and important changes. This approach is structured and goal oriented, using a broad repertoire of interventions, as well as understanding of the reciprocal relationships in a family, to promote change. Strongly associated with this model is deShazer's (1991, p. 113) miracle question: "Suppose that one night there is a miracle and while you were sleeping the problem that brought you to therapy is solved: How would you know? What would be different? What will you notice different the next morning that will tell you that there has been a miracle? What will your spouse notice?" Another special feature of this model is the use it sometimes makes of an observing team who give feedback, messages, and clues to the counselor and the family. Solution-focused brief family therapy advocates short-term counseling, typically 6–12 sessions. Because of its emphasis on health and rapid resolution of problems, it has appeal.

This model also has some ideas to offer the Wood family. The miracle question, in particular, can help the family to identify times both before and after Olivia and John's marriage when family members felt happier and interacted more successfully. Both Olivia and John have coped with serious difficulties in their lives; John dealt with the death of his first wife and being a single parent while Olivia, too, experienced loss and the challenges of being a single parent to a demanding child. Coping strategies that helped them through those times can be mobilized now.

Constructivist and Narrative Approaches to Family Counseling

Several pioneers in family counseling, including Adler and Satir, took a phenomenological perspective, emphasizing the importance of family members' views of the world. Solution-focused and other modern approaches to family therapy have built on this concept and assume a constructivist position that views reality as "multiperspectival" (Becvar & Bccvar, 1993, p. 297). Each family member has his or her own understanding of the family and language to describe the family. Constructivist counselors emphasize epistemology, the process of knowing and describing the social construction of reality (Amatea & Sherrard, 1994). They collaborate with their clients, speak their language, and accept their perspectives, seeking the logic and wisdom in their lives. Change is promoted by shifting those perspectives and modifying language so that resources and solutions emerge.

Narrative therapy, currently very important in family counseling, has built on these concepts (Eron & Lund, 1996; White, 1995). Narrative therapy suggests that people's lives are directed by how they think about, interpret, and organize their experiences and memories to develop a narrative of their lives. In treatment, counselors become co-authors rather than problem-solvers, helping people tell their stories and replace nonhelpful stories with alternate and more empowering ones. Metaphors, circular questions, externalizing of problems, deconstruction of stories, note-taking, restatement of stories, and other strategies enhance treatment.

OTHER MODELS OF FAMILY COUNSELING

The most important models of family counseling have been reviewed earlier in this chapter. Additional information on many of these approaches also is contained in Chapter 7. However, several other models, including psychodynamic family counseling and the Milan approach to counseling with families are mentioned here briefly.

Milan Systemic Family Therapy

Developed by Mara Selvini Palazzoli and her colleagues in Milan, Italy, and by Penn and Hoffman in the United States, this is an epistemological approach that integrates strategic and behavioral techniques (Boscolo, Cecchin, Hoffman, & Penn, 1987; Selvini Palazzoli, 1988). Repetitive sequences, feedback loops, and coevolution in families, in which each person affects others, receive particular attention. Using techniques such as circular questioning, rituals, and prescriptions (often that the parents take a vacation together, away from their children), this model involves extended sessions and observers who provide feedback to the therapists.

Psychodynamic Family Counseling ─────────────────────────────

Freudian theory is the basis for this approach to counseling families, developed by Nathan Ackerman, Kirchner and Kirchner, Scharff and Scharff, Harville Hendrix, and others. The goals of this approach are to increase ego strength and insight in order to reduce negative interactions based on early experiences and relationships. Techniques include a detailed history taking, with emphasis on family of origin, free association, use of transference and countertransference, exposing family secrets, questioning, observing defenses, interpretation, and working through. This approach continues to have appeal and usefulness for many counselors and families.

Many other approaches to family counseling are in use or are emerging including:

1. *Multiple Family Group Therapy*—This approach combines a small number of families in group therapy. Describing this approach, Thorngren and Kleist (2002, p. 168) stated: "Putting families together in a group provided more social support and opportunities for expanded awareness than the counselor could ever offer each family on a one-to-one basis." Combining elements of narrative, constructivist, interpersonal, and psychodynamic counseling and education, this approach helps families develop new strengths and perspectives.
2. *Filial Therapy*—Developed by Garry Landreth, this approach "trains parents to be therapeutic agents with their own children through a format of didactic instruction, demonstration play sessions," at-home practice, and supervision (Watts & Broaddus, 2002).
3. *Multisystems Approach*—Particularly relevant to cultural minority and lower socioeconomic families, this approach intervenes with families on many levels, including individual, family, extended family, friends, church and community, social service agencies, and other outside systems (Brown, 2002).

EXAMPLES OF TREATMENT PLANS FOR FAMILIES ─────────────────────

Nearly all of the treatment approaches discussed here have something to offer the Wood family, although some are more useful than others. Treatment planning for families is a flexible process that involves assessing family dynamics, determining appropriate modes of treatment, and integrating that information with the skills and preferences of the counselor. The last section of this chapter provides a CLIENT MAP for a family and also gives readers descriptions of three additional families for use in practicing treatment planning.

Treatment Plan for the Schwartz Family

The Schwartz family includes Denise, age 35, Peter, age 37, and Jeffrey, age 4. Both Denise and Peter were raised in the Jewish faith but neither currently has strong religious or spiritual beliefs. This is the first marriage for Denise and Peter. Their first child, a boy they named Jeffrey, was born 1 year after the marriage. Jeffrey died of a genetic disorder when he was 18 months old. Their second child, who Denise insisted be named after their first child, was born about 3 years later. Denise had a miscarriage between the two births.

Denise and Peter met in college and married after a courtship of nearly 5 years when Peter completed law school. Denise works part-time doing telemarketing from home, but spends most of her time caring for Jeffrey. She is overprotective, seems sad, and is very concerned about her marriage. She suspects Peter of having an affair. Peter works full-time as a lawyer, and seems tense and preoccupied. Denise was the oldest child in a large, enmeshed family. Peter was the youngest of three, with two older sisters. His mother abused alcohol and his father, who was in the military, was away from home for long periods of time.

Jeffrey presents with unpredictable behavior; he vacillates between aggressive acting out and clinging overdependence. The family sought counseling at the suggestion of Jeffrey's preschool teacher. Denise hopes that counseling also will improve her relationship with Peter.

Diagnosis of Family Members

Denise:

Axis I.	300.4 Dysthymic Disorder, moderate
Axis II.	Dependent Personality Traits
Axis III.	None reported
Axis IV.	Marital conflict
Axis V.	60.

Peter:

Axis I.	300.02 Generalized Anxiety Disorder, mild
Axis II.	Obsessive–Compulsive Personality Traits
Axis III.	None reported
Axis IV.	Marital conflict, pressure at work
Axis V.	62.

Jeffrey:

Axis I.	312.9 Disruptive Behavior Disorder NOS
Axis II.	V71.09 No Mental Disorder on Axis II

Axis III. None reported
Axis IV. Conflict in parents' marriage
Axis V. 55.

Case Conceptualization

This family presents with problems of loss, marital conflict, a child's disruptive behavior, and poor communication. Both Denise and Peter have been diagnosed with Personality Traits. Denise is experiencing moderate and long-standing depression, while Peter struggles with pervasive anxiety. They seem to be repeating some transgenerational patterns; Denise overfunctions as the caretaker while Peter has withdrawn, both physically and emotionally. Peter had been the center of attention as a child and during his courtship of Denise. He now is having difficulty with Denise's absorption with Jeffrey and her depression since the death of their first child. This family is in stage three, the family with young children. Role changes and maintaining the spouse relationship, common challenges in this stage, are particularly difficult for this couple. Denise and Jeffrey seem enmeshed, not surprising in light of the family history. Peter has been all but cut off from the family system and may have formed intimate relationships outside of the home. Family members have divergent communication styles. Peter tends to be Super-reasonable; Denise, both Blamer and Placator; and Jeffrey is a Distractor. Communication is limited and often incongruent. Secrets may further impair communication. Family values also are in conflict; Peter's values tend to be material while Denise emphasizes parenting. Both Denise and Peter come from European Jewish backgrounds; this is a source of commonality. Extended family is a resource and assists with babysitting and finances. Neither Denise nor Peter has clear and positive self-images; both have an external locus of control. This, as well as other factors, has made it difficult for them to establish a strong marriage and cope with their losses together. As a result, they have become distanced and disapproving of each other. They do have many strengths. They have stayed together despite great loss, they are verbal and intelligent, they once had a loving and rewarding relationship, and both are motivated to make a good home for Jeffrey.

Objectives: Short/Medium Term

1. Increase time Denise and Peter spend together as a couple as measured by self-report.
2. Reduce the frequency of Jeffrey's aggressive behavior and increase his independence as measured by the Behavior Assessment of Children inventory.

3. Reduce Denise's depression and Peter's anxiety as measured by the Beck Depression Inventory and the Beck Anxiety Inventory.
4. Enable couple to grieve and discuss their losses openly as measured by a 1–10 scale.
5. Improve ratings of marital happiness and security as measured by a marital satisfaction inventory.

Assessments

Scale to measure marital happiness, Beck Depression and Anxiety Inventories, baseline measure of Jeffrey's behavior, Behavioral Assessment of Children inventory, marital satisfaction inventory, medical evaluation of Jeffrey.

Clinician

Clinician should have experience in helping families deal with loss and grief.

Location

Outpatient counseling in a private practice, community mental health center, or family counseling agency.

Interventions

Treatment initially will emphasize a communications (Satir) approach, then integrate cognitive behavioral and structural interventions. The communications model will help the couple express and understand their feelings, develop congruence in their communications, and increase their self-esteem. This model can help them regain closeness and facilitate their grieving for their losses. Once Denise and Peter feel more secure in the marriage and with themselves, cognitive behavioral techniques will be used to promote closeness in the couple and help modify Jeffrey's behavior. Structural interventions will help to restore the parental hierarchy.

Specific interventions, linked to objectives, include the following:

- Education, modeling and practice of communication styles, healthy communication (3, 4, 5)
- Identification and modification of distorted cognitions (3, 4, 5)
- Education on parenting skills, changing children's behavior (1, 2, 3, 5)
- Caring Days (1, 3, 5)
- Joining, unbalancing, restructuring the family system (2, 3, 5)
- Education on grief, facilitation of sharing of feeling about the death of their child (3, 4, 5) and the miscarriage

Emphasis

Although support is an important ingredient in counseling this family, they can handle a moderately paced approach that focuses them on their concerns.

Numbers

Family and couples counseling will be the primary modes of treatment.

Timing

Weekly 50-minutes sessions will be scheduled for approximately 6 months.

Medication

If rapid improvement is not evident in both Jeffrey's behavior and Denise's depression, they will be referred to a psychiatrist for a medication evaluation.

Adjunct Services

Family and couple activities that are pleasurable and rewarding are essential to this family. Peter and Denise will be encouraged to resume ballroom dancing lessons that they had enjoyed shortly after their marriage. Peter might benefit from involvement in an Adult Children of Alcoholics group, while Denise might join a support group for mothers of young children.

Prognosis

Prognosis is good to very good for accomplishment of objectives via this treatment plan. The couple is motivated and has many strengths.

Cases for Treatment Planning ────────────────────────────────────

The following three cases provide readers the opportunity to develop family treatment plans. Feel free to provide additional details on these families, as long as the added information is compatible with the written description of each family.

Case 1. The Stuart family consists of George, age 52, a school principal; his wife Jody, 52, a librarian; and their children, Susan, 20, Mark, 17, and Lucy, 12.

All three children were adopted. Susan and Mark have both been high achievers and are good athletes. Lucy is mildly mentally retarded. Her self-care is poor and she is in a special program at school. She is very attached to her father and to Susan and is hostile toward her mother. Jody wants to move ahead in her career and resents Lucy's caretaking demands. She has been encouraging George to send Lucy to a boarding school, which he is reluctant to do.

Case 2. Steve Stern, age 46, and Hector Alvarado, 35, have been living together for 5 years and view each other as life partners. Steve was married for 15 years before he met Hector; he has two children, Mari, age 12, and Howard, age 10. Hector would like the children to view him as a stepparent, but Steve has kept contact between Hector and the children to a minimum. His explanation is that his ex-wife would deny him visitation rights if she knew the truth about his relationship with Hector. The two also have cultural differences: Steve's background is European Jewish and Hector's is Latino. Steve is the oldest of two; Hector is a middle child in a family of five children. Hector works as an accountant and Steve is employed in sales.

Case 3. The Young family includes Arlene, 33, Fred, 35, Fred Jr., 14, and Bobby, 10. Arlene is very talkative and attractive, and expressed long-standing dissatisfaction with her marriage. Arlene has had a number of poorly concealed affairs, which have generally gone unnoticed by her husband. She recently prompted the family's decision to seek counseling by charging expensive furs and jewelry to her husband's credit card. Fred is a highly intelligent and successful business executive. He reported no awareness of marital difficulties until his wife's recent spending spree. He views that as the main issue and wants help in controlling his wife's money management. Fred Jr. is quiet and intense. He is a good student, well behaved and scholarly, but with little peer involvement. He was conceived on his parents' third date and was the reason for the marriage, although he is unaware of this. Bobby is cute, talkative, and manipulative. He is intelligent but does not do well at school. He is a leader among his peers and clearly is the favorite of both parents.

This chapter provided information on diagnosis and treatment of individuals and families. Chapter 9 presents information on diagnosis and treatment of groups.

Assessment and Treatment Planning for Groups

Since the 1960s, group counseling has been used extensively to meet a wide variety of educational and therapeutic needs. Counseling groups are used in schools, mental health settings, and business and industry to both ameliorate emotional difficulties and promote knowledge and healthy development. Many factors have contributed to the popularity of group treatment. The group offers an opportunity for a person to benefit from the insights, perspectives, role modeling, and feedback of other group members. Group participants can practice new ways of communicating and relating to others in a safe and helpful setting. Counseling groups can reduce isolation and create a sense of belonging. As clients interact with people who have similar problems, their own difficulties become more understandable and less frightening, which leads to better self-acceptance.

The Association for Specialists in Group Work (2000, p. 330), a division of the American Counseling Association (ACA), defined group work as "a broad professional practice involving the application of knowledge and skill in group facilitation to assist an interdependent collection of people to reach their mutual goals, which may be intrapersonal, interpersonal, or work related." Yalom (1995, p. 1) identified 11 curative or therapeutic factors in group counseling:

- Hope
- Universality, which normalizes concerns and responses
- Information
- Altruism; sharing of oneself to promote the common good of the group
- Corrective emotional experiences and working through of issues
- Development and improvement of social skills
- Modeling of positive behavior and coping skills
- Development of insight

- Group cohesiveness, facilitating bonding and support
- Catharsis
- Attention to existential issues, to promote responsibility for one's own life, recognition of aloneness, concerns about mortality, and the uncertainty of existence

These factors are associated with positive change in many treatment modalities, but have a particularly strong association with successful group counseling.

Beyond the therapeutic benefits of group work, economics also contributes to the popularity of group work. Many counseling settings must address a broad range of complex issues and serve a large number of clients with limited resources (staff, time, and money) (Brown, 1994). The group format offers a means for meeting this challenge.

This chapter provides information on the dynamics of counseling groups, member and counselor roles, and theories of group treatment. In addition, the DO A CLIENT MAP (introduced in Chapter 6) is applied to groups in this chapter to promote understanding of the diagnosis and treatment of counseling groups.

HISTORICAL DEVELOPMENT OF GROUP COUNSELING

Group counseling was initially used in the early 1900s. Each decade saw new developments in group counseling:

- In the 1920s, Alfred Adler encouraged the use of groups composed of parents, children, teachers, and counselors to improve family functioning and promote children's healthy development. Adler also suggested regular family meetings (family councils) as a way to air and resolve family concerns. Jacob L. Moreno, who initiated the use of psychodrama, was another important contributor to the early development of group counseling.
- In the 1930s, the founding of Alcoholics Anonymous launched the use of peer support groups to promote self-help, personal growth, and symptom reduction. Twelve-step and other support groups are now widely available and frequently used as an adjunct to counseling. The inception of group guidance in schools also contributed to the importance of group counseling.
- The 1940s witnessed the spread of training and counseling groups to business and industry with the advent of Kurt Lewin's training groups (T-groups) at the National Training Laboratory. T-groups, along with Wilfred Bion's Tavistock groups, focused attention on group dynamics and the power of the group to promote change in people seeking help with problems as well as those seeking personal growth.

- In the 1950s, family counseling, discussed in Chapter 8, provided yet another approach to using groups for counseling.
- The growth of the human potential movement during the 1960s had a powerful impact on group counseling; that decade witnessed the emergence of encounter groups, group counseling marathons, sensitivity training groups, and the important work of Eric Berne (Transactional Analysis) and Fritz Perls (Gestalt Therapy).
- The founding of the Association for Specialists in Group Work in the 1970s reflected counselors' widespread acceptance of group counseling.
- During the 1980s and 1990s, group counseling expanded and refined its focus, addressing the needs of multicultural groups and specific diagnostic groups.
- Now, in the 21st century, counseling groups have maintained their importance. Recent new developments include Critical Incident Stress Debriefing, a group approach to helping people cope with traumatic and other stressful incidents, and on-line chat rooms and support groups.

Group counseling has established its importance over the past 100 years. Although research on specific approaches and applications is still limited, the effectiveness of group counseling has been well established (Kivlighan, Coleman, & Anderson, 2000).

SKILLS OF THE GROUP COUNSELOR

Group counselors need a broad range of skills that include, but go beyond, skills associated with conducting effective individual counseling sessions. The following are some of the special skills required of group counselors:

- Ability to plan a group, recruit and screen members, and compose a group
- Group management and establishment of a safe, ethical, and productive group environment
- Knowledge of the stages of group development and ways to promote positive development
- Knowledge of group dynamics, member roles, and ways to encourage appropriate member involvement
- Understanding of the use of exercises and structured techniques to promote counseling goals
- Communication of helpful feedback and suggestions
- Ability to teach and model coping, social, communication, and other skills
- Effective ways to bring closure to sessions and treatment

INITIATING THE COUNSELING GROUP ━━━━━━━━━━━━━━━━━━━━━━━━━━━━

The first step in initiating a counseling group is developing a clear vision of the group. This entails identifying the purpose and goals of the group, the type of people likely to benefit from such a group, and group parameters such as cost, frequency, length of each meeting, and whether the group will be open or time-limited. An informed consent statement should be developed, including confidentiality and other guidelines designed to promote protection and respect of group members.

Once counselors have completed these preliminaries, they are probably ready to recruit and screen members for the group or to take over leadership of a preexisting or preformed group. The preformed group often is found in organizational settings where counselors are called in to provide consultation services, perhaps promoting cohesiveness and productivity in a group of employees. A preexisting group is one that has been meeting with a leader who is leaving the group and passing it onto another counselor. Usually, however, counselors have the flexibility to construct a counseling group based on their own predetermined criteria.

These predetermined criteria typically include the following:

1. *Number of Members*—The ideal number of participants in a counseling group is 7 or 8, according to Yalom (1995), with a desired range of 6–14. When groups are too small (four or fewer), members feel pressured to perform or contribute, and the opportunities for interaction are diminished. On the other hand, when groups are too large, some members may feel discouraged from participating, while a subgroup of members may dominate the group (Gladding, 2003). The optimal number of members should be determined primarily on the basis of the number of leaders, the ages of participants, and the goals of the group. For example, a bereavement group for young children probably should be relatively small, while a personal growth group for college students could be larger.

2. *Nature of Concerns and Goals*—The goals of the individual participants should be compatible with those of the group as a whole to increase the likelihood that the group will become a supportive and unified system. A counseling group typically has one or more important objectives such as helping people cope with abuse or develop assertiveness. That primary objective usually determines the desired degree of homogeneity in the group. Greater homogeneity in background and concerns usually leads to greater cohesiveness and member involvement. A homogeneous group may be especially useful when members need primarily support or help with common problems (Gladding, 2003). On the other hand, a heterogeneous group reflects the outside world and so can serve as a useful vehicle for trying out new ideas and behaviors.

3. *Relevant Demographic Characteristics*—Demographic factors often are important in group membership. Limiting membership to one gender, age group, or cultural group can increase counseling effectiveness. For example, women who experienced childhood sexual abuse usually are treated in a same-gender group. Developmental issues such as retirement might be best addressed in a group of people in midlife or older. Executives with career and employment issues may derive the most benefit from a group composed of upper-level managers. Bowman (1993) suggested that ethnic homogeneity in counseling groups is most effective in addressing issues related to racial identity development. Screening of group members should take into account characteristics such as age, gender, and background in order to create a group whose members are likely to be cohesive and helpful to each other. In addition, counselors usually should ensure that the group has no outliers (e.g., one man in a group of women, one adolescent in a group of people in midlife) who might feel uncomfortable and detract from the work of the group.

4. *Relevant Personal Characteristics*—Not all people are appropriate for group counseling, so screening for suitability is essential. People who are extremely hostile or aggressive, in poor contact with reality, severely depressed, highly suspicious, very shy and withdrawn, or in a crisis usually are not good candidates for group counseling. Appropriateness for the group also needs to be assessed in light of the composition and goals of the group. For example, people with Borderline Personality Disorders typically are not well suited to membership in a heterogeneous therapy group. However, they may well benefit from a homogenous group in which Dialectical Behavior Therapy is used (Linehan, 1993).

5. *Financial Circumstances*—Potential members' finances must be reviewed if there is to be a fee or if eligibility for membership in the group is contingent on meeting low-income guidelines.

ILLUSTRATIVE CASE STUDY

The use of an example can clarify the process of initiating and leading a counseling group, as well as the nature and importance of some relevant variables. The example used throughout this chapter is a group formed by Sandra Surber, a counselor who specialized in helping people cope with chronic and life-threatening illnesses. Many of her clients were women coping with breast cancer. Through individual counseling with these women, Sandra learned that the immediate aftermath of treatment was a difficult time for these women. Fear of recurrence increased, complicated by fatigue and other side effects of their treatment. They had difficulty reassessing their priorities, finding the support they needed, and moving ahead with their lives.

Sandra decided to offer a counseling group that would address the needs of these women. Criteria for participation included the following:

- Participants were women who had been diagnosed with breast cancer; who had completed surgery, radiation, and/or chemotherapy in the past year; and who did not have metastatic (advanced) cancer.
- Participants were motivated to participate in the counseling group.
- Participants seemed able to function successfully in a group, manifesting no severe emotional disorders, hostility, or fear of group interaction and demonstrating at least adequate communication skills.
- Participants who were already in individual therapy and also wanted to participate in group therapy were required to authorize communication between their two counselors as well as obtain the approval of their individual counselor for their participation in the group.

To promote ample opportunity for communication as well as cohesiveness and self-disclosure, Sandra limited the group to eight members. She decided that the group would meet for eight sessions and would not admit new members during that time.

Sandra then planned an outreach program to recruit group members. She distributed announcements to area oncologists and cancer treatment programs and posted flyers at local libraries and markets. When Sandra received a telephone inquiry from a potential group member, she conducted a preliminary interview via telephone and then invited each woman who met the basic criteria to meet with her individually to learn more about the group. Before the personal interview, each woman completed a brief demographic and medical history form and a mood checklist. The first eight women who seemed suitable constituted the group. Others were either given referrals or were put on a waiting list for the next counseling group.

IMPORTANCE OF MOTIVATION

The members of a group, especially a preformed group, may have widely varying levels of interest in treatment. Some members may be motivated to seek treatment, but unwilling or hesitant to express themselves in a group setting. Some may focus on the group leader and disregard or resist input from group members. Those who are in the group involuntarily, such as people who are court-referred or referred by their employer, may be reluctant to engage in the group. Counselors need to obtain an accurate reading of people's interest in counseling so treatment planning can take account of possible barriers to effective treatment.

During the screening interviews, Sandra tried to determine the level of applicants' motivation. Several women were there at the urging of their partners or physicians. One woman expressed strong reluctance to discuss her "intimate information" with others but said that several people told her she "must participate in a group to insure survival." Clarification of the nature of the group, as well as the women's motivation, helped both Sandra and the potential participants decide whether they and the group were a good match.

GROUP ENVIRONMENT

Consideration of the group's environment includes an exploration of the members' home base (community, work setting, or school) and the environment in which treatment will be provided. Of particular importance is an examination of factors that might promote or inhibit the success of the group. For example, if the group is conducted in a school or corporate setting, the institutional climate, including the level of trust in the organization, may affect the success of the group.

The women in Sandra Surber's group all lived in a suburb of a large metropolitan area. This was a culturally and economically varied area where most people were accustomed to diversity. The group reflected that diversity, although Sandra was careful not to include individuals who were very different from the rest of the group. For that reason, a woman in her early 20s and a woman who had recently immigrated to the United States were referred to more appropriate sources of help.

GROUP DEVELOPMENT

Counseling groups go through a series of developmental stages. These stages have been described with slight differences, but with remarkable consistency, by group stage theorists (Gladding, 2003; Kormanski, 1988; Yalom, 1995). The following stages characterize groups:

Stage 1: Orientation and Exploration—The primary task of the initial stage is orienting the members to the counseling group and establishing the structure and goals of the group. The group leader reviews the informed consent statement and emphasizes the importance of confidentiality, respect, boundaries, the time schedule of the group, and other procedural and ethical guidelines. Members' roles and responsibilities are described and the leader might teach and model helpful and supportive ways to give and receive feedback.

During this initial stage, members usually introduce themselves and share relevant information about themselves. An exercise to promote involvement and disclosure is used often. Leaders usually make extensive use of reflection, link group members via similar experiences and statements, and encourage all members to play an active part in the group.

Sandra followed all these procedures in her initial group session. Because of the nature of her group, she emphasized the importance of support and sought to normalize feelings of anger, guilt, and fear, common among people coping with cancer. To initiate dialog and to start the group on a positive and empowering note, she asked each member to introduce herself by briefly describing two experiences or personal qualities that made her proud of herself. Once some initial rapport had developed among the members, Sandra suggested that each member tell the story of her diagnosis and treatment to focus the group on its goals and build cohesiveness.

Stage 2: Transition Stage—Some sources divide this stage into two parts. Gladding (2003, p. 199), for example, breaks the transition stage into "storming" and "norming." Indeed this stage includes both conflict and the emergence of shared group guidelines and feelings of cooperation.

Increased anxiety, defensiveness, anger, and struggles for control and dominance in the group often characterize this stage. Some members may enjoy the conflict, while others may withdraw, give advice, or engage in caretaking to reduce conflict and protect themselves and others. This can be a challenging stage for both group leaders and members. Counselors must control the environment of the group to be sure members are not emotionally harmed. To accomplish this, counselors typically focus on process and on the present, giving feedback and suggesting ways members can deal effectively with the tension and ambiguity of this stage.

In successful groups, the tension eventually abates as members establish their roles and their place in the group. Group goals and norms typically are revisited and clarified. Cohesiveness develops and the group becomes an eager and collaborative unit.

Stage 3: Working Stage—This typically is a period of productivity and harmony among members who have successfully negotiated the transition period. Self-disclosure increases as members feel safer in the group and become more caring and supportive toward each other. Both individual and group goals are accomplished.

Stage 4: Consolidation and Termination—This stage usually focuses on summarizing, interpreting, and consolidating the experience of the group. Members process their time together, celebrating closeness and success, planning for continuing gains beyond the life of the group, and typically feeling both sadness and pride as they say goodbye and the group ends.

GROUP DYNAMICS

Group dynamics change and evolve over the life of a group. The following list reflects important aspects of group dynamics and questions to facilitate consideration of each aspect:

1. *Cohesiveness of group*—How close-knit, committed, and involved are the group members?
2. *Level of trust*—Are the members able to take risks and self-disclose appropriately? To what extent are they able to move beyond superficial

conversation to deeper levels of interaction? Do they focus their trust solely on the group leader or do they trust other members as well?

3. *Nature and degree of communication*—How openly do members communicate? Who communicates with whom? Are alliances and subgroups evident? What styles of communication characterize each member and the group as a whole? For example, do the group members communicate well in cognitive areas but have difficulty sharing emotions?

4. *Group decision-making style*—Is it democratic or authoritarian? Are decisions made efficiently or laboriously? Are decisions often revisited or are they enduring?

5. *Formal and informal roles assumed by members*—What styles of participation are typical of the group members? What patterns of influence are exerted by group members? Do some members dominate group interactions? Who has leadership roles and functions? Do some members play supporting roles? Are some rescuers or scapegoats? What is the structure and hierarchy of the group?

6. *Rules and norms of the group*—What expressed and implied policies and procedures guide the operation of the group? For example, most groups have rules and norms that influence when members arrive, attendance, the nature and amount of self-disclosure and feedback, the power of the designated leader, and the topics considered in meetings.

7. *History of treatment*—What counseling interventions have been used previously with this group? What impact have they had? History is of particular significance to counselors who are working with a group that is already formed or functioning, such as a counseling group that is being transferred to a new counselor, a peer support group seeking professional intervention, or a group that was formed in another setting (e.g., a work group or a classroom group).

PLANNING THE TREATMENT

Once the needs and dimensions of the group have been assessed through interviews, questionnaires, observation, or other means, counselors can plan the treatment. This will be illustrated here with the DO A CLIENT MAP, which includes the following elements: Diagnosis, Objectives, Assessments, Clinician, Location, Interventions, Emphasis, Numbers, Timing, Medication, Adjunct Services, and Prognosis.

Diagnosis

The first step in treatment planning is understanding the needs, concerns, strengths, and weaknesses of the group members. Initially, the counselor may have had a general description of group goals and membership. However, screening interviews provide specific diagnostic and descriptive information about participants. Determining whether any of the participants has a severe mental disorder or symptoms and behaviors that might undermine the group goals is especially important.

Sandra viewed the eight people who arrived for the first group session as an appropriate group. Although they varied in terms of age, ethnicity, and educational and employment backgrounds, their commonalties seemed more significant than their differences. All had completed treatment for breast cancer within the previous 6 months. The women were apprehensive about a recurrence of their disease, worried about the impact of their illness on their families, and struggling to deal with physical changes, fatigue, and other side effects of their medical treatments. Several expressed a need to reassess their priorities and one was very angry about her illness and her medical treatment. None of the women had incapacitating mental disorders and none presented a danger to themselves or others. However, some were experiencing Adjustment Disorders, one had a General Anxiety Disorder, and one had a Dysthymic Disorder.

Objectives

Objectives for counseling groups depend on the overall nature and purposes of the group as well as the needs of the individual members. Whether the general purpose of a group is to be psychoeducational, preventive, problem-oriented, or growth promoting is important in determining objectives. Group counselors often assume an active role in goal setting, suggesting appropriate and shared objectives based on information provided during the assessment process. Group members can then process these tentative goals and refine them as needed.

The group of eight women who had completed treatment for breast cancer had elements of all four types of groups. Sandra planned to present some information on the usual impact of breast cancer and ways to cope with the disease (psychoeducational). She wanted to help the women deal with depression, anxiety, and other symptoms that resulted from their medical experiences (problem-focused), to prevent the emergence of additional symptoms (preventive), and to help the women use their medical experience as a catalyst for reevaluating and improving their lives (growth-promoting).

With Sandra's guidance, the group agreed on the following objectives:

- To better understand and learn to cope with fear of recurrence
- To better understand and learn to cope with the side effects of breast cancer and its treatments
- To learn ways to enhance their physical and emotional health
- To improve self-image and feelings of self-worth
- To reassess priorities, increase hope and optimism, and establish goals for a rewarding future.

Assessment in counseling groups refers to the individual members as well as to the group as a whole. Both qualitative and quantitative approaches to assessment can help counselors design a treatment plan for a counseling group.

Qualitative Approaches to Assessment

Many tools are available for assessing the dynamics and needs of a group. Intake interviews generate information on individual goals, expectations, history, motivation for treatment, stressors, and strengths. Observation of participants during the initial interview can yield important data for diagnosis and treatment planning. Questionnaires administered during the intake process can also help counselors identify common member concerns and needs.

As the group progresses, journals, shared with the counselor (and sometimes with other members), can provide information on the progress of the group. That information may facilitate accomplishment of individual goals and can also help shape treatment and record progress.

For Sandra, the initial telephone call, the applicant questionnaires, and the screening interview all gave her understanding of participant needs and goals. Particularly useful was information on the questionnaire related to the participants' histories and goals, as well as information regarding their medical diagnoses, treatment, and side effects.

Quantitative Approaches to Assessment

Quantitative measures, used cautiously, also can add information on the diagnosis and evaluation of a counseling group. An example is the Fundamental Interpersonal Relations Orientation questionnaire (FIRO), which has been used to measure interpersonal behavior of group members. This instrument profiles the individual on the basis of three interpersonal needs: control, inclusion, and affection (Yalom, 1995). The Social Support Inventory (McCubbin, Patterson, Rossman, & Cooke, 1982) measures social support in many types of groups (Carty, 1993). Pregroup and postgroup administration of instruments like these can measure change.

Group counselors have a challenging role. They must attend to three dimensions of their groups: the group as a whole, the individual members of the group, and the interactions among the group members. The following lists some of the many roles of the group counselor:

- Information-giver, orientor, coordinator
- Program developer and planner
- Goal and standard-setter
- Initiator
- Facilitator
- Gatekeeper
- Observer
- Supporter and encourager
- Role model
- Compromiser and harmonizer
- Analyzer and interpreter

Co-leadership can bring a positive dimension to the group experience, although that can increase both the cost of counseling and the complexity of the leader's role. In the group setting, effective communication and relationship skills manifested by co-leaders can provide a useful model. By sharing the task of group management, co-leaders can more effectively balance the demands of attending to the group members, their interactions, and the entire group.

Location

Whenever possible, group counselors should attend to environmental factors that might influence the quality of the experience. The location of the counseling group should be one that is likely to maximize attendance and promote a sense of comfort and belonging. It also should have appropriate facilities, including a room large enough to accommodate the members. If counselors think that a particular client group will feel uncomfortable, stigmatized, or inconvenienced by meeting at a mental health facility, group meetings might be scheduled at area churches, schools, libraries, or community centers. In addition, the location should be convenient, with ample parking as well as access to public transportation. The availability of facilities and personnel for child care may facilitate attendance at the group.

Physical comfort should be taken into consideration; such annoyances as uncomfortable chairs, extreme temperatures, and poor acoustics can inhibit the therapeutic experience. Counselors should be sure that the group setting is a relaxed and comfortable environment that communicates security and privacy.

Sandra held the counseling group in a large room at her private practice offices. She deliberately avoided institutional settings because members might then associate the counseling with their medical experiences. The room was decorated in soft colors and had Impressionist prints on the walls. Chairs and sofas allowed participants to sit close to others or to have some distance. For the first meeting, healthy snacks and fruit drinks were available in the waiting room to convey a welcoming atmosphere and reduce tension.

Interventions

The overall theoretical framework for leading a counseling group usually is initially determined by the primary purpose of the group. *Psychoeducational groups* typically provide didactic information and skills training. Assertiveness training groups and anger management groups are primarily educational in nature. *Therapeutic groups*, also known as *problem-oriented* or *remedial groups*, focus primarily on alleviating symptoms and mental disorders by changing emotions, thoughts, and behaviors. For example, people with Eating Disorders typically benefit from the modeling and support offered in groups like this. *Preventive groups* typically target at-risk populations and provide information and skills that will help people avoid difficulties in the future. Such groups might help single parents learn to take better care of themselves and their children or might help adolescents living in high crime areas to develop ways to handle peer pressure. Finally, *personal growth groups* aim to help people without significant emotional difficulties to further improve their knowledge and skills. Colleges offer such groups to freshmen to help them make good use of the college experience.

Many theories of group counseling have been developed. These are discussed later in this chapter. As discussed in Chapter 6, counselors should have a rationale for the treatment approach and specific interventions they use.

Because Sandra's counseling group combined elements of all four types of groups, she used a broad range of interventions. Her primary theoretical framework was cognitive-behavioral therapy, an approach that has proven its effectiveness in helping people cope with cancer (Moorey & Greer, 1989). Because Sandra saw her task as providing a combination of education and counseling, she planned a format that included a variety of interventions including didactic presentations, exploration and modification of dysfunctional thoughts, sharing of emotions and experiences, brainstorming to generate ideas, role-playing, and goal-setting exercises.

Emphasis

In terms of counseling groups, emphasis indicates how structured and directive the group will be; how much of the focus will be on remediation rather than prevention and growth; and how much attention will be paid to the past, the present, and the future. The individual members, as well as the objectives and theoretical framework for the group, help to determine emphasis.

Numbers

The size of the group and member roles (discussed earlier) are other elements to be considered. Gladding (2003) described member roles in terms of three categories:

- Group Building and Maintenance Roles such as facilitator, gatekeeper compromiser, follower
- Group Task Roles such as information-giver and -scckcr, coordinator, evaluato□
- Negative Social-Emotional Roles such as aggressor, blocker, rescuer monopolist.

Building and maintenance roles and task roles are clearly essential for the effective operation of the group, while the negative individual roles must be addressed by the leaders and the members. Ideally, the group should have a balance of members in building, maintenance, and task roles and no members in negative roles.

Timing

The timing of group counseling, which includes the length and frequency of sessions and the duration of treatment, is an important aspect of the treatment plan. Most groups meet for 1.5–2 hours at a time. Generally, a session of less than 1 hour is too short to accomplish much work. However, the group's productivity usually diminishes after 2 hours, and the discussion may become tedious and exhausting (Yalom, 1995). Most groups meet once a week in order to maintain continuity and cohesiveness and facilitate scheduling.

Deciding whether a group should be open or closed to new members after the first session is an important aspect of planning group counseling. A group that allows for a flow of members entering and leaving can provide stimulation and vitality, as well as flexibility. Promoting group cohesiveness and trust can be more difficult in an open group than it is in a group whose membership is stable and whose duration is specified. A closed group also is more likely to maintain continuity of issues and relationships. However, it may be difficult to maintain a closed group over an extended period of time. As months pass, some members may leave the group, and the diminished size of the group may inhibit its effectiveness (Yalom, 1995). Counselors must decide whether open or closed groups are more likely to accomplish their goals.

The length of a closed-membership group generally depends on the nature of the members' concerns. Groups meeting to assist participants in coping with a life crisis such as loss of a job or relationship might be of short or medium duration, meeting for less than 6 months. Groups focused on long-standing and severe concerns, such as childhood abuse or an Eating Disorder, might meet for a much longer period. The duration of the group may be specified at the outset or it may be left open.

Sandra's counseling group met once a week, on Saturday mornings, from 10 a.m. to 12 noon, for 8 weeks. She believed that this amount of time would allow the participants to develop trust, establish some new communication skills and patterns of interaction, receive support and information, acquire new strategies for coping with their medical diagnosis and its impact on their lives, and establish individual goals. Sandra also thought that having a foreseeable end to the experience would motivate participants to use their time productively.

Medication

Medications and dietary supplements are often used in addition to counseling. Although counselors are not able to prescribe medications, they can make referrals to psychiatrists of clients who seem likely to benefit from medication and can take note of possible side effects in members taking medication. Group counselors should be aware of the medications taken by the members and have knowledge of possible medication side effects.

Adjunct Services

Counseling groups can provide a safe environment for trying out new behaviors, interacting with others, and developing heightened awareness of oneself and others. However, the time spent in group represents a small percentage of the person's week. Thus, counselors often suggest outside activities and resources to reinforce progress and continue the development of skills and insights acquired during counseling.

Homework assignments or suggested tasks are a useful means of extending the therapeutic experience. These may be recommended to specific members of the group or to the entire group. Suggestions can come from the group leader or may arise from the members' interactions. For example, the group might suggest that a member speak with a particular person or try out a new behavior and report back on this action at the next group meeting.

Bibliotherapy is a widely used adjunct to counseling. Issues that emerge during a group session may be explored further through outside reading. Often counselors develop their own printed materials for psychoeducation.

Journal keeping also can be an effective means of extending the therapeutic group experience. Writing in a journal following group sessions can help people reflect on what happened in the session, make it meaningful to them, and bring closure to that experience.

Some group counselors develop questionnaires or logs in which members record their reactions to the group session. This provides a structured format that helps members to remember, reflect on, evaluate, and record feelings or thoughts that they were unable or unwilling to share during the group session. This activity provides information that is not only useful to participants but also helpful to counselors.

Self-help or support groups are another useful adjunct to group counseling. Generally leaderless and of low cost, these groups provide an opportunity for people to continue the work they began in counseling and to obtain practice and reinforcement of skills learned. Overeaters Anonymous (OA), Parents Anonymous, and job clubs are examples of self-help groups.

Reading about ways other people coped with cancer was an important adjunct to Sandra's counseling group. In addition, group members decided to embark on a fitness program in which each member identified goals relevant to her exercise and eating habits.

Prognosis

The prognosis for success in a group depends, to a great extent, on the counselor's attitude and how that is conveyed to the members. Counselors can "plant a favorable prognosis" (Kottler, 1994, p. 62) by preparing the members to expect a positive experience. From the first telephone contact through the screening interview and the initial group meeting, counselors have rich opportunities to instill an expectation of success in members' minds. During sessions, counselors can further facilitate a positive prognosis by drawing the group's attention to progress and encouraging the members to support and reinforce each other's gains.

EVALUATION

Evaluation of group counseling provides data on treatment effectiveness and facilitates improvement and enhancement of services. In addition, funding sources often require that mental health agencies demonstrate that they have met their goals in order to receive continued funding. Evaluation of counseling groups is particularly important if similar group experiences are planned in the future or if similar client groups need services. Evaluation then can be used not only to assess the effectiveness of a particular program of interventions but also to guide the development of future programs.

Several approaches are available for evaluating the impact of group counseling. An overview of some of these is provided here. In addition, knowledge of research methodology or the help of a research consultant can ensure the selection of valid procedures. Having specific and measurable objectives facilitates the evaluation process. Assessment of the success of counseling groups usually can best be accomplished by the use of a control group that can be compared with the treatment group. This might occur if treatment could not be provided to all of the potential members of a group experience; those people not yet served can then comprise a control group. Pre- and posttreatment evaluation of both groups can determine whether the treatment group improved significantly more than the control group. However, the investigator should be cautious in drawing conclusions and would need to determine the comparability of the two groups.

Because the development of control groups is difficult, the effectiveness of counseling usually is evaluated in light of the objectives established for the group. This can be done via administration of inventories or questionnaires before and shortly after the group experience. A third administration of the instruments might occur in a follow-up, some months later, to provide information on the persistence of changes over time. Standardized inventories, with demonstrated reliability and validity and norms based on groups similar to the one receiving treatment, typically provide the most trustworthy information. Sources discussed in Chapter 4 can help counselors select appropriate instruments. In addition, counselors often gather information on participants' subjective reactions to the interventions used and impact of a counseling group. To accomplish this, a counselor-made questionnaire tailored to the group may be informative despite its lack of reliability and validity. For groups with poor reading or writing skills, oral interviews, group discussion, or follow-up telephone interviews can prove useful.

The perceptions of people outside of the group also can provide useful information on the impact of the group experience. In a school setting, for example, counselors might ask teachers whether they have noted any behavioral, interpersonal, or academic changes in students involved in counseling groups. Another approach to evaluation involves obtaining data on demonstrated behavioral changes. Observation of students and review of their academic records are examples of this. While the cause-and-effect relationships between the treatment and these changes may be difficult to determine conclusively, such data can be strongly suggestive of the value of the group.

The evaluation of Sandra's group involved the use of three instruments. The Profile of Mood States (McNair, Lorr, & Droppleman, 1992), used before and after the counseling experience, provided a brief standardized quantitative measure that had demonstrated value in assessing the moods of people coping with cancer. In addition, Sandra developed a questionnaire, to be used at the conclusion of counseling, that asked members to evaluate many aspects of the experience on a series of Likert scales. A follow-up survey, tailored to the nature of the group and mailed about 6 months after the conclusion of treatment, provided additional information. Subjective reactions to the strengths and weaknesses of the counseling experience also were elicited during the group discussion in the last meeting.

TREATMENT MODELS FOR GROUP COUNSELING ━━━━━━━━━━━━━━━━━

Treatment approaches to group counseling include models developed for individual counseling and then adapted to group settings, those developed for both individual and group counseling, and those developed primarily or exclusively for group settings. This chapter reviews all of these but focuses primarily on approaches that are best suited for use in counseling groups.

Chapter 7 reviewed many theories of individual counseling. All of them, especially person-centered counseling, behavioral counseling, reality therapy, rational emotive behavior therapy, gestalt therapy, Adlerian counseling, and psychodynamic psychotherapy, also have been used in group treatment. Although some adaptation of those models occurs when they are used with groups, the approaches remain basically the same. Consequently, the application of those approaches to group counseling is discussed only briefly here. Readers are referred to Chapter 7 and to textbooks focused on group counseling for additional information on the nature and application of those models. This chapter does not seek to teach these approaches to the reader but, rather, to review their salient characteristics and discuss their use in the process of diagnosis and treatment planning.

Models Commonly Used in Both Individual and Group Counseling ━━━━━━

An impressive array of theoretical approaches used for group counseling is available. In addition, eclectic or integrated models of counseling facilitate treatment planning that draws on multiple treatment approaches in systematic and planned ways. Whether they view themselves as "eclectic" or are committed to a specific treatment model, group counselors need an understanding of the broad range of approaches to group counseling.

Cognitive Group Counseling

Cognitive counseling was initially developed for individual treatment but is well suited for group work. This approach assumes that people have the potential to be both rational and irrational and the capacity to understand their own thinking. Changing their dysfunctional thoughts will change how they feel and what they do. Cognitive group counseling provides the opportunity for people to explore their thoughts and beliefs along with other group members, to receive feedback, and to try new ways of thinking, feeling, and acting. Additionally, the group provides members with a safe setting in which to observe examples of faulty thinking in other people, thus facilitating their efforts to identify and modify dysfunctional thinking patterns in themselves.

This approach is especially useful when working with people who have good verbal skills, at least average intelligence, and the ability to identify thoughts, feelings, and behaviors. It often is used in combination with behavioral techniques to treat depression and anxiety or mild situational disorders. Cognitive group therapy has been found effective in treating such diverse concerns as child sexual abuse (Watson & Stermac, 1994), weight control (Lewis, Blair, & Booth, 1992), anxiety disorders (White, Keenan, & Brooks, 1992), anger and violence (Towl, 1994), and marital difficulties (Montag & Wilson, 1992). In general it is not appropriate for people who are psychotic or in a state of crisis.

Cognitive counseling provided the theoretical basis for the counseling group of women who had been diagnosed with breast cancer. Helping these clients examine and change their dysfunctional thoughts about cancer and its impact on their lives led to corresponding changes in emotions and behaviors. This approach also helped the women to clarify their priorities, establish goals, and plan realistic steps to achieve them.

Rational Emotive Behavior Therapy

Like cognitive counseling, REBT focuses on thoughts and the relationships among thinking, feeling, and behavior in an effort to modify peoples' views and beliefs about events and situations and help them lead more rational lives. REBT is a directive, active, and didactic approach that seeks to minimize self-defeating thoughts, help people acquire more realistic and tolerant perspectives, and change emotions and behaviors. Extensive use is made of exercises and homework to accomplish these goals.

REBT has been used in groups for remediation, prevention, and personal development. Albert Ellis, its originator, promoted the use of REBT to foster a positive atmosphere in classrooms (Ellis & Dryden, 1997). Ellis also conducted demonstrations of REBT in groups of over 100 people. REBT has been used in marathon sessions of up to 36 hours and in open-ended and closed-ended weekly counseling groups. In group counseling, REBT tends to be leader-centered, focusing on the concerns of one memeber at a time, with group members serving as auxiliary counselors.

Behavioral Group Counseling

Behavioral counseling focuses on current undesirable behaviors and establishes treatment goals that are specific, concrete, objective, and measurable. Based on learning theory, it emphasizes behavioral change strategies such as contracting, modeling, behavioral rehearsal, self-monitoring, and reinforcement rather than insight or exploration of feelings. Counselors tend to be structured and use teaching, demonstrations, goal-setting and other strategies to facilitate change. The goal-oriented nature of behavioral group counseling facilitates assessment of both group impact and participant progress.

Behavioral counseling lends itself well to group settings. The presence of other members provides sources of feedback and reinforcement, while the microcosm of the group environment gives people a safe arena for trying out new behaviors. Typically, behavioral counseling groups are composed of people with similar behavioral concerns, such as Eating Disorders, phobias, weak social or life skills, anger management, or self-destructive habits, so that opportunities for behavioral rehearsal, modeling, group support, and social rewards and consequences are maximized.

Reality Therapy

Behavioral in nature, reality therapy as developed by William Glasser is based upon the assumption that people are fundamentally self-determining (Glasser, 1998; Wubbolding, 2000). This approach focuses on people's strengths and sense of responsibility as reflected in their present behavior. Active and directive, reality therapy seeks to ameliorate behavioral problems and improve relationships. Reality therapy has been widely used in schools as a way to promote self-esteem (a success identity) in young people and to help them learn realistic and responsible ways of meeting their needs (Glasser, 1986).

Reality therapy has great versatility in its application to group work. With its emphasis on accountability, action, and thinking, this approach can foster rapid change. Its effectiveness has been demonstrated in treating at-risk or troubled youth (Cominskey, 1993), people who misuse substances (Honeyman, 1990), and others who have not achieved rewarding and responsible lives.

Person-Centered Group Counseling

The underlying assumption of this model is that people have the potential for growth and self-determination. This potential can be facilitated through counseling that enhances self-esteem and promotes personal congruence, self-acceptance, and self-actualization (Rogers, 1970). The group counselor models and communicates the core conditions of warmth, caring, genuineness, empathy, acceptance, and positive regard. The counselor also emphasizes active listening and rarely uses exercises and assignments. The person-centered approach is not problem-centered or goal oriented but, rather, focuses on relationships, feelings, and perceptions.

Carl Rogers, the founder of this approach, popularized the use of encounter groups and personal growth groups. These groups proliferated in the 1960s and 1970s and sometimes still are used today. Person-centered counseling groups usually are designed for relatively healthy people, whose primary goals are to heighten self-awareness and improve relationships. These groups focus on the present, and they are relatively open and unstructured (Yalom, 1995). Person-centered group counseling has led to the growth of Parent Effectiveness Training, person-centered play therapy, and community groups, which are designed to build cohesiveness as well as to enhance self-exploration and facilitate multicultural communication.

The person-centered approach lends itself well to a group setting; participants in these groups can receive acceptance and develop genuine, caring, and congruent relationships not only with their counselors, but with the other members of the group. These groups provide a safe climate and models of open and honest communication.

This approach is appropriate for people with mild adjustment and situational difficulties, especially those involving problems of self-esteem and self-confidence, stage-of-life issues, and establishment of goals and direction. Its strength is in its underlying sense of optimism. Well-functioning, motivated clients who are not in crisis are most likely to benefit from this approach. Sandra integrated elements of person-centered group counseling into her treatment plan in order to promote a sense of safety and enhance self-esteem. However, this approach by itself did not offer the structure needed by Sandra's clients.

Gestalt Therapy

Gestalt Therapy, developed by Fritz and Laura Perls, is an active, present-oriented, holistic approach that seeks to integrate all aspects and polarities of a person's life. It assumes that solutions to problems are within the self; the goal of counseling is to promote awareness and remove obstacles to solutions. The Gestalt model offers a variety of techniques and exercises, including the empty chair, use of body language, dialog with parts of the self, dream work, role reversal, and homework to facilitate this process (Zinker, 1991). Gestalt group counselors also serve as teachers, models, catalysts, and activists in the group.

The Gestalt model is used in both group and individual counseling. Even in groups, however, the focus of counseling tends to be on the behaviors of individual members (Shaffer & Galinsky, 1989). Nevertheless, the presence of group members can promote self-awareness and vicarious learning. Often, having a member make the rounds, go up to all of the group members and announce or demonstrate an important insight or behavior, emphasizes the significance of that statement or behavior. The presence of others sometimes increases the threat posed by Gestalt counseling, an approach that can involve pressure and confrontation. However, the threat can be diminished by the support of the group and the freedom it affords members to chose their levels of participation in the group. People who are reluctant clients and those who engage in excessive intellectualization and rationalization are particularly likely to benefit from feedback provided in Gestalt counseling and from seeing aspects of themselves in other members.

The Gestalt approach is most appropriate for use with relatively healthy, high-functioning people who display difficulty in accessing feelings and who have mild-to-moderate emotional and behavioral disturbances. This approach can help people to take control of their lives and their feelings. However, it requires skillful use because of the directive and creative role of the counselor.

Adlerian Group Counseling

Alfred Adler developed the Adlerian approach, also known as Individual Psychology. Adlerian group counseling is insight oriented. It is predicated on the notion that, although a life script is developed during childhood, it can be changed over time. Counseling is goal-directed and focuses on strengthening the person's ego and sense of empowerment.

According to this theory, people are primarily social beings, motivated by social forces and striving to achieve certain socially determined goals. Thus, the counseling group is a logical setting for Adlerian therapy, providing a social context for goal attainment.

The Adlerian group counselor is active and interpretive. This approach is useful for addressing parent–child problems, acting-out behaviors, marital difficulties, career concerns, impaired self-confidence, and relationship problems. It is an optimistic, encouraging, empowering and nonjudgmental approach. Adlerian groups are geared primarily toward fairly high-functioning, insightful clients. Because of its emphasis on the person-in-the-environment, the Adlerian approach is particularly well suited to working with multicultural groups. Systematic Training for Effective Parenting (STEP) is based on Adlerian principles.

Psychodynamic Group Counseling

An extension of Freudian psychoanalysis, psychodynamic group psychotherapy tends to be an analytical, insight-oriented, directive, long-term treatment model. It assumes that dysfunctional behavior is an adaptive response to inner pain originating in childhood (Rutan & Stone, 1993).

The group setting provides excellent opportunities for fostering insights and understanding. The anxiety and discomfort created by being in a group of strangers can stimulate regression, transference, and defense mechanisms. By observing these phenomena, the counselor can assist participants in recognizing and interpreting their own responses, thereby gaining understanding of their reactions—within and without the group environment. The group offers a safe environment for emotionally charged interchanges and therefore can help participants to understand and consciously change their characteristic responses. Going around the group and eliciting free associations is a useful strategy associated with this approach.

Psychodynamic group counselors tend to alternate between the role of detached expert observer of group process and the role of emotionally engaged participant whose affect is available for observation by the members. The counselor uses this role duality to suggest to members responses that might not otherwise be apparent to them. The counselor also uses the safety of the group environment to become an object of transference, enabling members to observe, interpret, and discuss emotions and reactions that, in other environments, might be too frightening, embarrassing, or threatening to acknowledge.

Psychodynamic group counseling has been used in a variety of situations. People working through issues relating to trauma benefit from this approach, as do people with other long-standing concerns (Friedman, 1994; Kanas, Schoenfeld, Marmar, & Weiss, 1994). This model also has been used to modify defense mechanisms, promote development, and treat Eating Disorders.

Brief Therapy Groups

Brief therapy groups can encompass a broad range of goals, including support, social skills training, cognitive-behavioral change, or psychoeducation. This model is not new, but has come into widespread use in the 1990s and the 21st century, as economic factors play an increasing role in the delivery of mental health services. However, brief therapy groups are not merely shortened versions of traditional therapy groups, but rather adopt strategies of brief solution-focused therapy in determining specific and measurable goals, maintaining a present time orientation, and attending to planning and efficient attainment of goals (Yalom, 1995).

Brief therapy groups can be appropriately used to deal with an acute life crisis, such as job loss or bereavement; a developmental crisis, such as adjustment to college or retirement; or with a particular symptom, such as binge eating (Yalom, 1995). Brief therapy groups focus primarily on interpersonal rather than intrapersonal concerns (Klein, 1993).

Existential Group Counseling

Like existential counseling with individuals, this approach has few techniques and is more a way of thinking about helping people than a treatment system. Treatment focuses on helping people develop self-awareness, take responsibility for their lives, control their anxiety, and create more meaning in their lives. Counselors contribute greatly to the process via authenticity, use of self-disclosure, and involvement in the group process. Sharing powerful fears, such as fears of death and aloneness, and discovering that others have similar fears can be very healing and can empower people to address their inherent fears and live a rewarding life (Yalom, 1995).

Fears of death and aloneness, as well as questions about the value and future of their lives, troubled many of the women in Sandra Surber's group. Expressing these fears, and hearing others verbalize the same fears, was very helpful to the women. It normalized their reactions and enabled them to manage their fears enough so that they could move past them and find ways to make their lives meaningful.

Models Used Primarily in Group Settings

While the treatment approaches discussed in the previous section are direct outgrowths of theories developed initially for individual counseling, other models have been developed primarily for use in group counseling. These models assume that the group format is the ideal environment for helping people.

Transactional Analysis

Transactional analysis (TA) was developed by Eric Berne in the 1950s and nearly always is conducted as a group experience (Berne, 1961). The approach focuses on helping people first to change their feelings and then to change their behaviors. According to TA, each person identifies with one of the following positions: I'm ok, you're ok; I'm not ok, you are ok; I'm ok, you're not ok; or I'm not ok, you're not ok. The second position is thought to be the most common. TA's underlying philosophy is everyone is okay and is lovable and capable of growth and self-actualization. TA counseling seeks to help participants believe, "I'm ok, you're ok."

TA theorists, strongly influenced by psychoanalytic thinking, identify three ego states: parent, adult, and child. The child embodies creativity, joy, and spontaneity; the parent includes the conscience, as well as traditions, beliefs, and values needed to guide daily functioning; and the adult is the assimilator, the rational evaluator, and decision-maker. Everyone has and needs all three ego states. Counseling helps people become aware of these ego states and draw on them appropriately and in balanced ways.

TA also pays attention to transactions between people (especially between group members and group counselors), strokes and injunctions (praise and criticisms) between members, analysis of ego states, games (repetitive, self-destructive, often dishonest patterns of behavior), and scripts or blueprints for life (Seligman, 2001b). TA groups also help people develop rewarding and productive life scripts and contracts to make positive life changes.

TA groups tend to be leader centered, make considerable use of instruction and exercises, emphasize long-term treatment, and focus on one person at a time (Gladding, 2003). Leaders use education and interventions to move the group forward while providing protection as well as permission for people to change. TA is often combined with redecision therapy, which draws heavily on Gestalt therapy (Goulding, 1987). TA is used with a broad and heterogeneous client group, but seems best suited to use with people who are verbal and motivated, not in crisis or danger, and who seem likely to benefit from a structured, leader-centered experience. Such people might be experiencing long-standing depression or anxiety.

Psychodrama

Psychodrama was introduced in the United States in the 1920s by Jacob L. Moreno and has been further developed by his wife, Zerka Moreno, as well as other followers (Goldman & Morrison, 1984). This creative approach enables participants to act out problems or difficult episodes in their lives, resolve those interactions via psychodrama, and try out new and more effective methods of behavior and interaction (Battegay, 1990). The group counselor, acting as director of the drama, works with a protagonist and members of the audience to create the targeted situation and reenact it in a healthier way. Following the enactment, group members provide feedback to the protagonist and relate the drama to themselves and their concerns. This process can release inhibiting and dysfunctional feelings; provide catharsis, insight, and resolution; and help people lead more responsible and rewarding lives.

Psychodrama may be used as the predominant mode of treatment in a small group, as a demonstration in front of a large group, or as an occasional mode of individual or group treatment along with other approaches. Because the psychodrama can be geared to individual needs, it is suitable for use with a wide range of people and is only contraindicated for those who are so confused or overwhelmed by emotions that they cannot function as participants in the drama. This approach is particularly useful for elderly people (including those with some dementia) (Huddleston, 1989; Martin & Stepath, 1993); people who have experienced assault or childhood abuse (including those diagnosed with Dissociative Identity Disorder) (Altman, 1992; MacKay, 1989); people with Substance Use Disorders (Duffy, 1990); and work groups involved in problem-solving (Gillis & Bonney, 1989). It can be used effectively with children, adolescents, and adults.

T-Groups

Also termed training groups, T-groups were developed by Kurt Lewin and colleagues at the National Training Laboratories (NTL) in Bethel, Maine, in the 1940s. T-groups, an outgrowth of person-centered counseling, were widely used in the 1970s but their use has declined since. T-groups focus on the present and on process. This model assumes that people learn best by being objectively and directly confronted with observations of their behavior and how it affects others (Yalom, 1995). T-groups are used to address specific organizational problems or issues, such as leadership effectiveness, communication skills, and problem-solving in organizations. The group provides an environment in which participants can experiment with new behaviors and try out new ideas, and has been referred to as "therapy for normals" (Yalom, 1995, pp. 490–491).

Skillful group leadership is essential in this model. A poorly led group runs the risk of harming the individuals within the group and the system that houses the group. Particularly when the T-group model is used in organizational settings, caution must be exercised. The counselor or leader must have management's commitment to both the group process and the transference of new skills and strategies from the group to the real work of the organization. Otherwise, members who have risked self-disclosure may find themselves penalized rather than rewarded for their efforts.

Tavistock Groups

The Tavistock group approach was initiated in England by Wilfred Bion and further developed by A. K. Rice and Margaret Rioch. The Tavistock approach typically has been implemented at weekend or week-long institutes. Tavistock groups resemble T-groups in that they are designed to promote the personal and professional growth of people who are not suffering from significant emotional disorders. However, the structure of Tavistock groups and the leadership model they follow are quite different.

The primary emphasis of the Tavistock group is on members' relationships to the group culture (Yalom, 1995) and developing the members' abilities to function effectively in work groups. In this leader-centered model, the counselor is an observer and interpreter, with analyses often grounded in a psychoanalytic framework. The leader's role is an impersonal one, focused on the group as a whole. The leader's interpretations frequently result in the group members becoming initially demanding and dissatisfied. However, as the group becomes able to use its own resources and develops insight into group process, members' frustrations tend to lessen and they develop appreciation of the open and accepting qualities of the group environment.

Bion characterized the emotional pattern of a group according to the dichotomy of a work group or antiwork (basic assumption) activity. He further described three recurring emotional states that are a part of all group interactions: aggressiveness, optimism, and helplessness. Bion believed that group functioning is complicated by conflict, and that it is the task of the counselor and work group to expose, clarify, and work through those conflicts. This approach is controversial and is no longer widely used (Yalom, 1995).

Theme-Centered Interactional Method (Theme Groups)

Theme-centered counseling was developed primarily by Ruth C. Cohn. Typically conducted as time-limited, relatively short-term group experiences

(1–15 sessions), these counseling groups have a predetermined theme that is announced and briefly described by the group leader at the start of each session. Issues of autonomy and interdependence are particularly important to this approach as members explore their own thoughts and feelings and react to the theme as well as the input of the other members.

Theme-centered groups are structured by the leader and by the theme and take a positive and personal approach. Leaders tend to be genuine and empathic, drawing heavily on person-centered techniques, and keep the group working productively and focused on the theme. Members are encouraged to take responsibility for their own participation and learning during the sessions.

Although the theme-centered approach to group counseling never gained widespread use and attention, it is included because it is a flexible technique that offers a balance of structure and support. These qualities make this approach appropriate for use with a broad range of people, including severely disturbed clients who are not appropriate for treatment in most group settings. Theme groups that emphasize present-oriented and pragmatic concerns have been used in conjunction with other modes of counseling in day treatment centers and psychiatric facilities to promote interaction, symptom abatement, and development of clients' coping mechanisms.

GROUP COUNSELING IN CONTEXT

Counselors can apply the skills of group leadership to a variety of contexts. The group counselor usually is situated in mental health settings, schools, or organizations.

The Mental Health Group Counselor

Typically, the mental health counselor is employed in a private practice, a specialized or community mental health agency, or in a hospital. In hospitals, counselors may conduct groups for people with similar mental health or physical problems, for people about to leave the hospital and reenter the community, or for families and care-givers. In private practice and in agency settings, counselors may lead personal growth groups, heterogeneous counseling groups, or groups for people with similar concerns, such as people dealing with divorce, people who are HIV positive, and people with substance-related difficulties. Groups for elderly people may focus on life review, current events, increasing awareness of reality, and promoting motivation.

The School Group Counselor

Group counseling can be especially effective in the school setting because, as young people develop, they often look to their peers, rather than to adults, for acceptance, validation, and support (MacLennan & Dies, 1992). This format can be less threatening to youth than the prospect of developing a close relationship in one-to-one counseling with an adult. Group counseling in the schools can be preventive, growth promoting, psychoeducational, or problem-focused. Counseling groups, which provide peer support and modeling, can give adolescents a sense of belonging and can help them to separate and achieve independence from adults.

School counselors increasingly provide group counseling to address students' emotional and social needs. The following are common goals of group counseling in the school:

1. Helping children deal more effectively with specific problems or issues such as parental divorce, bereavement, bullying, peer pressure, social discomfort, college and career choices, and relationships
2. Offering support and role models
3. Providing relevant information on such issues as adolescent development, the impact of drugs and alcohol, and sexuality
4. Teaching new skills related to communication, study, socialization, leadership, stress management, self-management, assertiveness
5. Promoting children's understanding of themselves and others
6. Facilitating transitions, as from middle to high school and then to college or work

School counseling groups tend to be shorter and smaller than general counseling groups (Shechtman, 2002). They may meet for an hour or less and may only have 5–7 members in a group that will meet for 8–12 sessions. Groups sometimes are limited to only one gender, depending on the topic and the age of the participants. Cognitive behavioral therapy usually is the treatment approach used in school counseling groups but expressive-supportive groups are also useful.

In addition, school counselors increasingly offer counseling groups to parents. These groups may address specific needs or may be designed to help parents deal with their children's educational, career, personal, and social needs.

Counselors in Organizational Settings

Counselors are involved in group work through a variety of roles in business, government, and industry settings. Among these counselors are human resource administrators, career specialists, vocational rehabilitation specialists, consultants (internal and external), trainers/educators, and EAP (employee assistance program) treatment providers. Counseling groups can be especially effective in treating work-related problems such as stress, "workaholism," harassment, lack of assertiveness, and weak leadership skills. More information on counselors in organizations is provided in Chapter 10.

ROLES AND STYLES OF THE GROUP COUNSELOR

The roles of group counselors are diverse, varying according to style of leadership, nature of group, and purpose of the role. The literature identifies three broad styles of leadership:

- Authoritarian: group is leader-centered, leader gives advice, structures group process.
- Democratic: group is member-centered, leader makes suggestions but process is cooperative.
- Laissez-faire: leader gives little or no structure to the group.

Group leaders have certain functions, regardless of the types of group. These functions include organizing and structuring the group, providing information, developing a positive therapeutic alliance, promoting accomplishment of group tasks, facilitating appropriate member involvement and interaction, fostering healthy group development and dynamics, and bringing the group to a close. Exactly how a particular leader performs these functions depends on the goals of the group, the appropriate leadership style for that group, and the group members. Every group is a different and challenging experience, with new opportunities for growth for both members and leaders.

In addition to the traditional counseling roles of the group leader or facilitator, counselors interested and skilled in group counseling have a wide variety of opportunities and settings open to them. These include the following.

The Counselor as Fund-Raiser

Today's counselors must be skillful not only in clinical methods and administrative functions, but also in generating the funds needed to conduct their groups. These funds may be generated through grant writing, through lobbying government officials, through marketing programs to potential clientele, and through providing fund-raising programs and services. For many counselors, fund-raising is an unexpected but important new role. In an era of increasing budgetary constraints, counselors in all contexts must be aware of fiscal needs and resources and be creative in generating funds to sustain their work.

The Counselor as Mediator

Group counselors may take on the role of mediator between individuals in a group or between groups within an organization. In many situations, including families, schools, businesses, and governmental agencies, group counselors are increasingly mediating disputes, and teaching and facilitating conflict management.

The Counselor as Teacher/Trainer

Group counselors can teach interpersonal as well as self-management skills within a group context. For example, many school counselors train peer counselors. They also work with school faculty and staff, conducting diversity training, helping them identify and address bullying, and offering other psychoeducational training to school personnel. Counselors in corporate settings or human services agencies also train their clients as well as their colleagues in such skills as assertiveness, time management, and conflict resolution.

The Counselor as Human Resource Specialist

Counselors providing human resource management functions have an increasing role in organizations. These counselors may facilitate employee development or design human resource development programs, including training, psychoeducation, coaching, and mentoring programs. The related role of organizational development specialist is discussed further in Chapter 10.

The Counselor as Supervisor

Counselors may supervise clerical and administrative staff, students, and other counselors and mental health professionals. The role of supervisor usually combines teaching, management, and clinical abilities. Supervisors need to possess skill in active listening, problem-solving, giving feedback, communication, strategic planning, and evaluation. The role of supervisor is quite different from that of counselor, primarily because of its more evaluative and directive nature. This role shift may be disconcerting if unanticipated. Training in counselor supervision can alleviate some of the floundering that might accompany a role shift from counselor to supervisor.

OVERVIEW OF GROUP COUNSELING

With some exceptions, group counseling, especially as the primary or sole method of treatment, is most suitable for people who are in reasonably good contact with reality; who have cognitive, behavioral, or emotional concerns rather than specific situational problems; who are not severely anxious, depressed, or deficient in interpersonal skills; and who can benefit from overall personal development. Group counseling helps people develop trust, increase self-awareness and self-confidence, experience empathy for the needs and feelings of others, learn new behaviors and coping skills, improve their sense of identity, increase responsibility and effective reality testing, acquire a sense of belonging and acceptance, improve social and communication skills, modify troubling thoughts and feelings, and effectively address individual issues. Although group counseling is not helpful to everyone and is not simply a more efficient and economical variation on individual counseling, it plays an important role in the treatment of many people and can be particularly useful as an adjunct or supplementary approach to individual or family counseling.

CASES FOR DIAGNOSIS AND TREATMENT PLANNING

The following brief cases are presented to give readers an opportunity to diagnose the needs of groups and develop treatment plans designed to meet those needs. Readers should feel free to fill in the gaps in these cases by adding information that is necessary for diagnosis and treatment planning, as long as that information is congruent with the information already presented.

Case 1. You are a counselor at an urban university that has experienced multiple incidents of reported rapes and dating-related sexual violations. You have decided to conduct a counseling group for people who have reported these incidents and also would like to include in the group other people who may have experienced but not reported similar incidents. Describe how you would go about setting up the group and the plan you would follow in conducting the group. Be sure to consider issues of member selection and protection, confidentiality, and leadership roles.

Case 2. As a counselor at a community-based organization, you have observed recently that many middle-income professionals in their 40s and 50s have been seeking financial assistance due to job loss and subsequent difficulty in locating employment. You have decided to apply for a grant from a local charitable organization in order to provide group counseling services to this population. Write a plan for the counseling services you would provide. Include in your plan the specific information you would need to present in your grant proposal, following the slightly revised version of the DO A CLIENT MAP format below.

- Diagnosis and statement of need
- Objectives
- Assessments and evaluation plan
- Clinician and other staff required
- Location
- Interventions and services offered
- Emphasis
- Numbers
- Timing
- Money required (budget)

- <u>A</u>djunct services
- <u>P</u>rognosis

Case 3. In the middle school where you are a counselor, several teachers have indicated that they are having difficulties with students from single-parent families. These difficulties have been diverse, ranging from acting-out behaviors to frequent absenteeism and withdrawal and, in one case, a suspected Eating Disorder. Indicate how you might help these students via group counseling. Develop a plan that considers group objectives, member recruitment and selection, theoretical approach, numbers, timing, and how the group counseling will be provided within the context of the school.

Case 4. You are a counselor at a community mental health center. Your community has experienced forest fires that destroyed homes and caused the deaths of several residents and fire fighters. The whole community has been adversely affected by this, including those who were immediately affected by the deaths, those who lost property, and those who were indirectly affected by these experiences. Develop a multifaceted plan to help your community recover from this disaster. Your plan should include group interventions aimed toward remediation (problem resolution), prevention, and psychoeducation.

10

Counseling For Career and Organizational Development

Shannon Peters, Brian J. Peters, and Linda Seligman

OVERVIEW OF CHAPTER

This chapter discusses counseling for career development and organizational development. Career counseling typically focuses on individual development, whereas organizational development seeks to improve the functioning of a business or other organization. Both types of counseling provide people with tools to face the multiple challenges of today's work environment and help them achieve satisfaction, purpose, and outstanding performance.

Introduction to Career Development Counseling

According to Gysbers, Heppner, and Johnston (2003), career counseling shares many of the same fundamental characteristics and qualities as other types of counseling. The relationship between counselors and clients is as central to career counseling as it is in other kinds of counseling. This is reflected in Swanson's (1995) definition of career counseling as "… an ongoing, face-to-face interaction between counselor and client, with the primary focus on work or career-related issues; the interaction is psychological in nature, with the relationship between counselor and client serving an important function" (p. 245). The main difference between career and other forms of counseling is that the presenting problem usually focuses on career or work-related concerns, with assessment and information giving used frequently. Of course, as with other types of counseling, the presenting problem is often not the primary issue. Many people find it safer to seek counseling for a career-related concern than for underlying personal-emotional issues, family-related issues, and other interpersonal issues.

You might now be asking, "So why have a separate type of counseling for career-related concerns if in fact it shares many of the same guiding principles as other types of counseling?" The answer is because career-counseling theory provides a basis for what career counselors do, how they do it, and why they do it. Treatment of career-related concerns requires specialized constructs and interventions based on knowledge gained from career development theory, research, and practice. Career counseling is distinguished by its capacity to connect people's personal world to the social and economic world (Collins & Watts, 1996). Gysbers et al. (2003) suggest that the terms "career counseling" and "mental health counseling" are ways to organize theory and research and clarify focus, not ways to limit what counselors do.

Introduction to Organizational Development

Organizational development (OD) is a term that is widely used yet difficult to define. In fact, organizational development consultants may not even have a clear definition of their work. The term "organizational development" has different meanings for different people. Broadly stated, organizational development is the process of facilitating planned change in order to enhance organizational systems, structures, strategies, people, and culture. Organizational development services are designed to meet the needs and goals of employees, leaders, work groups, departments, and entire organizations.

Organizational development experts, generally referred to as OD consultants or practitioners, provide consultation and intervention services to help organizations develop programs and processes that support and maintain positive change. In this chapter, the term OD practitioner is used; this term is most appropriate for counselors who practice OD work in conjunction with their role as counselors. Foley and Redferring (1987, p. 161) define OD consultants or practitioners as "organizational change agents using behavioral science theory, research, and technology to enhance congruence between structure, process, strategy, people, culture, and environment."

Often, counselors and OD practitioners and their colleagues in the field of human resources go separate ways (Thomas & Hite, 2002). This chapter encourages counselors to broaden their perspective and look at their clients from an OD perspective.

CAREER DEVELOPMENT

This section introduces readers to the field of career development. Included are a brief history of career development, a discussion of career concerns and the importance of their context, a review of important theories of career development, information on career counseling with diverse populations, and an overview of professional development and settings for career counselors.

History of Career Development Research, Theory, and Practice

The counseling profession grew out of the foundation that career and vocational counseling established. Unfortunately, along the way, career counseling came to be narrowly defined. Many misconceptions developed, including the following: career counseling separates the work and nonwork areas of people's lives; career counseling is time-limited; career decisions take place at only one point in life; career counseling lacks psychological depth; it focuses only on outcomes and methods and ignores process.

Prior to the 1900s, little assistance was available for people wanting help with career development. Knowledge about existing career opportunities resulted primarily from contact with family, friends, church, community, and school. Boys typically followed in their fathers' footsteps, often learning the trade of their fathers. The world of work for girls meant helping their mothers and learning to care for home and family. Little literature existed prior to the 1900s on career development and guidance.

During the late 1800s and early 1900s, many people moved from rural to urban areas, which provided more diverse work opportunities. The industrial revolution of that period brought with it poor working conditions, employment of children, and depersonalization of workers. The vocational guidance movement that evolved at that time sought to improve living conditions and quality of work life and to encourage workers to believe that they actually had career choices. Early models of career counseling provided a way for people to sort out their choices. Research conducted predominantly on white, middle-class males suggested that people benefited from these early approaches to career counseling (Brown, 2003).

A movement to promote career development was born, led by Frank Parsons, known as the father of career counseling. In 1908 Parsons opened the Vocational Bureau of Boston with the purpose of helping people learn about different careers. In 1909 he wrote his famous book *Choosing a Vocation*, reprinted in 1967. The first professional organization for practitioners interested in career development, the National Vocational Guidance Association, was formed in 1913. In 1984, it became the National Career Development Association. The US Department of Labor published the first edition of the *Dictionary of Occupational Titles* (*DOT*) in 1939. (Its classification system was not replaced until 2001, with the advent of O*NET.)

Beginning in 1939, when E. G. Williams published *How to Counsel Students*, career counseling theories sprang up rapidly. The 1950s was a particularly rich time for advances in career development theory and counseling. Ginzberg, Ginzberg, Axelrad, and Herma (1951) published *Occupational Choice: An Approach to General Theory*, which presented the first theory of career development. Donald Super (1957) published the second and perhaps most influential theory of career development in

The Psychology of Careers. Anne Roe formulated the first personality-based theory of career development in 1956 in her book *The Psychology of Occupations.* The groundbreaking work of John Holland (1966) focused attention on theories of vocational choice. Countless other contributions to career development theory exist, some of which are discussed later.

Factors Enhancing Development of the Field

Since the inception of career counseling in the early 1900s, many historical events have contributed to the development of this field. Among these are:

- World War I, which necessitated assessment and testing procedures such as the Stanford-Binet Intelligence Test to facilitate job placement of people in the military;
- the 1917 Smith-Hughes Act federal grants for nationwide vocational education programs;
- the Solder's Rehabilitation Act of 1918, creating a vocational rehabilitation program for disabled veterans;
- the 19th Amendment, giving women the right to vote;
- World War II, which resulted in much of the male work force serving in the military and the need for women to fill the many open jobs;
- the programs established in 1945 to help veterans return to civilian life;
- the loss of jobs by many women when the men returned from war;
- the increasing level of skill required by industry, leading more people to attend college;
- the 1954 *Brown v. Board of Education of Topeka* decision in which the Supreme Court agreed that segregated schools are "inherently unequal" and must be abolished;
- the 1957 launch of Sputnik by the Soviet Union, leading to the National Defense Education Act. This provided funding to school systems for strengthening instruction in science, mathematics, foreign languages, and other critical subjects; counseling and testing services; training institutes in colleges; student loans and fellowships; and education for technical occupations necessary to national defense;
- the Rehabilitation Act of 1973 and its subsequent amendments that made a high priority of assisting people who are disabled people to find competitive employment;
- the Civil Rights Act of 1964 was enacted, broadening availability of educational and occupational opportunities;
- the Career Education Incentive Act 95-207 of 1977, which stated that education should be seen as preparation for work;

- the 1998 Workforce Investment Act, which provided a national employment system designed to meet both the needs of businesses and of job seekers;
- the 1999 Ticket to Work and Work Incentives Improvement Act designed to assist people with disabilities receiving SSI and SSDI via training and support that would enable them to obtain employment.

Each period of history brought with it new career-related challenges. Among these are changes in the nature of work; increased diversity of race, ethnicity, gender, and age in the work force; technological advances that affect skill development; globalization of the economy; loss of job security and downsizing; and violence in the workplace (Swanson & Gore, 2000). Career counseling, research, and theory continue to evolve and expand in response to these and other changes.

CAREER DEVELOPMENT AND CONTEXT

Just as the field of career counseling has developed in response to contextual changes, so do people's career concerns and development. Career counselors can best understand their clients by taking a comprehensive and holistic view of their concerns. According to Wolfe and Kolb (1980, p. 3), "Career development involves one's whole life, not just occupation. As such, it concerns the whole person ... in the ever-changing contexts of his/her life. The environmental pressures and constraints, the bonds that tie him/her to significant others, responsibilities to children and aging parents, the total structure of one's circumstances are also factors that must be understood and reckoned with. In these terms career development and personal development converge. Self and circumstances evolving, changing, unfolding in mutual interaction constitute the focus and the drama of career development" (p. 3). This dynamic definition of career development takes into account the many factors that play a critical role in people's life-career development.

Career Concerns and Context

Career-related concerns are inherent in the career development process. Cantor, Acker, and Cook-Flanagan (1992, p. 644) defined career concerns as "those tasks that individuals see as personally important and time consuming at particular times in their lives." The nature of these concerns usually is linked to contextual factors such as time (life stage and historical era), life circumstances, and roles. Career concerns come at different stages of development, ranging from the adolescent who is choosing a college to the person in midlife planning for retirement. Some career concerns arise from life transitions that can come by choice or are thrust upon people, such as being laid off from a job or needing to provide for a growing family.

Anderson and Niles (1995) examined the concerns that adults present when seeking career counseling. They found that many adults are dealing with such broad issues as uncertainty, ambiguity, low self-efficacy and self-knowledge, and deficits of occupational information. Anderson and Niles (2000) found that people in career counseling discussed general concerns in addition to the career-related concerns for which they sought counseling. Because work plays such a significant part in the lives of most people in our culture and is so interrelated with other aspects of their lives, career and general concerns tend to intersect (Anderson & Niles, 1995; Krumboltz, 1993).

Campbell and Cellini (1981) studied career concerns of adults and developed the Diagnostic Taxonomy of Adult Career Problems. This taxonomy reflects the great breadth of career concerns and includes the following problem areas:

1. Problems in career decision-making (e.g., getting started; information gathering; generating, evaluating, and selecting alternatives; planning implementation).
2. Problems in implementing career plans (e.g., characteristics of the individual and characteristics external to the individual).
3. Problems in organization/institutional performance (e.g., deficiencies in skills, abilities, and knowledge; personnel factors; and conditions of the organization/institutional environment).
4. Problems in organization/institutional adaptation (e.g., initial entry; changes over time; interpersonal relationships).

Aubrey and D'Andrea (1988) studied the people's midlife career concerns and found the following issues to be most common: shifting personal values; downsizing and job loss; dissatisfaction; interpersonal conflict; coping with technological advances and the need to keep skills current; and stress, competition, and relocation. Other concerns include being underemployed, entering or reentering the labor force, and the impact of age and fluency in English on career development.

CAREER COUNSELING SKILLS

These diverse concerns highlight the need for counselors to possess a wide range of knowledge and skills in order to address the variety of needs that today's clients present. Career counselors should have knowledge of mental disorders, their identification and treatment; career resources and assessment tools; conflict resolution and ways to address ambiguity and uncertainty; technology; ethical standards and practice; and multicultural counseling (Brown & Lent, 2000). In addition, career counselors need to demonstrate understanding of human development and of career development. They need to have respect for the complexity of human, social, and global issues; commitment to promoting career development; understanding of client's needs; ability to coordinate resources for meeting those needs; and respect for the worth, dignity, uniqueness, and potential of all people. Career counselors need to help clients expand their understanding of themselves; set priorities; establish short- and long-term life career goals; plan effectively; explore and understand the work of world; compare their work-related needs, plans, desires, and expectations to options available in the labor market; and achieve their career goals.

THEORIES OF CAREER COUNSELING AND DEVELOPMENT

As is evident in the previous sections, career counseling and development are multidimensional, involving interacting contextual and personal variables in ever changing environments. Most models of career counseling endorse an individualized approach in which clients' needs dictate interventions and assessment tools designed to facilitate their career development. The most significant theories of career development and counseling reflect the complex mix of environmental, social, cognitive, emotional, and behavioral factors that predict and impact people's career-related choices, satisfaction, and performance. This section provides an overview of some of the career development theories that influence current practice.

Trait and Factor Theory

Trait and factor theory stems from the early work of Frank Parsons. His premise was that the best way to choose an occupation is to know oneself and the world of work and then make a connection between the two. This approach follows a three-step procedure: (1) assess a person's traits; (2) assess the requirements of current occupations as well as labor market information; and (3) match person with an occupation. The significance of knowing oneself has long been recognized as one of the key constructs in career counseling.

In 1939, E. G. Williamson expanded the trait and factor theory by using assessment instruments to measure people's traits as well as the traits required in certain occupations. The major assumptions underlying this approach are that people's traits and occupational traits can be matched and that close matches are positively correlated with occupational success and satisfaction. This theory views career development as static rather than developmental; it does not recognize that interests, values, abilities, and personalities change.

Personal Environment Correspondence Theory

Lofquist and Dawis (1991) developed the Personal Environment Correspondence (PEC) theory. This theory takes into account the dynamic relationship of people to work environments and proposes the existence of a strong relationship between job satisfaction and work adjustment. People bring their personalities and requirements to the work environment, while the work environment has its own characteristics and requirements. For people to succeed and be satisfied, the person and the work environment need to be congruent. According to PEC theory, career counselors, therefore, should facilitate matching of workers' personality traits, needs, values, interests, and abilities with the requirements, characteristics, and reinforcers of the work environment.

The process of work adjustment can happen in both active and reactive modes. The active mode occurs when workers attempt to change the work environment. The reactive mode occurs when workers attempt to change themselves so that they correspond better with the work environment. Today this theory seems quite valuable given the constantly changing work environments. Career counselors need to assist clients to acquire skills and develop work habits that match the needs of evolving work environments, but people also need to choose contexts with which they are congruent.

Holland's Typology

Holland (1992) believes that people are attracted to certain occupations because of their personality types. These types stem from both genetics and background. According to Holland's theory, six personality types and six kinds of work environments exist in Western culture. Both personality and work environments can be categorized into realistic, investigative, artistic, social, enterprising, and conventional types. The interaction of personality and work environment determines satisfaction, stability of choice, and persistence. The goal of Holland's approach is to enhance knowledge of the self and of occupational requirements and environments in order to help people acquire a clear vocational identity.

Holland proposed the concept of differentiation, that people vary as to how clearly their personalities are represented by each of the six types. Consistency is the degree of fit between a person's personality type and that person's current or intended work environment. Holland focused on the three types a person and work environment most closely resemble upon assessment. People who resemble several types equally with no clear type preference tend to have difficulty making career decisions.

Holland represented the six types with a hexagon (see Figure 10.1). Types that are nearest to each other on the hexagon are considered to be more congruent than

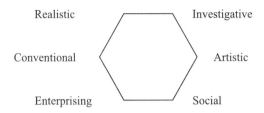

Figure 10.1. Holland's hexagon.

types that are at opposite sides of the hexagon. Rounds and Tracey (1996) found strong evidence to support the cross-cultural usefulness of Holland's Typology.

Holland suggested that having a clear vocational identity, defined as the "possession of a clear and stable picture of one's goals, interests, and talent" (Holland, 1992, p. 5), was essential to positive career development. Holland developed the Self-Directed Search (SDS) and the Vocational Preference Inventory (VIP) to measure these constructs. A person's scores on these assessment instruments suggest the sort of career counseling and choices that will be helpful.

Life-Span Life-Space Theory

Super's (1957) theory of Life-Span Life-Space is a theory of career development that emphasizes the importance of the changes that people go through as they mature and develop. Super recognized that this process of career development is complex, affected by many internal and external factors.

One factor viewed as very important in this approach is self-concept. Super viewed work as the expression of people's self-concepts and believed that self-concept had a strong impact on career development. Self-concept is defined as both the internal personal view of the self and the view of the self in a situation or unique context in which one develops and lives.

Super's Career Development Theory

This theory holds that career development is a lifelong process that proceeds in stages. The five major stages of career development are: (1) growth (birth to age 15); (2) exploratory (ages 15–24); (3) establishment (ages 25–44); (4) maintenance (ages 45–64); and (5) disengagement (65+). As people progress through these developmental stages, they negotiate developmental tasks along the way; these includes crystallization, specification, implementation, stabilization, and consolidation. The completion of these tasks is linear in nature but people can cycle and recycle through each task or group of tasks before moving on. This segment of Super's theory is referred to as Life-Span. According to Super, career maturity involves both attitudinal and cognitive factors and is defined as the readiness to master the developmental tasks of a stage of career development (Swanson & Gore, 2000).

The Life-Space segment of Super's theory focuses on people in relation to others and the different roles (e.g. child, parent, citizen, leisurite) people simultaneously inhabit throughout life. Super emphasized that people give different degrees of salience to each role at various points in their development. Finding a balance among roles is difficult, but success in one life role tends to facilitate success in other life roles. This, too, is an aspect of career development.

Career Patterns

Most of Super's ideas were derived from The Career Pattern Study, a longitudinal study that tracked the career development of a group of adolescent boys, beginning in 1951 and lasting until they were 36 years old. The study confirmed Super's theory that people move through life in predictable stages, linked to age.

Super's research also identified career patterns, determined by socioeconomic factors, mental and physical abilities, personal characteristics, and opportunities. This study provided evidence of the following four career patterns for men: (1) Stable—person skips the trial period and goes from school to stable job, staying until retirement; (2) Conventional—person progresses from initial employment to trial position to stable employment; (3) Unstable—person progresses from trial to stable to trial with establishment delayed or inhibited by occupational changes; and (4) Multiple Trial—person makes frequent occupational changes, making establishment difficult. Super's research also identified seven career patterns for women: (1) Stable Homemaker—person has little meaningful employment experience; (2) Conventional—person has brief employment interrupted by full-time home making; (3) Stable Working—person enters occupation after education and work remains the primary focus; (4) Double Track—person combines employment with homemaking; (5) Interrupted—person is employed, then focuses on childrearing with significant time out of labor force before returning to employment; (6) Unstable—person shifts from home to work to home to work; and (7) Multiple Trials—the same as men's multiple trial pattern.

Of course, career patterns for women have changed since Super's initial conceptualization with many mothers in the work force, men choosing to stay at home and care for children, and dual-career families. However, these patterns are still helpful when assisting clients in examining alternatives.

Career Maturity

For Super, career maturity involved successful negotiation of the stages of career development and successful balancing of multiple roles. Savickas (1997) agreed with Super's concepts, but proposed changing the term career maturity to career adaptability, or "readiness to cope with changing work and work conditions" (Savickas, 1994, p. 58). Career adaptability includes planning, exploration, information, decision-making, and reality orientation.

Circumscription and Compromise Theory

Gottfredson's Theory of Circumscription and Compromise examines how people narrow their career options and make choices along the way. Compromise is defined as adjusting one's career choices due to limiting factors, such as job market statistics (Gottfredson, 1981). Circumscription involves limiting one's view of acceptable occupations based on cognitive maps of occupations including the prestige of the occupation and its congruence with one's gender and social class (Gottfredson, 1996).

Gottfredson states that people's self-concepts are made up of social aspects (sex type, gender, and socioeconomic status) and psychological aspects (values, personality variables, and intelligence), with social aspects generally having a greater influence on people's choices. Gottfredson proposed that people progress through the following four developmental stages during circumscription: (1) orientation to size and power (ages 3–5); (2) orientation to sex roles (ages 6–8); (3) orientation to social valuation (ages 9–11); and (4) orientation to internal, unique self (beginning at age 12). As they progress through the developmental stages, people add more criteria to their preferences for an occupation.

Gottfredson found that people unnecessarily circumscribe their career options and, as a result, sometimes sacrifice fulfillment of their internal selves in order to meet their expectations regarding job prestige and appropriate gender choices (Brown, 2003). The goals of this approach include helping people develop self-concepts that integrate subjective and objective aspects of the self and prevent or reverse unnecessary restriction in people's early career development. Accomplishment of these goals can facilitate people's efforts to make good matches of their internal selves with realistic career choices.

Decision-Making Theory

Many of the career-related decisions people make have a significant impact on other areas of their lives such as life-style, choice of friends, leisure activities, and place of residence. Gati and Asher (2001) define career decision-making as the process people engage in when they search for career alternatives, compare them, and then make a choice. Career decision-making, therefore, includes the person who makes the decision, the possible alternatives, and the person's selection criteria. Making career decisions is often a complex task with too many alternatives, too much information, and too much input from others. This can lead to feelings of discomfort, anxiety, and confusion, although some people negotiate this process effortlessly (Osipow, Walsh, & Tosi, 1980).

Tiedeman & O'Hara (1963) decision-making model focuses on the decision-making process more than on the outcome of the decision. This model links career development theory to other psychological theories such as Erikson's developmental stages. According to Tiedeman, what makes decision-making difficult is the challenge of integrating the need for individuation and the need to remain connected to society. Successful accomplishment of this integration requires differentiation and sound self-awareness (Miller-Tiedeman & Tiedeman, 1990). Tiedeman viewed this struggle for integration as a lifelong process.

Decision-making entails progressing through a series of stages:

- Exploration (pondering a course of action and reflecting on aspirations, abilities, and interests within the societal context)
- Crystallization (continued assessment of alternatives leading to stability of thought)
- Choice (definitive goal is selected and behaviors identified, to promote goal attainment)
- Clarification (developing confidence in the choices)
- Induction (progression toward integration of individuation and social purpose)
- Reformation (assertive action to promote the self-view in relation to others)
- Integration

The first four stages involve anticipation, while the final three stages promote implementation and adjustment to the occupation.

THEORETICAL CONCEPTS OF THE PROCESS OF CAREER DECISION-MAKING

This chapter now focuses on theories that help people negotiate the career decision-making process. Sampson (1981) found that often people's dysfunctional thoughts regarding themselves and the world of work inhibited readiness to make career decisions. Lack of readiness can also reflect an unwillingness to take responsibility for making a decision or a lack of confidence in the ability to make wise decisions.

Some theorists hypothesize that there are critical points in people's lives when they make choices that greatly influence their career development such as choices of schools, initial jobs, and occupational changes. Other decision-making theorists are more concerned with ongoing choices across the life span. Decisions people make are influenced by their awareness of the choices that are available to them and their knowledge of how to evaluate those choices.

Hansen's Integrative Life Planning

Hansen's Integrative Life Planning (ILP) emphasizes the integration of the mind, body, and spirit (Niles & Harris-Bowlsbey, 2002). The ILP model proposes six developmental tasks for adults including finding work that needs doing, weaving the roles of life into a meaningful whole, connecting family and work, valuing pluralism and inclusivity, managing personal and organizational transitions, and exploring spirituality and life purpose.

Cognitive Information Processing Perspective

Peterson, Sampson, and Reardon (1996) developed the Cognitive Information Processing (CIP) perspective. According to this model, the ultimate goal of career counseling is facilitating the growth of information-processing skills and enhancing clients' capabilities as career problem-solvers and decision makers. The attributes that contribute to this process are self-knowledge, cognitive skill, and healthy emotional functioning.

The CIP perspective views career development and decision-making as ongoing processes, involving continual growth, learning, and change. Counselors help clients with these processes by enabling people to identify their needs, develop relevant knowledge and skills, and use information in career problem-solving and decision-making. According to this theory, use of the following sequential procedure can improve cognitive processing, facilitate decision-making, and lead to solutions of career-related problems. This sequential procedure includes:

1. Communication—the problem is examined by identifying the gap between the current situation and the desired outcome.
2. Analysis—the causes of the problem and barriers to closing the gap are identified.
3. Synthesis—possible courses of action are examined by first generating all possible solutions and then narrowing down the choices to the most feasible alternatives.

    4. Valuing—chosen alternatives are prioritized according to the client's value system, taking into consideration costs and benefits to the client's world.

    5. Execution—implementation of first-choice alternative is planned and implemented.

After the plan is executed, clients revisit the communication phase to determine whether the gap has been closed and the problem solved. If counselors and clients agree that the work has been successful, clients can move onto the next problem or gap. If not, clients must recycle the process with the new information they acquired about themselves and their options.

Values-Based Theory

Brown's (1996) values-based theory suggests that most people's motivations and behaviors stem from their values. According to this theory, interests do not play a major role in career choice; rather, it is values, developed through interaction of inherited characteristics and life experiences, that are the primary determinant of career decisions.

Helping people clarify and prioritize their values is fundamental to this approach. Value clarification goes beyond matching traits and interests to work environments and focuses on the meaning that people place on work and other life experiences. People must choose the values that define who they are and what sort of life they want to lead (Cochran, 1997). Making these decisions can be difficult for people who lack cognitive clarity or have conflicting values, because such decisions require that one value be sacrificed for another more highly prized value. If people understand their values and have value-based information they will be more likely to make effective decisions. Asking people what they want out of life and a career is one way to help them understand what they value. This can be an especially useful approach to understanding clients from cultural backgrounds that value commitment to family values more than finding a rewarding career. The role of counselors is to help clients clarify what values are important to them and find ways to express their values through their work as well as through other aspects of their lives (Niles & Bowlsbey, 2002; Patton & McMahon, 1999).

This theory suggests that no decision is made in isolation. In light of this, career counselors need to take into account clients' diagnoses, mental status, interpersonal concerns, and other important aspects of their lives and make appropriate referrals as needed.

Learning Theory of Career Counseling

Krumboltz (1979) developed the Learning Theory of Career Counseling (LTCC). He proposed that social learning exerts a powerful influence on career decision-making and development. Social learning refers to the knowledge and attitudes that people acquire from role models, experiences and behaviors that are rewarded and reinforced, and messages they receive from family and society.

LTCC includes many concepts that reflect current thinking about career development. It views career decision-making as a lifelong endeavor that must be learned. It emphasizes that there is no one right occupational choice for a person. The theory recognizes the impact of people's background and beliefs on their career choices and development. Finally, it encourages people to expand their capabilities and interests and prepare for changing work tasks, thus empowering them to be active participants in their own career development.

Planned Happenstance theory, based on Krumboltz's LTCC, is designed to help clients by facilitating the generation of meaning, recognition, and incorporation of chance events into their career development (Mitchell, Levin, & Krumboltz, 1999). Indecision, usually seen as undesirable, is viewed according to Planned Happenstance as a realistic mindset for a chaotic, constantly changing world. People are encouraged to act on curiosity and be open-minded about themselves and their options. Rather than waiting for chance or fate to occur, people learn to maximize the likelihood of chance happenings by actively exploring all options.

Social-Cognitive Theories

This theory incorporates learning theory, as well as the role of cognitive factors, in determining career decisions. The theory also draws on Bandura's (1986) social-cognitive theory and the self-efficacy theory of Hackett and Betz (1981). Hackett and Betz (1981) and Lent and Hackett (1987) contributed to this theory by applying social learning theory to the field of career counseling. According to these theorists, three related social-cognitive variables (self-efficacy beliefs, outcome expectations, and personal goals) interact in a dynamic and reciprocal way with aspects of the individual (gender and ethnicity, environmental issues, and learning experiences) to determine career decisions, development, and performance.

Self-efficacy, outcome expectations, and personal goals are important concepts for career counselors. *Self-efficacy* is the belief people hold in their ability to successfully complete a given task. People tend to attempt tasks at which they feel they will succeed at and avoid tasks at which they believe they will fail. Factors that contribute to people's sense of self-efficacy are prior accomplishments, seeing others like themselves succeed at the task, and being told they can accomplish the task. The belief people have about the outcome of a specific behavior is referred to as *outcome expectation*. *Personal goals* reflect a commitment to action steps to achieve a given outcome. Personal goals organize and guide behaviors. Together, self-efficacy and outcome expectations promote career-related interests. Interests, in turn, influence personal goals and goal-oriented actions. Finally, the outcome of the actions determines whether self-efficacy is strengthened or weakened. Through this process, people are able to make decisions and reach goals.

Using this theory, career counselors help clients by enhancing self-efficacy, promoting realistic outcome expectations, and teaching goal-setting skills. Niles and Harris-Bowlsbey (2002) suggested that this theory can address problems of performance and persistence in overcoming obstacles, as well as modify dysfunctional beliefs that contribute to low self-efficacy.

Other Relevant Theories

Many other theories of career decision-making and development have been advanced. Some of these, like narrative career counseling and constructivist career counseling, reflect the application of general theories of counseling to the career arena. Others were developed specifically for career counselors. Although an exhaustive presentation of these approaches is beyond the scope of this book, the theories that have been reviewed reflect the importance to career counselors of concepts of development, self-image and self-efficacy, goals and values, learning experiences, integration, and the personal characteristics and context of the client.

CAREER COUNSELING WITH DIVERSE CLIENTS

In an increasingly diverse society, counseling for career development must address the "effects of social and economic barriers such as economic hardship, immigration disruption, and racial discrimination on the career behavior of ethnic minority individuals" (Leong, 1996, p. 550). Career counselors need to know clients' worldviews and contexts in order to make appropriate interventions.

Blustein (1994) defined context as "that group of settings that influence developmental progress encompassing contemporary and distant familial, social, and economic circumstances" (p. 143). All behavior, including career development, occurs within a cultural context. "Individuals are shaped through the differential exposure that occurs according to gender, race/ethnicity, sexual orientation, socioeconomic status, and disability—factors that help to form people's environments and their life experiences, as well as their responses to the environment" (Swanson & Gore, 2000, p. 248).

Recent research has investigated groups of people whose career development may differ from the groups that have received most of the research attention— middle-class, able-bodied, heterosexual, Caucasian males. Initially, research focused on between-group differences. The next step in research was to focus on within-group differences, that is, variation or naturally occurring differences among people within the same group. Currently, diversity issues are being incorporated into career counseling theory and practice, with contextual issues viewed as especially important in career development. A currently debated issue is whether it is necessary to develop separate theories of career development for multicultural clients or new theories that are broad enough to include all groups (Harmon, 1997; Leong & Brown, 1995; Meara, 1997).

Leong (1996) developed an integrative model of career development that suggests that counselors need to attend to three dimensions of people's personality and identity: the universal, the group, and the individual. All three are of equal importance and should be viewed as dynamic. Leong and Serafica (2001) proposed that this theory could be combined with other theories of career development to make them culturally valid.

PROFESSIONAL DEVELOPMENT AND SETTINGS FOR CAREER COUNSELING

The National Career Development Association (NCDA), a division of the American Counseling Association, is the leading professional association specifically for career counselors. According to NCDA, career counselors have many roles including individual and group counseling; clarifying life/career goals; administering and interpreting objective and subjective inventories to assess abilities, aptitudes, interests, values, and personality; identifying career options; encouraging exploratory activities; utilizing career planning and occupational information systems; promoting better understanding of the world of work; facilitating improved decision-making skills; assisting in development of individualized career plans; teaching job-search strategies; assisting in resume writing; helping resolve potential conflicts on the job; promoting understanding of the integration of work and other life roles; and helping people who are experiencing job stress, job loss, and career transitions (Zunker, 2002). Many tools, such as objective and subjective inventories, are available to assist career counselors in their practice. The Internet has greatly expanded the number of resources available to career counselors; these include labor market information and trends, job-search websites, occupational information, and information on resume writing.

School and college counselors, vocational rehabilitation counselors, career counselors in community settings and private practice, counseling psychologists, teachers, social workers, placement specialists, employee assistance counselors, and others help people with career and educational issues. OD practitioners, discussed in the next section of this chapter, also deal with career-related issues. An overview of a career counseling case study in the context of an organization is presented in the last section of this chapter, illustrating the work of both career counselors and OD practitioners.

ORGANIZATIONAL DEVELOPMENT

Counselors have a broad array of clinical skills that can be used not only to help individual clients with their difficulties but also to solve organizational challenges and problems. Counselors have excellent interviewing skills, know how to ask clear questions, and understand people well (Harmon, 2001). Counselors have empathy and insight. They can facilitate group and family sessions and are used to dealing with diversity. Counselors help clients develop awareness, generate alternatives, and create the motivation to take action. All of these skills are essential for OD practitioners as well as for other types of counselors.

The opening sections of this chapter provided a definition of OD. This section (1) provides a brief history of OD; (2) examines key theories of OD; (3) summarizes the process of OD; and (4) discusses the connections between the OD process and the counseling process.

History of Organizational Development

The beginning of interest in and attention to people in organizational contexts is often attributed to Frederick W. Taylor, whose writings led to improved recognition and productivity for industrial workers in the early 1900s (Newstrom & Davis, 1993). Lillian Gilbreth and Whiting Williams followed Taylor's work with publications emphasizing the importance of the human side of work. Smither, Houston, and McIntire (1996) attribute the birth of OD to psychological studies conducted in the 1920s and 1930s at the Hawthorne plant of the Western Electric Company. In the famous illumination study at that plant, researchers found that workers improved their productivity every time the researchers paid attention to them.

The actual term OD can be traced to group counseling, more specifically the T-group (Smither et al., 1996). In the late 1940s, the Research Center for Group Dynamics sponsored intergroup relations workshops (T-groups) under the direction of Kurt Lewin. Throughout these sessions, participants shared feedback on the behavior of group members. Many organizations instituted T-group programs with the goal of raising employee productivity and morale by improving communication between employees.

OD emerged in the late 1950s and 1960s out of theories of group dynamics and planned change (French & Bell, 1999). Argyris (1957), Likert (1961), McGregor (1966), and other mid-20th-century writers pointed out that much evidence suggested that organizational practices affect mental health. The "human relations movement" called attention to dysfunctional aspects of management and advocated more people-oriented styles of management that addressed the social and psychological needs of employees. Each decade, more literature appears on organizational dynamics in an attempt to understand, predict, and control the effect the workplace has on people's lives and vice versa (Foley & Redfering, 1987).

Theories of Organizational Development

OD practitioners, like counselors, base their practice on a theoretical foundation that guides their work with clients. OD practitioners use this foundation to plan and implement change programs in an organizational context. Current theories of OD demonstrate the complex mix of environmental, social, cognitive, emotional, and personal factors that impact workers and workplaces (Thomas & Hite, 2002). This section provides an overview of theories for thinking about planned change in OD efforts.

Kurt Lewin's Three-Stage Model of the Change Process

This chapter previously mentioned Kurt Lewin's work with people in T-groups. Lewin also developed a model that can be used to understand the change process in organizations. Lewin suggested that change is a three-stage process (Schein, 1987):

1. *Unfreezing:* Creating motivation and readiness to change.
2. *Changing through Cognitive Restructuring:* Helping clients to see, evaluate, and react differently based on a new point of view.
3. *Refreezing:* Helping clients to integrate the new point of view.

Lewin stressed that in making efforts to change, the "field," or organization as a whole, must be taken into account, including both its psychological and nonpsychological aspects (Smither et al., 1996). OD practitioners study the organization as a systematic web of relationships, not as discrete parts. In this respect, the morale of one supervisor can affect the morale of a staff, which will affect the quality of the organization's products and customer service.

Systems Theory

Systems theory views organizations as systems in open exchange with their environments. Complex human variables such as values, roles, and attitudes all play an important part in the connection between organizational systems and their external environments (Smither et al., 1996). The use of the term "system" implies interdependency, interconnectedness, and interrelatedness among elements in a set that constitutes an identifiable whole or gestalt (French & Bell, 1999). Smither et al. (1996) stated that organizations are a special type of open system; organizational roles are tied together by a network of communication that allows people in an organization to operate as a single organism. Any OD effort changes a whole system, not just any single component or part. For example, providing coaching to a leader to empower employees can contribute to the development of an organizational culture that supports increased productivity, higher employee satisfaction, and greater customer satisfaction.

Murray Bowen's Family Systems Theory

Bowen's family systems theory, discussed earlier in Chapter 8, is a systems theory about the family and the larger social systems of which their members are a part (Comella, 1996). Bowen's theory focuses on the family as a functional unit, addressing the process of mutual influencing and interdependency within the unit (Fox, 1996). An organization can also be viewed as a functional unit, as can the department and work groups within the unit. Bowen's theory differs from general systems theory in the OD literature because of its focus on the organization as an emotional system. For example, Bowen stresses that responses are affected by the level of anxiety experienced within the system and the system's ability to tolerate the anxiety.

Behavior within an organization may be an automatic response rather than a conscious choice (Fox, 1996). For example, an employee may respond to a poorly communicated organizational change by unconsciously resisting organizational policies, by coming in late, or by not completing required paperwork. Emotional forces can support or undermine policies, procedures, plans, and initiatives (Kerr, 1996). Bowen's theory reminds OD practitioners that dilemmas in organizations are human dilemmas.

Wiseman (1996), who extends the concept of the emotional process to the internal forces within OD practitioners, suggests that OD practitioners see their role as providing assistance to a system while also managing their own emotional reactions to the organization. Bowen's theory can help OD practitioners think about, rather than simply react to, the emotional process in both the organization and themselves. OD practitioners then can help the leaders and staff of an organization deal with their own emotions, become more aware that change and adaptation are a natural and necessary part of all systems, and come up with creative solutions that are beneficial to both the individual and the organization.

Organizational Development and Counseling

As organizations recognized the counseling needs of employees, Employee Assistance Programs (EAPs) were established (Zunker, 2002) in the early 1940s. EAPs provide counselors another role in organizations. EAPs have proven effective in assisting employees with problems of daily living and are essential to helping an organization both meet its productivity goals and take responsibility for the welfare and success of the employees (Balgopal, 1989). EAPs provide employees and organizations with many types of assistance, including mental health and wellness programs.

Peters (2000) noted that EAP counselors are a valuable asset to organizations and should not work in isolation. An important goal of EAP counselors should be to establish strong and continued rapport between the EAP and the systems within the organization including the human resources department, the Equal Opportunity Employment (EEO) office, the union, the health unit, and the different levels of management.

The Organizational Development Process

The scope of some EAPs has expanded to include OD services, but these are often limited to trainings that introduce such elements of OD as team building and dealing with change. OD interventions, on the other hand, are generally long-term and systemic efforts (French & Bell, 1999). The OD program usually begins when leaders identify a problem within their organization and seek help to address the problem. Leaders may turn to the human resources department or EAP to request services and then may be referred to OD consultants or specialists. Leaders meet with OD practitioners to explain the problem and look at potential solutions. The OD practitioners prepare a proposal that outlines the tasks, deliverables, and costs. Leaders review the proposal and decide whether there seems to be a good fit between their organization and the consultant and program being recommended.

Engaging in organizational change can be a daunting and sometimes unpredictable process. Leaders and managers often wonder where to begin, what to take into account, how to overcome resistance, and how to ensure that the changes made will be successful. OD practitioners help organization members create plans, improve processes, assess training needs, implement change, and deal with the anxiety around the process. Just as counselors partner with the individual client, OD practitioners partner with the client organization to provide support from beginning to end. OD practitioners:

- Seek to understand each work group or organization's unique needs in order to determine the most appropriate interventions.
- Develop a project plan, including goals and objectives, timelines, and deliverables for each step of the process.
- Provide support that is needed to keep the project moving and implement changes.
- Maintain frequent communication with key personnel within the organization so there are no surprises.

- Solicit feedback from key personnel in order to monitor the process and ensure that the plan and services match the specific needs of the organization.
- Help the organization evaluate the results of the OD effort and develop internal programs to support the changes and address additional needs.

Key to the successful OD effort is to never underestimate the time and cost commitment for both the practitioner and the client. Similarly, OD practitioners should be sure never to promise more than they can deliver. As counseling professionals and human beings, OD practitioners are often eager to please and make changes that will improve people's lives. However, they must be cautious and establish clear goals and expectations with the client. Wiseman (1996) stressed that the role of the OD practitioner is to "think" systems and to provide knowledge about how systems function, not to provide answers.

Assessment

Once the organization's leaders and the OD practitioners have an agreement to work together, a thorough assessment is the next step. One of the most fundamental practices in conducting an OD effort is making a proper diagnosis of organizational problems (Smither et al., 1996). It is not enough to have been told by leaders or management, for example, that employees have low morale or communications problems. These statements may be correct from their perspective. However, staff problems are generally symptomatic of larger systemic issues such as management practices or an organizational culture that does not adequately promote employee satisfaction or performance.

There are two main approaches to conducting the assessment: interviews and surveys. A thorough and well-conducted assessment using either or both of these approaches assists OD practitioners in gaining a clear understanding of employees' perceptions of key facets of the organization, including but not limited to such variables as leadership, supervision, diversity, feedback, and ethics. This assessment will help in:

- Focusing groups on development needed to create high-performing teams
- Helping employees identify attitudes that inhibit job growth and satisfaction
- Providing comprehensive data for problem-solving and improvement initiatives
- Identifying strengths that can be celebrated by the organization
- Monitoring employees' satisfaction and identifying trends.

Interviews. Interviews are a primary source of information for most OD practitioners. Counselors can use their skills to form an empathic relationship with interviewees that increases the likelihood of honest reporting and responses. Interviews can serve the valuable purpose of providing employees with an opportunity to express their concerns and frustrations and feel heard. The drawback to interviews is that the process can be time consuming for large employee groups. Group interviews can streamline the process, although sometimes one-to-one interviews are preferred.

Individual Interviews. Individual interviews vary in duration but usually last at least 1 hour. In the interviews, employees are asked a series of questions that are usually prepared in advance and included in an interview guide that was reviewed by key personnel involved in the project. OD practitioners prepare the interview guide with questions developed in collaboration with the key personnel who initiated the OD intervention. Typical questions for a work group include:

- What are the strengths of this work group?
- How would you describe communication in your work group?
- What would you like to see as a result of this process?

The degree to which the questions are structured depends on the importance of making comparisons among employees' responses and drawing inferences about specific topic areas (Smither et al., 1996). The more structured the interview, the more the interviews can be compared to each other to draw valid conclusions about the group being assessed. A structured interview is especially useful for helping novice OD practitioners to reduce their anxiety, gather relevant data, and structure their time effectively.

OD consultants may begin an interview by briefly talking about their own experience and credentials, their role in the current OD process, the purpose of the interviews, and guidelines for confidentiality. A clear understanding of the OD process reinforces employees' sense that they are influential in the effort and engages them as allies. Confidentiality is maintained by reporting themes that come up with employees rather than reporting or quoting specific details, unless employees agree that it would be beneficial to disclose some particular piece of information. Unlike clinicians, OD consultants focus the interview on issues pertinent to the work environment, not to people's personal lives. Information gathered should be relevant to the assessment and improvement of the organization rather than the individual. OD practitioners may refer employees to the EAP or other resources if personal issues are affecting their performance within the organization. At first, this may seem incompatible with counselors' usual roles. However, boundaries should be maintained between mental health counseling and OD. OD practitioners should be careful to avoid clinical terminology such as *diagnose*, *analyze*, or *treat*, as this may cause employees to feel like they are being questioned by a therapist, which is inappropriate in an OD effort.

Group Interviews. An alternative to the individual interview is the group interview or focus group. Focus groups may be used in place of, or in conjunction with, individual interviews as a more cost- and time-effective option. In focus groups, OD practitioners act as facilitators and pose questions to the group. Observing the group dynamics in itself can provide a wealth of data about communication, conflict, and intensity of feelings within the organization.

Interviews are often the sole assessment tool when working with a very small number of employees or when very broad open-ended questions are most useful (Smither et al., 1996). However, surveys may be used along with or instead of interviews.

Surveys. OD practitioners use two main types of surveys: customized surveys and standardized surveys. Information obtained from interviews may be used to develop customized questionnaires or surveys. Customized surveys are designed for a specific client organization. However, they have limited validity and reliability if they are not carefully constructed by survey experts. Standardized organizational and team climate surveys are available from testing companies and have normative data so that comparisons can be made between one organization and those on which the survey was normed. These surveys typically are easily administered and scored and have extensive data on validity and reliability. Standardized surveys help "take the temperature" of the organization or work group and provide quantitative data that can be powerful when interpreted back to the organization.

Feedback: Findings and Recommendations

Once OD practitioners have gone through the assessment phase, the next step is to create a report that summarizes findings and makes recommendations regarding ways to address problematic issues. This report is first reviewed with leaders and other key personnel involved in the OD effort. Often there will be some results that are difficult for leaders to hear as they relate to issues surrounding leadership. Counselors use their clinical skills to develop trust and instill hope during this phase.

A summary of the results can be provided next in a feedback session to the entire staff. OD practitioners and organizational leaders agree on a format for the session, often facilitated by the OD practitioner. Plans to implement improvement initiatives are far more likely to occur when management shares assessment results with its workers (French & Bell, 1999). Sharing the results with employees can be very effective in communicating that problems expressed have been heard and providing employees with a sense of ownership in the change effort.

During this stage, goal setting for the OD effort begins. Three basic rules of setting goals are recommended: (1) make the goals specific, (2) make the goals attainable, and (3) make the goals measurable (Gibson, Ivancevich, & Donnelly, 1982).

The Intervention Process

Smither et al. (1996) define the intervention as the procedure the OD practitioner uses, after diagnosing an organizational situation and providing feedback, to address the identified organizational problems. At this point, the OD practitioner should develop a framework of steplike procedures so that progress can be monitored and the program can be revised as needed (Foley & Redfering, 1987). The following are some of the major types of OD interventions that are used to address organizational needs.

Team Building

A variety of team-building programs have been designed to improve the productivity of existing teams, educate team leaders, and give new teams the right start. Counselors' communication skills are important in their role as OD practitioners. These skills can help them acquire useful insights into organizational group dynamics, provide hope for improvement to team members, and apply solution-based strategies. Team-building programs help team leaders and members achieve the following goals:

- Identify team strengths and weaknesses
- Clarify issues facing the team
- Understand different communication and conflict resolution styles
- Identify problem-solving and decision-making skills
- Understand behaviors under stress
- Empower the team and team leader
- Balance the need for individuality and togetherness
- Develop an action plan for maintaining continuous improvement

Leadership Coaching and Management Skills Training

OD practitioners can help leaders develop and fine-tune their leadership skills to maintain high performance in the workplace. OD practitioners work collaboratively with leaders to evaluate essential leadership competencies and design individually tailored feedback and action-oriented coaching programs. Counselors often have a great deal of insight into the interpersonal skills required to assist leaders to foster creativity, innovation, and renewal in their organization. These programs help leaders better understand:

- How leadership style and communication impacts a person's ability to lead
- How to coach employees to enhance performance
- The role of emotions in the workplace

- Ways to supervise difficult employees
- Career and life planning
- How to promote career and life planning

Organizational Planning and Change Management

OD practitioners collaborate with organizational members to create plans, improve procedures, assess training needs, and implement change. In this way, OD practitioners help the organization to accomplish the following:

- Evaluate and build on organizations' strengths
- Analyze the environment for workplace trends and opportunities
- Identify the internal and external barriers to the success of organizations' vision
- Determine how current systems can change to support a strategic direction
- Communicate the plan to employees

Training

Training is essential to help employees to develop competencies and adjust to new demands precipitated by organizational change (French & Bell, 1999). While training alone does not make an OD effort, the OD process itself often suggests the need for additional training. Counselors have experience informing, explaining, and educating, and therefore can provide training (Harmon, 2001). Counselors who focus on issues dealing with work life often provide training on stress management, dealing with difficult people, and other topics that relate to the workplace.

Leaders within an organization may contact OD practitioners requesting training to solve organizational dilemmas. However, practitioners should do an assessment of the nature and history of the problem and the desired outcome goals before agreeing to offer training. Often, training is seen as a quick fix to a problem. In the long run, however, interventions focusing on assessing and altering organizational structure and policies may be more cost effective than traditional training interventions that are mostly educational in nature (Korman, 1994). Employees' awareness of the existing problems, along with feelings that they have no control over work situations, can lead to increased stress and dissatisfaction and a need for interventions that go beyond education.

Evaluation

The extent to which goals of the OD effort have been achieved should be assessed throughout and at the conclusion of the effort. Practitioners should be aware that leaders who initiated the effort may perceive the evaluation as a potential threat;

if it is shown to be unsuccessful, they may fear that they will be blamed for its failure (Smither et al., 1996). OD practitioners should ensure that the evaluation measures are determined, as much as possible, prior to or early in the process of intervention and reflect the goals of the overall intervention. Porras and Berg (1978) have proposed that OD practitioners focus evaluation on two key areas of organizational life: (1) the OD effort's effects on social interactions such as trust and communication and (2) the effort's effects on organizational outputs such as productivity, quality, job satisfaction, and turnover.

CASE ILLUSTRATION IN ORGANIZATIONAL DEVELOPMENT

This section presents a simplified case illustration of an OD effort. The case summarizes the OD process, including career development interventions provided to an employee.

Kick-Off and Assessment

Reports of declining employee morale, conflict within work groups and between the three work groups and their supervisors, and employee performance problems led a newly appointed manager of a division within the company to seek the help of an OD practitioner. The manager and the OD practitioner spoke at length on the telephone and then met in person. The manager was motivated to address the identified issues and agreed to have the OD practitioner conduct a thorough assessment, including the administration of a standardized organizational survey and individual interviews of all 35 staff members. The OD practitioner also met with representatives of the Equal Opportunity Office and the union to develop customized survey items that assessed staff perceptions of the right to exercise employee rights and the ability to address areas of concern with supervisors and management.

The following central themes were identified in the surveys and interviews:

1. Employees enjoy their work.
2. Employees believe that the work they do is important.
3. Employees trust the division manager and are cautiously optimistic about the initiative to improve the work environment.
4. Employee morale is declining as a result of autocratic leadership by team supervisors.
5. Employees do not feel free to approach work group leaders with problems due to their autocratic leadership styles.
6. Employees do not feel a sense of teamwork within their respective work-groups and across work groups in the division.

7. Employees are not held accountable for paperwork, which often needs to be redone by supervisors or a select group of high-performing employees.
8. Employees expressed frustration with the way paperwork was processed.
9. Employees want better communication within the division and expressed anger that regular staff meetings were not there.

The OD practitioner summarized the assessment in a meeting with the division manager and recommended a comprehensive 6-month OD program that included the following elements:

• Individual feedback sessions for the three work group supervisors.
• Feedback session for staff to report assessment results and introduce the follow-up phase of the OD effort.
• Group and individual coaching for the work group supervisors.
• Team-building programs for each work group and the division as a whole.
• The formation of a process improvement team, composed of nonsupervisory staff members who would develop recommendations to improve the paperwork processing and set up a system of division staff meetings. This team would meet biweekly for the duration of the OD effort and be facilitated by the OD practitioner.

Intervention

During the next 6 months, all of these services were implemented. The initial feedback sessions with the work group supervisors met with the most resistance and unease. Supervisors tended to blame the employees for not being motivated and not following procedures. All three supervisors were coached on the following:

• Application of a variety of motivational theories and leadership styles
• Giving and receiving criticism and praise to enhance employee performance
• Understanding emotions in the workplace

By developing rapport with the supervisors in the individual sessions and establishing rapport among the supervisors in the group sessions, both supervisors and employees reported much improved satisfaction and performance in the division. The supervisors agreed that the most valuable tool they acquired was developing their nonjudgmental listening skills so that employees felt encouraged to go to them with more information.

Team-building sessions for the individual work groups and the division as a whole focused on exploring:

• Preferred work styles

- Communication and conflict resolution styles and techniques
- Individual and team action plans for continuous improvement

The process improvement team developed recommendations for a new system to process paperwork within the division and a weekly and monthly staff meeting schedule. These recommendations were then proposed to the rest of the division staff, the work group supervisors, and finally the division manager for review. Implementation occurred with only minor revisions. Enabling all employees to have an impact on decision-making in the management of work significantly contributes to both employee satisfaction and overall organizational effectiveness.

Throughout the process, the OD practitioner worked closely with the division manager and established a high level of rapport and trust. The division manager reported stress stemming from new roles and responsibilities. The OD practitioner recognized multiple symptoms of anxiety in conversations with the manager about both work and family life. The OD practitioner suggested that the manager talk to the company's EAP counselor about ways to deal with the stress. The division manager followed through on this recommendation and reported a significant reduction in stress as a result of practicing some basic stress-reduction techniques.

Evaluation and Follow-Up

Many positive changes were evident at the conclusion of the OD effort. Errors in paperwork processing were significantly reduced. Staff meetings, led by work group supervisors and a revolving staff member, were held on a regular schedule. This resulted in reports of improved communication throughout the division as well as enhanced feelings of empowerment in staff members. The work group supervisors were amazed at the results of the group problem-solving process. The amount of informal complaints to the EAP office and union were significantly reduced as staff grew increasingly comfortable working out problems among themselves and with their supervisors.

At the end of the OD program, the division manager agreed to administer the standardized organizational survey 1 year after the initial administration to quantitatively evaluate the success of the program. The OD practitioner and the division manager also agreed on a third phase of the program in the form of an annual retreat that would include team-building and group problem-solving components.

Conclusion

Few professions equip people with the skills necessary to perform effectively as an OD practitioner as well as in the field of counseling. Carey and Varney (1983) identified interpersonal skills and perceptiveness as the critical skills predicting the success or failure of an OD effort. Counselors possess interpersonal skills and perceptiveness related to both their training and, quite often, to their basic personality. Finally, although the transition from "couch to corporation" may be a natural one, counselors who are interested in working as OD practitioners must be committed to putting in long hours learning about organizations and the numerous ways to diagnose and treat the organization and its employees (Martin, 1996). With some homework, the willingness to take a risk, and with an open mind, counselors can help both organizations and their employees to self-actualize and reach their goals.

CASE ILLUSTRATION OF CAREER DEVELOPMENT COUNSELING ──────────

Despite improvement in the organization described previously external economic pressures resulted in organizational restructuring, which threatened the jobs of middle management. The OD practitioner recommended that the organization contract with a career counselor to provide outplacement services. As part of the outplacement services, individual career counseling was offered to all middle managers. This section provides a case illustration of career development interventions with Claude, a middle manager in the organization.

Claude, an Asian American male in his early 30s who is a computer programmer, was referred for career counseling by his family physician, who felt that some of the client's complaints about lower back pain and headaches could be stress-related. Although Claude did not initially agree with this idea, he was tired of the back pain and headaches. While refusing personal counseling, he agreed to career counseling since it was being offered to all middle managers at his company. His girlfriend, who had a very positive experience in counseling, convinced him to "give it a try." Claude saw career counseling as a reasonable option because he had become increasingly concerned about the future of his career.

Claude reported that economic events had forced his company to begin an organizational restructuring process that would probably include eliminating his position. Claude had started working at the company immediately upon graduating from college 11 years ago. At the outset of the restructuring process, he was assigned a new supervisor. His supervisor tended to be a "micromanager" and continually made unreasonable demands upon both Claude and his colleagues. According to Claude, the supervisor seemed unable to tolerate even the slightest deviation from her way of doing things. Claude reported that things had gotten so bad, he was considering a complete career change to the fields of training or teaching, "something different" as he put it. At the same time, Claude stated that he had always enjoyed being a computer programmer (Holland Code: IAR) and he seemed well-suited for the job. In fact, Claude was an accomplished professional and because of both his competence and creativity, he had been offered positions by a number of rival companies.

When the career counselor explored Claude's concerns with him, the career counselor learned that Claude was a quiet person who has not communicated the extent of his occupational upset to anyone. In fact, he was so troubled by events in his organization that his work performance had suffered and he had recently been criticized by his supervisor for missing some company deadlines. Over the past 6 weeks, Claude had missed a few days of work because of his back pain; he admitted that this has slowed company progress on an important project. Now, the decision to leave or stay no longer appears to be up to Claude; he expects to be laid off soon.

Planning the Treatment

Upon completion of the intake forms, interview, and review of client information, the treatment planning process began. The following elements of the treatment plan are reflected in the DO A CLIENT MAP format, presented in Chapter 5: Diagnosis, Objectives, Assessment, Clinician, Location, Interventions, Emphasis, Numbers, Timing, Medication, Adjunct Services, and Prognosis (Seligman, 1998).

Diagnosis

Claude is being laid off from his current job. He is now forced to look for new employment. His recent absenteeism is a sign of problems in his organization. Claude's dissatisfaction with his job results from the reorganization in his company and his personality differences with his new supervisor rather than because his occupational field is incongruent with his personality and interests.

Objectives

1. Expand the client's self-knowledge and awareness of the world of work.
2. Clarify the client's knowledge of occupations and occupational preferences and dislikes.
3. Improve Claude's ability to deal with stress.
4. Establish an action plan built on the client's strengths and life planning.
5. Help the client find more rewarding employment.

Assessment

Given Claude's desire to change his occupation, it seems appropriate to explore his interests. In college, Claude completed the Self-Directed Search (SDS). The results indicated that his Holland Code was IAR. This code suggests that

Claude's personality type is congruent with the following categories of occupations: (1) Investigative-scientific and some technical; (2) Artistic-artistic, musical, and literary; and (3) Realistic-skilled trades, technical and service. Claude's Investigative and Realistic personality style are congruent with his current work environment, although his Artistic interests seem untapped. Since the results of the test are now 12 years old, Claude's counselor decided to readminister the SDS as well as administering the Strong Interest Inventory (SII) to Claude.

Claude's support system also needs to be assessed. Changing careers is often a stressful point in one's life; social support has been found to be a predictor of a client's ability to cope effectively with stress (Peters, 2000). The support Claude receives from his girlfriend is a possible resource for him in the future.

Clinician

Claude related well to the counselor, a 40-year-old male, and felt comfortable disclosing feelings related to his difficulties with his female supervisor. The counselor will need to take into consideration cultural issues when working with Claude. For example, Asian Americans often have difficulty describing personal achievements and limitations, so the counselor will have to encourage Claude to practice assertion and communication skills, both within the counseling setting and in the work environment (Zunker, 1990).

Location

The location for Claude's career counseling is an office located in the building of Claude's company. There is little stigma associated with employees utilizing this service, as it is being offered to all middle managers at the company. It is convenient for Claude to attend sessions that will increase the likelihood of his following through with services, especially given his initial reluctance to seek counseling.

Interventions

Claude's counseling is based largely on the culture-centered, person-environment approach of Holland but is also an eclectic approach in that it includes other elements that have been found to promote successful outcomes in career counseling clients. The elements of the intervention, linked to objectives, include:

- Use subjective and objective assessment to identify occupational interests and work environments in which the client feels most comfortable (1, 2, 5).
- Help Claude to explore his expressed interests and occupational preferences to confirm or disconfirm his desire to pursue a radical career

change. Fully explore his rationale for choosing the other fields he mentioned. Let him know that the Holland Code for the fields he mentioned is social and enterprising. This does not seem to fit with the results of his previous assessment or with his personality. They are on the opposite side of the hexagon from the codes he recently received on the SDS. Explore with Claude the possibility that he might have picked those fields out of frustration, without really exploring them fully (1, 2, 5).

- Make a list, with the client, of companies that he is interested in exploring further (4, 5).
- Encourage Claude to conduct informational interviews with chosen companies to gain a better understanding of the work, work setting, supervisory structure and style, benefits, and other attributes of each particular company (1, 2, 4, 5).
- Improve client's coping skills and stress management techniques to help him during this period of increased stress and transition. Address client's feelings of failure and sadness at having to make this change (1, 3).

Emphasis

Sessions will be structured and directive. However, development of trust and rapport in the client–counselor relationship is important. When helping clients deal with change, help them see the positive side of change—change as opportunity. It is also important to normalize the client's discomfort by letting the client know that reorganization has become a problem for many people in our society at this time.

Numbers

Individual career counseling sessions will be conducted with Claude.

Timing

Claude will be seen for weekly 50-minute sessions. The contract for career counseling services is for a maximum of 12 sessions. The pacing of the sessions can be rapid given Claude's urgent presenting concern and fairly high level of functioning. If more career counseling is warranted at the time of completion of the 12th session, a referral will be provided to Claude.

Medication

A referral to a psychiatrist for a medication evaluation is not indicated at this time.

Adjunct Services

1. A referral may be made to a specialist for Claude's back pain and headaches.
2. Claude will be provided the name of the person in the human resource department who is responsible for talking to employees about severance packages, 401K plans, and other relevant benefits.
3. Claude will be encouraged to attend networking meetings of the professional associations of which he is a member. Networking continues to be a significant resource for developing job leads and marketplace information.
4. Social and recreational activities will also be suggested to Claude to help him manage his stress.

Prognosis

Given the nature and relatively brief duration of Claude's presenting concerns, his resources, his positive work history, and his motivation to find more rewarding employment, his prognosis appears to be excellent.

Documentation, Report Writing, and Record Keeping in Counseling

In recent years, the counseling profession has witnessed a strong and growing emphasis on accountability, professionalism, and ethics. This has led to an expanding need for counselors to document and substantiate the value of their work. However, according to a study of counselor preparation conducted by Prieto and Scheel (2002, p. 11), "...a search of professional counseling literature databases indicates that the role of case documentation and record keeping—one of the most common activities that counselor trainees engage in, and an activity that directly reflects trainees' conceptualization of clients' needs and difficulties—has not received the attention it deserves." Most would-be counselors enter the field because of their interest in working with people; the prospect of maintaining records and documenting their work may conflict with their interest in interpersonal interactions. Done properly, however, written records of the counseling process can enhance the treatment process, accelerate progress, expand availability of services, and provide protection to both counselors and clients. For counselors of the 21st century, maintaining clear, comprehensive, and accurate records of their work is a necessity.

Written documentation, reports, and records of the counseling process can accomplish the following goals:

1. Provide clients with information on the counseling process and on their rights and responsibilities.
2. Protect client confidentiality.
3. Help counselors organize and remember information and develop sound treatment plans and interventions based on that information.

4. Provide direction to the counseling process, thereby increasing client motivation.
5. Facilitate authorization for treatment and third-party payments.
6. Ease transfer of a client from one counselor to another.
7. Transmit information on a client.
8. Track progress, record homework tasks, and ease transition from one session to the next.
9. Facilitate revisions in treatment plans if progress is stalled or clients have achieved their goals.
10. Protect the counselor in the event of a lawsuit or other challenge to competence by demonstrating that appropriate treatment has been provided.
11. Facilitate supervision and case conferences.
12. Provide a written record at the termination of counseling that can be helpful if the client returns for counseling at a later date.

Two types of counseling documentation, a write-up of an intake interview and a treatment plan, have already been discussed in this book. This chapter will present information on other documents prepared by and for counselors, including referrals for assessment, assessment reports, requests for treatment authorization, consent to treatment/professional disclosure statements, requests for information, progress notes, midtreatment evaluations and requests for authorization of additional counseling sessions, safe-keeping contracts, transfer summaries, written reports for case conferences, and closing reports.

ASSESSMENT REFERRALS AND REPORTS

Counselors frequently request, write, and receive psychological or psychometric reports on the testing or assessment of clients. Sometimes the assessment process involves writing two reports. One is written to the psychometrician (usually a psychologist or psychiatrist) by the client's counselor or caseworker, requesting and explaining the need for an assessment. The other, written by the psychometrician, provides information on the assessment, including an analysis of any test results and responses to questions posed at the time of referral.

Wolber and Carne (1993, p. 1) wrote of psychological reports

Probably no other form of evaluative reporting provides the mental health practitioner with a comparable in-depth view of the subject. A well-written psychological report can clarify personality dynamics and explain overt behavior. It is capable of providing answers to differential diagnostic issues and pointing a finger at possible etiology. A good psychological report can explain to the reader the effects of the interaction of cognitive and intellectual factors upon personality. The psychological report can provide an "x-ray" of the personality, depicting dynamic factors at a level below the manifest personality or overt behavior of the subject.

A well-constructed psychological report provides for a normative comparison concerning the functioning of an individual and an integrated and coherent presentation of relatively objective data. Hypotheses and recommendations can be formulated from the information provided. Often major treatment and placement decisions are based on the findings and recommendations of the psychological report.

Assessment reports usually are based on a combination of test data, interviews, and observations. Psychological or assessment reports usually are more analytical and interpretive than reports based solely on intake interviews. This is appropriate because the inventories most often used have been studied extensively, and their interpretation has been validated by empirical research. Such reports should respond to the referral questions and enable mental health professionals to better understand and help their client.

Wolber and Carne (1993) described typical psychological reports as three or four single-spaced pages in length. These reports generally are written in the third person and should be person-focused rather than test- or theory-focused (Groth-Marnat, 1990). Usual components of a psychological report include identifying information on the client, the reason for referral, presenting problems, assessment instruments used, background information on the client, behavioral observations during the assessment, the client's intellectual and cognitive functioning, personality dynamics (emotional, intrapsychic, and interpersonal), diagnostic impressions, recommendations, and a summary (Wolber & Carne, 1993).

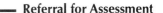 **Referral for Assessment**

Sometimes counselors feel stymied by clients' lack of progress, confused about the nature of their difficulties, uncertain about their diagnosis, or simply in need of more information. At such times, counselors might refer clients to a psychologist or psychometrician for testing and evaluation. (See Chapter 4 for additional information on the testing process.)

When making such a referral, counselors often prepare brief referral reports, providing information on the person to be assessed and the reason for the referral. This helps the psychometrician develop rapport with the client and select those tests and inventories that are most likely to yield needed information and provide answers to the counselor's questions. The following summarizes the items typically included in a referral report:

- Identifying information on client (e.g., age, ethnic/cultural background, occupation)
- Presenting problems
- Reason for referral (referral questions)
- Brief overview of client's background (development, health, family situation, educational and occupational history)

- Treatment history
- Summary of previous psychological and psychiatric evaluations
- Client's attitude toward the assessment process

The following report includes information typically provided when requesting an assessment. The next section includes the test report prepared in response to this referral.

THE CENTER FOR COUNSELING AND CONSULTATION
PSYCHOLOGICAL REFERRAL

Client: Edwin (Ed) Ables   *Counselor*: Joyce Waters, M.Ed., LPC

Presenting Problems

Edwin (Ed) Ables, a 9-year-old White male in the fourth grade at Watkins Mill Elementary School, was brought to counseling by his mother, who has custody of Ed and his 12-year-old sister. Ms. Ables reported that since she and her husband divorced 2 years ago, Ed has become hostile and disobedient, both at home and at school. In addition, his academic performance has declined considerably and he is now performing below grade level.

Reasons for Referral

- To assess Ed's level of intelligence and academic abilities
- To provide insight into the dynamics of Ed's behavioral changes
- To determine the diagnosis
- To facilitate treatment planning

Background

Until 2 years ago, Ed resided with his biological parents and sister, who is 3 years older than he. Although Ed's interest in school varied, depending on the subject, he received above-average grades and did not present behavioral problems, either at home or at school. When his parents divorced 2 years ago, Ed's mother gained custody of the children. Ed's father travels extensively on business and, although he has maintained contact with the children, sees them infrequently and irregularly. Ed's mother is employed as a lawyer who works full-time. Both children have been in daycare and after-school programs from an early age.

Ed's physical development reportedly has been normal and he has had no serious illnesses. He has several male friends in his neighborhood, but lately they have been withdrawing from him.

Treatment History

Ed has been seen for one counseling session with his mother and two sessions of individual play therapy. During all three sessions, he spoke little and avoided interaction with this counselor. He evidenced little interest in the play materials except for a model airplane that he took apart and put together repeatedly. His apparent reluctance to engage in counseling led to this referral for psychological testing.

Previous Test Results

No previous psychological assessment of Ed has been conducted.

Attitude Toward Assessment

Ed may manifest some resistance to the assessment process but, with some encouragement, can probably be persuaded to cooperate. (End of referral report.)

The Assessment Process

In the past, doctoral level psychologists generally conducted evaluations. However, counselors are increasingly conducting assessments, especially when information is needed on career development, family dynamics, or potential for rehabilitation. Most counselors are not trained to administer projective tests and individual intelligence tests. However, a battery of tests can be compiled, consisting entirely of tests commonly used by counselors, to provide a comprehensive picture of a person's overall functioning and answer most referral questions. The following sections provide two evaluation reports, an assessment of Ed completed by a psychologist, and an evaluation of another client, completed by a counselor, to illustrate both types of assessment reports.

Although people can be assessed without a referral report or any guidance from their counselor, that is unusual. In such cases a comprehensive test battery, assessing the following areas, might be administered.

1. *Intellectual and Academic Abilities*—The Stanford–Binet Intelligence Scale or one of the Wechsler Intelligence Scales often is used to measure intelligence, while such tools as the Wide Range Achievement Test provide information on academic skills.

2. *Personality*—Psychologists typically use a battery of projective tests, including the Rorschach Test, the Thematic Apperception Test, the House-Tree-Person, and perhaps a sentence completion inventory. Both psychologists and counselors also assess personality through objective inventories such as the Minnesota Multiphasic Personality Inventory, the Millon Clinical Multiphasic Inventory, the California Psychological Inventory, the Beck Depression and Beck Anxiety Inventories, and other inventories discussed further in Chapter 4.

3. *Perception and Organicity*—The Bender Visual Motor Gestalt Test (Bender Gestalt) is frequently used to provide information on these areas as well as supplementary data on personality dynamics and intellectual functioning.

Measurement of career-related interests, aptitudes, and values usually is not part of a comprehensive assessment unless the counselor requests such information or the psychometrician believes that such information would be particularly important to the referring person or agency.

The referral report for Ed indicated that information was needed in the following areas of functioning: personality, behavior, interpersonal relationships, intelligence, and abilities. The referring counselor also requested further understanding and treatment guidelines for Ed's current behavioral, academic, and attitudinal changes. A report of the psychological evaluation of Edwin Ables follows. It is organized according to a typical framework.

ASSESSMENT REPORT PREPARED BY A PSYCHOLOGIST

Client: Edwin (Ed) Ables   *Psychologist*: Clayton Chang, Ph.D.

Date of birth: October 17, 1994   *Date of evaluation*: May 5, 2004

Tests administered: Wechsler Intelligence Scale for Children
                                          Wide Range Achievement Test
                                          House-Tree-Person
                                          Bender Visual Motor Gestalt Test
                                          Thematic Apperception Test
                                          Rorschach Test

Reason for Assessment

At the time of the evaluation, Edwin (Ed) Ables, a 9-year-old White male, was being seen for outpatient counseling by Joyce Waters, LPC, who referred Ed for an assessment. Information was requested on Ed's intellectual functioning and academic abilities as well as on the dynamics, diagnosis, and treatment of Ed's current behavioral, interpersonal, and academic difficulties.

Background

The client was brought to the evaluation by his mother, who reported that Ed had been fighting and arguing at school, misbehaving at home, and experiencing academic difficulties. Ed is in the fourth grade and resides with his mother and sister, age 12. Ed's parents divorced approximately 2 years ago and Ed has infrequent contact with his father. Ms. Ables reported that her own relationship with Ed is inconsistent and vacillates between arguing and getting along well. She perceived Ed as feeling "torn between his parents" and stated that he was having difficulty coping with their divorce. She also reported that Ed manifested some social problems and tended to play with younger children in the neighborhood rather than socializing with his peers, who lately have avoided contact with him.

Impression of Client

Ed was well groomed and casually, though appropriately, dressed. He is of average height and weight, looks approximately his stated age, and presents a positive appearance. Ed initially appeared reluctant to engage in the assessment process. He refused to remove his hat and coat and spoke little to the examiner at the outset. As the evaluation progressed, Ed became more engaged in the process. He gradually established a satisfactory degree of rapport with this examiner and participated fully in the assessment after the first 20–30 minutes of conversation.

Assessment of Abilities

On the Wechsler Intelligence Scale for Children, Ed achieved a verbal IQ score of 101, a performance IQ score of 118, and a full-scale IQ score of 109, placing him in the average range of intelligence. However, the disparity between Ed's verbal and performance scores is significant and probably reflects a mild learning disability that affects his reading abilities. This should be investigated further. The test protocol reflected considerable subtest scatter, suggesting that Ed's intellectual abilities have not developed smoothly and probably have been adversely affected by both emotional and learning difficulties.

Ed's intellectual strengths include his grasp of spacial organization and his capacity for visual motor coordination. He has a good grasp of planning, anticipation, and cause and effect relationships. He has sound judgment and clearly is aware of socially appropriate ways to behave. In fact, he may sometimes be excessively conventional or conforming.

Ed's grasp of verbal concepts and his verbal skills are relatively weak. Arithmetic problems, presented verbally, also presented difficulty for him. Ed was easily distracted and sometimes gave up prematurely on tasks. On the other hand, he enjoyed the challenge presented by some of the timed tests and became highly motivated and competitive when he was working against the clock. He generally worked quickly and was not careless in his performance.

The Wide Range Achievement Test was used to assess Ed's academic abilities. He did best on the arithmetic section emphasizing computation rather than problems. His arithmetic score was at the fifth grade level and in the high average range, while his reading and spelling scores were at the third grade level and in the low average range.

Although Ed's intelligence level suggests that he could perform satisfactorily in a regular classroom, the imbalance in his intellectual abilities probably makes it difficult for him to complete tasks that emphasize verbal skills and that do not involve clear and relatively brief time limits. He handles some tasks easily but has considerable difficulty with others; this may be frustrating and confusing to Ed. I suggest that his mother request an educational evaluation to determine whether special help or modifications in Ed's assignments might better accommodate the imbalance in his intellectual abilities.

Assessment of Personality

Ed is experiencing considerable anxiety and depression. Although he is capable of satisfactory impulse control, his acting-out behavior offers a way for him to alleviate depression and anxiety and so is rewarding despite its adverse consequences. Ed is an unreflective boy who has little capacity for insight or empathy. He tends to be action-oriented and prefers to deal with problems and emotions through activity rather than through discussion.

Ed experiences low self-esteem. He is concerned about his weak performance at school and perceives himself as incompetent and helpless. Although he wants to improve his academic performance, he does not know how to do this and so feels hopeless and pessimistic. Ed also perceives himself as different from his peers, viewing himself as strange and even menacing. His parents' recent divorce has contributed to these feelings, as does Ed's strong underlying anger.

In relationships, Ed prefers a dependent stance; however, when that is prevented, he distances himself and becomes angry and disappointed. This pattern is especially characteristic of Ed's relationship with his father, who bears the brunt of his anger. His mother, his sister, and his peers also are viewed as having let him down. Ed feels that his mother is pushing him away, possibly through her efforts to have Ed spend more time with his father. Ed is uncomfortable with this yet does not want to disappoint his mother.

At present, Ed is having some difficulty figuring out who he is and establishing satisfactory ego boundaries. Although he certainly has inner strengths, he feels as if he is on a road toward destruction and is aware that he needs some help.

Diagnosis

Axis I.	313.81	Oppositional Defiant Disorder, moderate
	300.4	Dysthymic Disorder, early onset, moderate
	315.00	Reading Disorder (provisional)
Axis II.	V71.09 No mental disorders on axis II	
Axis III.	None reported	
Axis IV.	Parents' divorce, limited contact with father, conflict with mother, declining academic performance, withdrawal of friends	
Axis V.	60.	

Recommendations

Both counseling and academic help are indicated. Although Ed may initially seem unwilling to accept those interventions, that reluctance is likely to diminish with time and patience because Ed is aware of his need for help. Although Ed does not manifest severe symptoms, the nature of his difficulties can negatively impact his future development if not ameliorated soon. Because Ed is not very verbal or insightful, he may have difficulty involving himself in talk therapy. Play therapy, providing both choices and clear limits, is more likely to be helpful, as is behavioral counseling, which could teach Ed constructive ways to express and manage his feelings of anger and frustration. Family counseling with Ed, his mother, his sister, and, if possible, his father also is recommended to help Ed cope with the impact of the divorce, express his feelings and concerns to his family, and establish more consistent contact between Ed and his father. An academic evaluation also is recommended to clarify the nature of Ed's apparent Learning Disability focused on verbal and reading skills. Subsequent tutoring and educational changes are likely to improve Ed's academic performance as well as his mood and self-esteem. (End of report.)

───────────────────────────────── **Psychological Assessment by a Counselor**

A licensed professional counselor wrote the following assessment report. It illustrates the use of objective tests of ability and personality, as well as information gleaned from an interview, to provide useful recommendations.

ASSESSMENT REPORT

Client: John Marino   *Counselor*: Clare Alvarado, LPC, CCMHC

Date of birth: February 3, 1986   *Date of evaluation*: June 5, 2004

Tests administered: Wechsler Adult Intelligence Scale (WAIS)
COPSystem (CAPS ability battery, COPS interest
inventory, COPES work values survey)
Millon Clinical Multiaxial Inventory

Reason for Evaluation

John Marino, an 18-year-old White Italian American male, was referred for an evaluation after his conviction for car theft. John is being considered for participation in a prerelease program that would provide him with job training and employment and prepare him for his release from prison in 6 months. However, during his interview for that program, John seemed withdrawn and depressed and had considerable difficulty in responding to questions. An assessment was requested to determine his suitability for the prerelease program and, if that were recommended, to provide suggestions as to how to help John succeed in that program and formulate sound future plans.

Background

At the time of his arrest, John was in his senior year of high school in a special education class. He was living with his mother and two younger brothers; the whereabouts of his father were unknown. John reported an interest in engaging in noncompetitive sports, such as in-line skating and biking, and in watching football and basketball games. He stated that he had dated little and had no close friends. He acknowledged occasional use of cannabis and alcohol prior to his incarceration. He does not have clear career goals but states he wants to complete high school.

Impressions of Client

John is a tall, slender man who appears his stated age. John initially gave a negative impression when seen for the assessment. He seemed disinterested in what was going on around him and was dressed in clothes that were soiled. John had weak verbal skills, volunteered little information about himself, and was difficult to engage in discussion.

Despite his initial negative reaction to the assessment process, John recognized that his suitability for the prerelease program was being assessed and he did cooperate with the evaluation. He expressed curiosity about the nature of the testing and often asked to have another chance or an explanation of tasks he had failed. John is a reasonably persistent worker with a satisfactory grasp of trial-and-error learning. His concentration and attention were satisfactory and he had little difficulty following directions. His short-term memory was above average. John worked at a satisfactory rate of speed on visual-motor tasks but slowed down considerably on tasks that called for verbalization or writing.

Abilities

On the WAIS, John achieved a verbal IQ score of 87, a performance IQ score of 86, and a full-scale IQ score of 85, placing him in the low average range of intelligence and between the 11th and 25th percentiles. This instrument yielded no evidence of learning disability or severe pathology. John does have weak academic skills, although he can read and perform simple mathematical computations. Despite his disinterested demeanor, John is aware of what is going on around him and what is expected of him, grasps situations fairly quickly, and can plan appropriate actions. However, he has little interest in academic pursuits. His fund of information and his vocabulary are particularly poor. He also has a low energy level.

John's scores on the Career Ability Placement Survey (CAPS) battery were consistent with his scores on the WAIS. All eight scores were below average, but his scores in mechanical reasoning, manual speed and dexterity, and spatial relations were relatively high (4th stanine), while scores in language usage and verbal reasoning were quite low (2nd stanine).

Personality

Assessment of John's personality yielded no evidence of severe emotional disorders but did highlight some areas of concern. John seems to be a guarded and suspicious young man who is well defended and resistant to self-disclosure. He tends to be rigid and constricted and has difficulty dealing with anger appropriately. He is a fairly passive person who wants to be liked but who has little genuine interest in other people. His social skills are weak and he is not interested in working on these skills in order to relate better to others. Some underlying depression was noted, but John seems to be masking and denying these feelings with a bland exterior. He does not seem to be troubled by significant anxiety.

Interests and Values

The COPSystem interest inventory suggested that John's strongest interests are in outdoor and skilled technology areas. Lowest interests were in arts, communication, and science. The COPS values inventory indicated that John valued privacy and being concrete and realistic; values such as aesthetics, social concern, and leadership were unimportant to him. These values are consistent with John's interests and abilities.

Diagnosis

Axis I.   311 Depressive Disorder Not Otherwise Specified, moderate
          305.00 Alcohol Abuse (provisional)

305.20 Cannabis Abuse (provisional)
Axis II.   V62.89 Borderline Intellectual Functioning
           Paranoid and Schizoid Personality Traits
Axis III. John reported having been treated for acne
Axis IV.   Incarceration
Axis V.   55.

Recommendations

John has more potential than is initially evident. He can profit from educational experiences and should be able to learn skills that will facilitate his employment. He can be motivated and hard working, although he needs to develop goals and direction, improve his life skills, and receive some occupational training. John probably would be most successful in a hands-on job in which he has clear direction but can work fairly independently, producing a visible product. One of the current opportunities at the prerelease center involves training and employment in bicycle repair; an option such as this may be well suited to John's interests, personality style, and abilities.

John seems to have the capacity and motivation to benefit from and successfully complete the prerelease program. Standards should be set for him that are realistic yet mildly challenging. Counseling is recommended to help him deal with personal issues, including his underlying depression and the conflict he seems to experience between his tendency to withdraw from others and his wish to be liked. Attention also should be paid to John's impulse control and his use of drugs and alcohol, probably a greater problem than John acknowledged. John is a young man with some motivation and strengths; counseling and occupational training at this time has the potential to make an important difference in his future. (End of report.)

CONSENT TO TREATMENT FORM

A consent to treatment form, also known as a professional disclosure statement or counseling agreement, has become an important and required part of an initial counseling session. This statement provides information on the counselor's training and areas of expertise and acquaints clients with rights, roles, and guidelines that are important in the counseling process. Typically, clients read this statement during the first counseling session and then discuss it with the counselor. Both client and counselor sign the document to indicate their agreement with its policies, and then the client receives a copy of the document as a reminder of its information. This statement provides protection for both clients and counselors; once it has been discussed and signed, neither can legitimately deny knowledge of the policies and procedures it contains.

The following information usually is included in a counseling agreement:

1. Counselor's qualifications, including degrees, where obtained, licenses, and certifications.
2. Counselor's theoretical orientation.
3. Counselor's areas of expertise and counseling services provided.
4. Information on counselor and client roles and responsibilities, how to best use the counseling process, and potential risks and benefits of treatment.
5. Clients' rights including sharing records with other professionals, participating in goal setting and treatment evaluation, asking questions, terminating treatment, and filing complaints.
6. Fees and billing arrangements, including when payments are expected, use of third-party payments, use of collection agencies if payments are not made, charges for sessions that are missed or canceled late.
7. Information on privileged communication and counselors' policies on confidentiality (typically supplemented by an accompanying notice of privacy practices required by the Health Insurance Portability and Accountability Act [HIPAA]).
8. Information on counselors' use of tape recording and note taking during sessions.
9. Policy in the event of an emergency.
10. Information on counselor's use of consultation with peers and supervisors.

Sample Consent to Treatment Form

COUNSELING AGREEMENT FOR CLIENTS OF DR. LINDA SELIGMAN

Welcome to the Center for Counseling and Consultation, a private practice directed by Dr. Linda Seligman. I appreciate your having selected me to provide counseling or other professional services to you. I will do all I can to offer you the highest quality care possible.

The purpose of this agreement is to provide you with important information about my background, the counseling process, your rights and responsibilities, and the policies of the Center for Counseling and Consultation (CCC). Counseling is more likely to be successful if we have a mutual understanding of the treatment process.

Information on Dr. Linda Seligman

I have a Ph.D. in Counseling Psychology from Columbia University. I am licensed as a Clinical Psychologist in Virginia and Maryland and as a Licensed Professional

Counselor in Virginia. I am certified in Eye Movement Desensitization and Reprocessing and am a Certified Clinical Mental Health Counselor (CCMHC). I am a member of the American Psychological Association and of the American Counseling Association. I have been the Director of the CCC since 1985 and a practicing counselor and psychologist for 25 years.

Professional Services

My practice includes adolescents, adults, couples, and families. I provide individual, group, and family counseling. I have particular expertise in counseling people who are coping with chronic and life-threatening illnesses, people with mood or anxiety disorders, people with relationship or self-esteem concerns, people with career difficulties, and people with a history of trauma, including physical or sexual abuse. My primary theoretical orientation is Cognitive–Behavioral. However, I am trained in and draw on a wide variety of other approaches including solution-focused brief psychotherapy, reality therapy, and psychodynamic psychotherapy.

In addition to psychotherapy, I offer coaching, supervision to other therapists, and psychological testing and assessment. I am also involved in teaching and consultation on diagnosis and treatment of mental disorders, professional writing, practice development, and other areas.

Counseling Process

Within the next few sessions, we will establish goals for our work together and will then plan a treatment that seems likely to help you achieve those goals. I have found counseling to be most effective if we work collaboratively; I expect you to come to our sessions on time, to complete any tasks we agree upon, and to do your best to talk about the concerns, behaviors, thoughts, and feelings that are bothering you. Although counseling usually results in positive changes in mood, behavior, relationships and other areas, it may also lead to unanticipated and unwanted changes. If anything about our counseling troubles or disappoints you, I strongly encourage you to talk about that in our sessions so that we can address your concerns.

Client Rights

You have the right to full information about your treatment and to play an active part in that treatment. You have the right to receive a copy of the code of ethics that I follow, to ask questions about the counseling process, to express your concerns, to obtain a second opinion, to terminate counseling, and to contact appropriate state and national professional organizations if you have doubts or complaints about our work together (provide contact information).

Confidentiality

Confidentiality, one of your most important rights, is maintained as part of the counseling process in accord with the ethical standards of my profession. Your written authorization is required for release of information or records, such as to your physician. Use of insurance forms to obtain third-party payments authorizes me to release information to your insurance company and to my billing service. Exceptions are made to this policy on confidentiality only in the event of court order, clear and imminent danger to you or another person, or suspected abuse of children, the disabled, or the elderly. An exception also can be made in the event of nonpayment of fees necessitating the use of a collection agency; that agency will not receive information on the content of our work but may need to receive dates of sessions and copies of your consent to treatment forms. In addition, I sometimes consult with peers but will not provide any identifying information about you in the course of consultation. Please be aware that I cannot guarantee confidentiality of information released to insurance carriers.

I take notes during sessions and occasionally tape record sessions, with clients' permission. These procedures help me obtain a deeper understanding of our work together and find effective ways to help you reach your goals. All notes and tape recordings are kept in locked file cabinets.

Policies Regarding Fees, Payments, and Cancellations

My current fee is $ --- for a 45-minute session unless I participate with your insurance company. Payment should be made at the beginning of each session. I will be glad to provide you with statements and to complete your insurance forms as needed. A charge of $25 per 15-minute segment also will be made for consultation by telephone. No charge will be made for brief telephone conversations to schedule, change, or confirm appointments.

If you need to cancel or change an appointment, please give me at least 48 hours notice. If that is not done, you will be charged for any missed appointments. Please be aware that insurance companies do not make payment for missed appointments. (You will not be charged for weather-related cancellations if area schools are closed due to the weather at the time of your appointment.)

Communication Including Policies for Emergencies

I will provide you with my telephone and pager numbers as well as my email address. Messages may be left on my voice mail at any time. I or one of my colleagues regularly check my voice mail and I will return your calls as soon as possible. In the event of a true emergency, you may call my pager number. If I do not return your call within 60 minute or you cannot safely wait up to an hour, please go to your nearest hospital emergency room or call your nearest community mental health center. I will also give you the telephone numbers of emergency services that you can access in the event you need immediate help. If you do not need an immediate response, you may contact me by email.

Please sign below to indicate that you have reviewed, understand, and are in agreement with the policies in this statement.

INTAKE QUESTIONNAIRES

Along with counseling agreements, many counselors give clients an intake or life history questionnaire to be completed early in the counseling process. Counselors can easily develop these forms to meet their needs. A brief intake form might ask for name, home, and work addresses, telephone numbers, email address, date of birth, insurance information, presenting concerns, medical conditions, medications, treatment history, names and ages of immediate family members, and person to contact in the event of an emergency. Suggestions for information to be included in longer questionnaires can be drawn from Chapter 5.

SAFE-KEEPING CONTRACTS

Dealing effectively with a client's suicidal ideation is one of the most challenging and important tasks of the counselor. Sometimes a written contract can facilitate that process. Although asking a client to sign a contract agreeing not to commit suicide may seem strange, this process communicates the counselor's concern as well as the seriousness of the situation and provides encouragement and alternatives. Steps for self-protection are listed in the contract, including sources of emergency assistance and activities that are likely to reduce suicidal ideation. Agreement is signed and dated by both client and counselor. The following safe-keeping contract provides a model for such agreements.

Sample Safe-keeping Contract

I agree that between now and July 1, I will not overdose on my medication, cut myself, drive in a reckless manner, or otherwise endanger my life. If I have thoughts about harming myself, I will instead follow the steps agreed to by my counselor and myself.

RELEASE OF INFORMATION

Counselors often find it helpful to communicate with people who are acquainted with or who have provided treatment to a client, for example, family members, teachers, school counselors, physicians, lawyers, or psychiatrists. Unless the client presents a danger or is a minor, a client's written permission should be obtained before counselors talk with anyone about a client or even acknowledge that a person is seeing them for treatment. The following is an example of a release of information form, used to obtain clients' written permission to disclose information.

Example of Release of Information

I authorize *(name of sending person or agency)* to release to *(name of receiving person or agency)* at *(address)* the following information: *(specify information to be released)* pertaining to myself or my child *(name of child)* for the following purpose: *(state reason for request)*. This authorization is signed with the understanding that the information will not be passed onto anyone else without my written permission and will not be used for any other purpose than that specified above. Authorization expires (maximum of 90 days from date of signing).
(Form should be signed and dated by both client and counselor.)

PROGRESS NOTES

Counselors are expected to maintain progress notes in nearly all mental health treatment programs as well as in private practices. Progress notes are entries made in clients' charts or files each time the counselor has a session or other significant interaction with a client.

Progress notes are particularly useful in settings where several mental health professionals are working with a particular client. In a psychiatric hospital, for example, a nurse, a family counselor, a psychiatrist, and a case aide all may have contact with a client in a single day. Different schedules and other commitments probably make it impossible for the four helping professionals to meet daily to share their perceptions of the client's development. Progress notes provide the vehicle for that communication.

Progress notes document the counseling process and help counselors demonstrate that they have been providing appropriate treatment. Progress notes facilitate gathering and recording relevant information and remind counselors of important goals, topics, and plans for the client's treatment. Progress notes are also a useful way for counselors to track progress, document changes, evaluate treatment effectiveness, and plan sessions. A quick review of the progress notes on a previous session helps counselors shift their focus from one client to another and refresh their memory of important issues, interventions, and suggestions.

Progress notes should be written soon after a session, telephone conversation, or other interaction to increase the likelihood of accurate recall. Notes should be clear, concise, and brief; focused on the client; and nonjudgmental. Counselors should sign and date each progress note.

STRUCTURED FORMATS FOR PROGRESS NOTES

Progress notes can be simply unstructured comments written in the client's record after each session. However, having a framework facilitates writing progress notes and make the notes clearer and more useful. Several formats are available for maintaining progress notes.

Cameron and Turtle-Song (2002) described a method that has been widely adopted. The acronym SOAP is used to identify the four categories that are covered in the progress notes:

Subjective—In this section, counselors briefly summarize their impressions of a session, perhaps considering the degree of progress made, the client's mood and perceptions, the client–counselor interaction, and the pace of the session.

Objective—This includes factual information as well as direct observations of the client's progress and behavior and information on the content and process of the session itself.

Analysis or Assessment—Next, counselors analyze and synthesize the implications of the subjective and objective material. Particularly important are comments on the relationship of the session to overall treatment goals.

Plans.—Finally, counselors focus on the future and list tasks that clients have agreed to undertake, anything the counselor needs to do to prepare for the next meeting with the client, and areas to be explored or considered in the next session. Long-range plans also may be included here.

The following is an example of a progress note, written according to the SOAP format:

5/18/04—Third individual counseling session held with Carrie Carter. (S) Carrie seemed more animated and talkative than in previous sessions. She was more comfortable discussing her relationship with George and described a pleasant afternoon they had shared, but she still felt pessimistic about their relationship. (O) For the first time, Carrie arrived on time for our appointment. She brought in her revised resume and had begun an exercise program. However, she continued to avoid discussion of her family of origin. (A) A cognitive behavioral approach to treatment, with some supportive interventions, seems to be effective. Carrie is mobilizing her resources and is beginning to take constructive action. Homework assignments (e.g., rewriting her resume) are particularly useful to her. (P) Progress should be reinforced and continued in career and physical fitness areas, with additional homework tasks suggested. Client also may be ready to examine her automatic negative thoughts about relationships and role-play a discussion with George about some of her concerns.

Another format for progress notes is the TIPP format, which includes the four categories illustrated in the following example:

9/20/05—Sixth individual counseling session with Debra Lee.

Themes/Topics—Debra talked with pride about gaining more balance in her life and being more effective at limit setting and reinforcement with her children. As planned, she wrote a letter to her mother-in-law, expressing the hope that they could maintain a positive relationship despite Debra's imminent divorce. Topics reflect ambivalence: excitement about building a better life for herself and fear that she will not be able to succeed as a single woman and mother.

Interventions—Progress since starting counseling was assessed using a 1–10 scale and was rated as follows: self-esteem—increased from 5 to 6, relationships with children—increased from 3 to 5, relationship with husband—still rated 2, mood—increased from 6 to 8. Examination and modification of cognitions were used in an effort to reduce Debra's minimization of her strengths. Reflection and reinforcement were used to consolidate and strengthen gains.

Progress/Problems—Debra's depression has lifted and her energy has returned. She is having more positive interactions with her children but still seems intimidated by her husband. In addition, she continues to be other-directed with her sense of self coming from her ability to help others.

Plans:

1. Administer Beck Depression Inventory, compare with initial administration.
2. Discuss assignment of writing descriptions of herself and her relationships, identifying both strengths and weaknesses.
3. Teach relaxation and assertiveness skills to help Debra cope with family conflict.

Progress notes tend to be fairly brief, often shorter than the examples presented here, but they should convey important information on sessions. Counselors with limited time may become perfunctory in writing progress notes and may view them as burdensome. Such attitudes may result in notes like "Ms. Carter was seen for counseling today. Session dealt with career and interpersonal issues." While such notes may satisfy an agency requirement, they are not helpful to either the counselor or to others working with a client. Brief but informative progress notes can be written in a few minutes. Whenever possible, counselors should use progress notes as an opportunity to reflect on a session and refine treatment planning.

Counselors should bear in mind that progress notes and other client reports may be subpoenaed by the courts and may be subject to review by the client. Consequently, counselors should avoid labeling or judging clients and avoid terminology that seems stigmatizing or unprofessional.

EVALUATION OF COUNSELING EFFECTIVENESS

Ongoing evaluation of treatment effectiveness is an important component of the counseling process. A progress review can reinforce gains, encourage client motivation, and facilitate improved treatment planning. A variety of circumstances may prompt a progress review:

1. The client may show little improvement or may feel dissatisfied with the counseling.
2. New areas of importance may come to light, as counselor and client develop rapport and the client becomes more open and self-aware.
3. One or more goals have been achieved and the counselor wants to solidify those gains and determine the next focus of treatment.
4. The insurance company providing third-party payments may request a progress report to determine whether continued mental health services are needed for a particular client.
5. A break in treatment may occur, perhaps because of a change in treatment providers, the client or counselor's vacation, or the client's decision to temporarily stop treatment.
6. Counselor and client may want to assess whether the client is ready to complete counseling.

All these and other circumstances call for an evaluation of progress and perhaps a reconceptualization of a client's diagnosis and treatment plan.

Informal Evaluations

Ideally, evaluation should be a continuous part of every counseling relationship, with the counselor reviewing the progress demonstrated at each session and counselor and client frequently discussing the client's growth. Such informal evaluations are important in ensuring that client and counselor are working together effectively and that the client is satisfactorily progressing toward established goals. Informal evaluations can facilitate more formal evaluations. A collaborative discussion of progress, built into a counseling session, is a useful way to reinforce progress, clarify goals, and determine whether changes are needed in a treatment plan. Some counselors conduct such formative evaluations on a regular schedule, perhaps every month, while others are spontaneous, waiting for appropriate times in the treatment process. Particularly appropriate times for a re-evaluation are a clear sign of progress (e.g., client's first social event as a single person); a setback (e.g., a perceptible increase in the client's level of anxiety); a noteworthy life event (e.g., the client's first day at college); calendar times such as the client's birthday, the start of a new year, or the first anniversary of the client's divorce; or when the client expresses unusually positive or negative feelings about the counseling process.

One way to approach such an evaluation is to use the client's initial treatment objectives as a starting point and make *lists of accomplishments, additional objectives*, and *strategies for goal achievement*. This process is usually most effective if the client takes the lead in developing the lists, with the counselor writing down the items and helping the client to generate and clarify ideas. Items should be specific and concrete and should be written in such a way as to make the list a meaningful reference point the next time such an evaluation is done.

The following is an example of such a formative evaluation, reflecting an assessment of progress after 3 months of counseling with Jane, a 58-year-old woman who sought counseling because of Agoraphobia and high anxiety:

1. Objective—Regain full mobility via use of car and subway.

   (a) *Baseline*—No driving or use of subway.
   (b) *One Month*—Could drive in her neighborhood, accompanied by another person.
   (c) *Three Months*—Can drive alone in neighborhood and can drive long distances with another person. Can take subway at times other than rush hours.
   (d) *Four-Month (future) objective*—Drive alone to visit mother, take subway during rush hour.

2. Objective—Return to work on a full-time basis.

   (a) *Baseline*—Has not been to work in 3 months.
   (b) *One Month*—Client is putting in 10 hours of work a week at home. Has been to office weekly to pick up and drop off work.
   (c) *Three Months*—Is working at the office 4 hours a day, 3 days a week.
   (d) *Four-Month (future) objective*—Expand office hours to 6 hours a day, 5 days a week.

3. Objective—Develop at least two friendships and two regular leisure activities.

   (a) *Baseline*—Had no contact with friends and no leisure activities other than watching television.

   (b) *One Month*—Initiated contact with two former friends. Began taking a daily walk.

   (c) *Three Months*—Signed up for a course in genealogy and has been gathering information about singing groups she might join. Has been to church twice. Continues daily walking and regular telephone contact with two friends.

   (d) *Four-Month (future) Objective*—Begin course in genealogy, go to church every week, have lunch with one friend, join a singing group.

   (e) *Strategies to Facilitate Accomplishment of 4-Month Objectives*— Progressive muscle relaxation, *in vivo* and imaginal desensitization, improvement of communication skills.

Such lists can help both client and counselor see that progress has indeed been made, can clarify areas where change is still needed, and can encourage the client to make those changes. Client and counselor should each retain a copy of the lists as the basis for future discussion.

Structured Interim Progress Reports

Sometimes, a more formal, extensive written evaluation of a client's progress is indicated for reasons previously described. In writing interim reports, counselors can usually assume that their readers have some knowledge of the intake report that was completed when the person began treatment. While information on that report may be summarized, it need not be repeated.

Typically, interim reports are fairly brief (longer than progress notes but shorter than intake reports). They are intended primarily to evaluate the client's progress in light of treatment objectives and to make recommendations for further treatment, if indicated.

Outpatient Treatment Progress Report

With the spread of managed care, counselors increasingly are required to prepare Outpatient Treatment Progress Reports (OTPR) to justify the need for continued counseling and obtain payment for their services. Typically, three to eight sessions are authorized by a managed care organization when clients inform the organization that they wish to seek counseling. If the client and treatment provider believe that the client's concerns have not been resolved within that initial batch of sessions, the counselor usually prepares and submits an OTPR, requesting additional sessions.

If an interim report is being prepared according to agency policy or in response to a request from an insurance company, a format for writing such a report probably will be provided.

The following example illustrates a typical format used by managed care companies. This report requests authorization for additional sessions for Sharon Miles, a 45-year-old woman.

Client: Sharon Miles   *Counselor*: Alma Burke, Ph.D., LPC

Date of birth: March 6, 1959   *Date of request*: August 5, 2004

Diagnosis

Axis I.   301.13 Cyclothymic disorder, moderate
Axis II.   V71.09 No diagnosis on axis II
Axis III. Obesity, high blood pressure, arthritis reported
Axis IV.   Marital conflict
Axis V.   58

Date of initial assessment: May 15, 2004   *Number of sessions since initial assessment*: 8

Clinical Condition (reasons for seeking treatment, current condition, severity, duration, impairment, previous treatment)—Presenting concerns included mood instability, depression, weight gain, physical problems, marital conflict, continuing grief linked to death of mother.

Background and Risk Factors—Client is an only child. Father died in a car accident when she was 4; he had history of alcohol-related problems. Mother had history of hospitalizations for depression and committed suicide. Client is married and has no children.

Brief Mental Status Examination (abnormal findings only)—Moderate depression and anxiety, mood instability, some impairment in behavior and judgment, but presents no danger.

Course of Treatment to Date, Progress—Individual cognitive-behavioral counseling has been the primary mode of treatment. Two sessions were held with the client and her husband. Referral for medication was made and Prozac was prescribed. Client's moods have stabilized and depression is somewhat reduced. Client has begun to address feelings regarding mother's suicide.

Current Symptoms and Level of Functioning—Client is functioning better at home; depressive symptoms and emotional outbursts have been reduced. However, she continues to experience low self-esteem, grief, inertia, and marital conflict.

Current Goals and Treatment Plan—Ms. Miles now is ready to address her marital difficulties and to increase her activity level. Cognitive-behavioral counseling and systems family therapy will be used to help her locate part-time employment, increase her activity level, become involved in a weight-control program, improve marital communication and satisfaction, further alleviate depression, and stabilize mood.

Criteria for Discharge—Ratings of self-esteem and overall satisfaction with life will be at least 6 on a 1–10 scale, client will engage in regular physical activity and will be participating in a weight-control program. Mood will be in the normal range on the Beck Depression Inventory.

Estimated number of additional sessions until termination of treatment—10.

TRANSFER SUMMARY

A transfer summary or report is designed to help counselors continue treatment of clients who had been in counseling with another therapist. It provides an overview of the client's treatment history, focusing on progress as well as continuing concerns, and suggests ways to work effectively with the client based on response to the initial treatment. Although some transition time usually is needed for clients to develop trust and rapport with a new counselor and to work through any feelings of anger and grief connected with the departure of the first counselor, transfer reports can reduce the difficulties inherent in such transitions, paving the way for the establishment of a sound counseling relationship. The following example illustrates a typical transfer report.

EXAMPLE OF TRANSFER SUMMARY

Client: Aaron Rudderman   *Counselor*: Doris Lopez, M.Ed., LPC, NCC

Presenting problems—Aaron Rudderman, a 51-year-old White Jewish male, sought counseling for help with depression, marital difficulties, and career concerns, and in coping with his diagnosis of Parkinson's disease. Mr. Rudderman's physical health began deteriorating about 3 years ago. Soon after, Parkinson's disease was diagnosed and he was placed on medication to reduce the symptoms of the disease. However, the client could no longer perform his job as a cab driver and could not engage in such physical activities as lawn care, car repair, and playing ball with his son, now 15. Depression and family conflict, probably present at a low level for many years, increased and led to suicidal ideation and talk of divorce.

Mr. Rudderman is diagnosed with a Major Depressive Disorder, late onset, with atypical features.

Nature of treatment—The client has been seen for 17 sessions of individual counseling and 5 sessions of couples counseling. A multimodal approach to treatment was taken because of the pervasive impact of the client's medical condition, although brief psychodynamic psychotherapy was emphasized in treatment in order to address client's depression and guilt related to anticipated rejection. This approach also was helpful in clarifying Mr. Rudderman's ambivalent view of his present situation. Part of him longs to be the helpless invalid, cared for and pampered by his wife, while another side of him sees all symptoms of his Parkinson's disease as psychosomatic, denying the genuine limitations he does have on his activities. Behavioral interventions were also an important part of treatment and helped to reduce depression and increase goal-directed activities.

Progress—Mr. Rudderman's depression has been reduced and his marriage seems stronger, although both areas need continued attention. He has formulated some future goals, based on a long-standing interest in the stock market, and currently is taking courses to become a financial planner. Client and his son have become closer and the client's self-esteem has improved. Better sleeping and eating habits, as well as appropriate weight gain, have been reported.

Recommendations—The next 6 months may be difficult for Mr. Rudderman since he will complete his training in financial planning and expects to seek employment. He needs help in maximizing use of his intellectual and physical abilities without setting unrealistic expectations for himself. Continued couples counseling can help to reduce his wife's tendency to be demanding and critical as well as the client's discouragement. Brief psychodynamic psychotherapy can continue to be helpful to this client, but his tendency to analyze and intellectualize excessively suggests that the psychodynamic approach should be balanced by some behavioral interventions. Behavioral counseling can also help him develop some realistic leisure activities.

Although Mr. Rudderman is out of crisis, he needs continued help for at least the next 6 months to progress in his marriage and his career and to establish a rewarding life-style in light of his physical limitations. He is expected to make the transfer to another counselor without much difficulty and has expressed enthusiasm about continuing his counseling.

CASE CONFERENCES

Some agencies have regularly scheduled case conferences in which staff members present cases and share perceptions and suggestions on those cases. These are not necessarily problematic cases (although this can be a useful way to get help with an impasse in counseling), but may represent a client with an unusual or interesting history or concern. Planning and writing notes in preparation for these meetings can increase their usefulness.

Case conferences generally are intended to be learning experiences for the presenter as well as for other staff members, although they also can be intimidating and anxiety-provoking for the presenter. Case conferences should not be a place for mental health professionals to belittle each other's work or flaunt their own accomplishments. Rather, they should be a place where colleagues collaborate to help each other provide more effective treatment. The counselor responsible for presenting at a case conference need not have all the answers about a client. In fact, case conferences usually are more interesting and productive if presenters have some specific questions about the dynamics, diagnosis, or treatment of the client being presented.

Case conferences vary, depending on the nature of the mental health facility, the client being presented, the style of the presenter, and skills and attitudes of the participants. Some conferences involve the staff in observing the client and counselor engaged in counseling, while at others clients attend part of the conference and speak to the participants about their concerns. Another approach to case conferences involves the counselor presenting an audiotape or videotape of part of a counseling session. In the most common format, the counselor simply provides information about a client and their work together. Regardless of the format of a case conference, presenters generally should provide the following information to the group:

1. Identifying information—client's name, age, education, occupation, cultural and religious background, family constellation, and other important demographic data.
2. Results of mental status examination.
3. Presenting and underlying concerns.
4. Diagnosis.
5. Brief overview of background and current situation—emotional and physical development, family of origin, current family, educational and occupational history, leisure activities, relationships, significant events.
6. Treatment history—history of mental disorders and emotional difficulties, previous treatment, duration and nature of present treatment, client attitude toward treatment, progress made.
7. Counselor's concerns/questions—diagnostic questions, confusing dynamics, treatment impasses, problems in the therapeutic alliance, and other questions about treatment planning.

Considerable similarity exists between an assessment referral report (discussed earlier in this chapter) and counselors' presentations at case conferences. That is because both have the same purpose: providing other professionals with enough information on a client so that they can help the counselor better understand and treat that client. In both the written report and the oral presentation, counselors should be concise and should not try to give a full picture of a person's background and treatment. Only material that is relevant and essential to understanding the client in light of the concerns of the counselor should be included. That process of selectivity should maximize counselors' chances of receiving the help they need with a case.

CLOSING REPORTS

The last reports to be reviewed in this chapter are closing or termination reports. These are prepared when a person discontinues counseling, regardless of whether the termination is a decision reached jointly by client and counselor or is a unilateral decision. Closing reports generally become part of clients' files at the mental health facility where they have been counseled so that, if they return for treatment, information is available on their difficulties, the nature of their treatment, and its impact. With the client's written permission, this information can also be released to medical or mental health personnel outside of the agency. Some counselors also prepare abbreviated versions of their closing reports to give to clients when they finish counseling. These may even be prepared in conjunction with clients and can serve as a means of reminding clients of their gains, reinforcing their progress, and establishing future goals and plans.

Closing reports typically are fairly brief, one to two pages at most. Although these reports usually include a brief review of the client's history and development, they focus primarily on the current treatment process. Typical closing reports state the client's diagnosis and describe the progress made, the interventions used, the impact of treatment, and the client's continuing difficulties and goals.

Closing reports can also yield quantifiable information for an agency on the people who are being treated, their diagnoses, the type and length of treatment provided, and the progress made. This can substantiate treatment effectiveness and indicate areas of high need.

An example of a closing report follows. Counselors can adapt its structure to their own closing reports.

EXAMPLE OF A CLOSING REPORT

Client: Miranda Santiago   *Counselor*: Everett Fox, M.A., LPC

Dates of counseling: 8/13/04–12/15/04

Presenting Concerns

Miranda Santiago, a 42-year-old Latina woman, sought counseling to help her cope with her stressful family situation as well as her anxiety and depression. At the time she sought counseling, Ms. Santiago was living in a two-bedroom apartment with her second husband, Carlos, to whom she had been married for 3 years; her daughter Mindy, age 18; and her mother Julia, age 78, who was in the middle stage of Alzheimer's disease. Ms. Santiago was providing full-time care for her mother and had little time or energy for Carlos and Mindy. Both had complained about this situation and were spending as little time at home as possible. Ms. Santiago was very concerned about her marriage and her daughter's behavior, but felt it was her duty to care for her mother as her mother had cared for her. Ms. Santiago was diagnosed as having an Adjustment Disorder with Mixed Emotional Features.

Background

Ms. Santiago was an only child. When she was 3 years old, her father was murdered in his bakery during a robbery. Her mother took over the bakery and, with little help, managed to support herself and her daughter. Ms. Santiago married for the first time at age 21. Her husband was in the military and was killed in an accident when she was 27 and her daughter was 3. Her mother, Julia, helped Ms. Santiago until Julia's health began to deteriorate. Julia has been living with her daughter for 2 years. Ms. Santiago married Carlos after a long courtship. He was aware of Julia's condition but did not expect his wife to bring her mother into their home.

Treatment History

Ms. Santiago was in a crisis when she entered counseling. She felt immobilized by stress and believed that she was being forced to choose between her mother, on one hand, and her husband and daughter, on the other. Ms. Santiago was seen for seven sessions of individual counseling and three sessions of family counseling with her daughter and husband. Brief solution-focused counseling was the primary approach to treatment. Objectives of counseling included reducing stress, anxiety, and depression; building on the client's strengths; improving family closeness and communication; and helping Ms. Santiago make decisions and take control of her life. Cognitive distortions were explored and modified and coping behaviors, including stress management, decision-making, and increasing rewarding activities, were taught. Counseling was both supportive and structured in nature, promoting expression of feelings as well as behavioral change.

Outcomes

Ms. Santiago responded well to treatment. Depression and anxiety abated quickly as she took steps to improve her situation and realized that her husband remained committed to their marriage. She gathered information on both her mother's condition and on residential programs that could provide care for her mother, visited programs that seemed appropriate, and is now making arrangements to place her mother in a residential program that met Ms. Santiago's criteria. In order to give herself time to gather this information, she located and made good use of a respite care program for people with Dementia. Ms. Santiago also began to use caregivers at home so that she could have more time with her husband and daughter. Family communication has improved, with family members using skills they were taught in family counseling sessions.

Recommendations

Despite the marked progress this client has made, Ms. Santiago recognizes she needs time to build her self-confidence, to facilitate her mother's move to a residential program, and to improve her family relationships. In addition, Ms. Santiago established long-range future goals for herself, including obtaining part-time employment, rebuilding neglected friendships, and taking a college course. A timetable, along with specific steps, was established to help her move toward these goals. The client thought she had the direction and motivation she needed and so decided not to continue counseling at present. However, a setback in her mother's condition or future family difficulties could necessitate additional short-term counseling. If Ms. Santiago resumes counseling, a structured, behavioral approach is recommended. To be effective with this client, such an approach should allow for client's self-expression but should not encourage extensive discussion of negative feelings or past difficulties.

From this report, another counselor working with Miranda Santiago would have some understanding of the client's background, strengths, and weaknesses, as well as information on the sort of counseling that is likely to be effective. Such information can ease the person's return to counseling and can facilitate the counseling process for both client and counselor.

FOLLOW-UP EVALUATIONS

A final procedure to be described in this chapter is the follow-up evaluation. Such evaluations involve contacting clients by mail or telephone some time after they have completed counseling in order to ascertain whether the gains made during counseling have been sustained (and perhaps even increased). A follow-up evaluation provides a way for counselors and agencies to monitor their effectiveness and is a vehicle for offering continued help to former clients who are experiencing difficulties.

Counselors who conduct follow-up evaluations of their clients are taking some risks. They may learn that they have not helped clients as much as they thought they had. Counselors may find that more work still needs to be done with people who seemed to be doing well a few months earlier. Clients may misinterpret the contact and try to transform a professional relationship into a personal one. Counselors who initiate follow-up contact with their clients should make their goals clear to the clients and should be prepared to offer them further assistance.

On the other hand, learning that clients are doing well can be very rewarding to counselors. The follow-up process can also be reassuring to clients, whether or not further counseling is indicated, and can facilitate their seeking help if it is needed in the future.

No generally accepted guidelines for follow-up evaluations have been established. Posttreatment evaluations should occur long enough after counseling to reflect persistence of change but not so long after that they seem inappropriate or overdue. A 3-month interval between termination and follow-up is common, but both longer and shorter intervals are appropriate, depending on the nature of the client–counselor relationship, the client's concerns, and the guidelines of the mental health agency. Informing the client at termination that a follow-up contact will be made can pave the way for that contact as well as encourage the client's progress.

No special format need be used for follow-up contact. Some agencies routinely send written questionnaires to clients, while others leave it to the discretion and preference of the counselors who can decide whether to contact clients and whether to use mail, telephone, or email for follow-up. Having a standardized procedure, such as a written questionnaire or structured interview, can streamline the follow-up process and facilitate the use of the information received from clients to demonstrate effectiveness and justify funding. Regardless of the format used, the posttreatment evaluation can be an excellent way for counselors to show that they are genuinely concerned about and committed to helping their clients and are, indeed, advocates of the lifelong process of personal growth and development inherent in the philosophy of mental health counseling.

12

Ethical and Professional Development for Counselors

In this next to last chapter of the book, we shift attention away from application of diagnostic and treatment planning skills. Our focus here will be on two other essential ingredients of the effective counselor: competence in ethics and wise choices in professional development. Without those ingredients, counselors seem unlikely to be effective, no matter how much knowledge they have about diagnosis and treatment planning. This chapter has two purposes: to familiarize counselors with the nature and importance of ethical standards and to promote understanding and advancement of their professional development.

———————— THE IMPORTANCE OF ETHICAL STANDARDS AND PRACTICE

Each of the mental health professions (e.g., counselors, psychologists, social workers, marriage and family therapists) has its own ethical guidelines, as do the National Board for Certified Counselors (NBCC) and the state licensing boards for the mental health professions. Although the various guidelines have considerable overlap and generally address similar issues, slight differences exist among the guidelines. The American Counseling Association (ACA) has two important documents that provide information on ethical behavior. The Standards of Practice, the briefer document, contains the minimal ethical behaviors required of counselors and is likely to be viewed by the legal system as reflecting the mandatory ethical standards for the profession. The Code of Ethics elaborates on the Standards of Practice and reflects what has been referred to as the aspirational standards, the highest level of ethical behavior. Both of these documents can be accessed online at http://www.counseling.org/resources/codeofethics.htm An additional useful resource is the *ACA Ethical Standards Casebook* (Herlihy & Corey, 1996).

Many important reasons exist as to why counselors should be knowledgeable about and adhere to the ethical code and standards of the ACA:

- The existence of a body of ethical standards enhances the power, credibility, and reputation of the profession.
- These guidelines offer counselors a conceptual framework to help them make sound decisions in ambiguous and challenging situations.
- Adherence to the ethical standards of one's profession can provide a strong defense if a counselor is accused of malpractice.
- Providing clients with an explanation of our most important and relevant ethical standards offers safety and predictability. This, in turn, helps them make better use of counseling and determine what information they want to share with their counselors.
- Similarly, counselors can be reassured by knowing that their work is guided by a set of standards formulated by a committee of knowledgeable peers and reviewed by the entire membership of their professional association.
- Violations of ethical standards can lead to serious negative consequences, including loss of licensure and certification and loss of membership in ACA, which can lead to loss of the ability to work in one's chosen field.
- Because knowledge of ethical standards is essential to effective counseling, examinations required for licensure or certification in counseling emphasize ethics.

GENERAL ETHICAL PRINCIPLES

The next section of this chapter provides specific information on the *ACA Code of Ethics* and *Standards of Practice*. Underlying these guidelines are the following five general ethical and moral principles (Herlihy & Corey, 1996):

1. *Autonomy*—Counselors respect people's freedom of choice and action. Counselors foster independence and empowerment and respect and prize diversity and differences.
2. *Nonmaleficence*—Counselors should do no harm and should always act in the best interests of their clients.
3. *Beneficence*—Not only do counselors refrain from doing harm, they are proactive in promoting good and helping others.
4. *Justice*—Counselors are fair and just in their professional relationships and interactions.
5. *Fidelity*—Counselors maintain their commitments to their profession and to their clients. They are reliable and responsible, nurture and sustain trust in their relationships, value and protect the therapeutic alliance, and are truthful and congruent in their communications.

Familiarity with and understanding of these five general principles can help counselors understand the specific ethical codes and standards and make wise decisions when a particular situation or dilemma is not specifically addressed in the *ACA Code of Ethics* and *Standards of Practice*. This understanding also can help them grapple effectively with the most challenging type of ethical issues, those that entail a conflict among two or more of these principles. For example, assume a counselor is providing marital counseling to a couple who initiated treatment due to the wife's infidelity. The husband believes the wife has ended her extramarital relationship and is intent on improving their marriage. However, the counselor accidentally encounters the wife at a restaurant, engaged in an ardent embrace with another man. Does the counselor respect the wife's right to engage in this relationship (autonomy), maintain her confidentiality in order to protect the therapeutic relationship (fidelity), or decide that the husband is being harmed by this deception and should be informed of the truth (beneficence)? Examples like this sometimes make sound ethical decision-making a challenging endeavor.

OVERVIEW OF *ACA CODE OF ETHICS AND STANDARDS OF PRACTICE*

The *ACA Code of Ethics* and *Standards of Practice* are divided into eight sections. Each of those sections will be reviewed and discussed here.

The Counseling Relationship

The *ACA Code of Ethics* (ACA, 1995, p. 1) states that counselors' primary responsibility is to "respect the dignity and to promote the welfare of clients" as well as to encourage their growth and development. This standard has many implications for counselors' conduct.

Counselors are charged with protecting clients and maintaining their welfare by promoting their freedom of choice in treatment, developing treatment plans that are likely to be effective, and using careful screening and other procedures to provide a safe environment during group counseling. Counselors should provide clients with clear information, preferably in writing, about the counseling process and procedures, with particular care exercised in describing use of computer technology. Counselors should only provide counseling when it is beneficial to clients and should ensure that clients whom the counselors believe they cannot help are referred to appropriate sources of help.

Respect for and appreciation of diversity is inherent in this ethical standard. Counselors must not discriminate against clients on the basis of culture.

Avoidance of dual relationships (e.g., client and student; client and family member) is important in maintaining a sound counseling relationship. Counselors are prohibited from engaging in sexual intimacies with former clients for at least 2 years after the termination of treatment. Similarly, care must be exercised when counseling clients who have family, social, business, or other relationship with each other outside of counseling.

Counselors need to establish a fee schedule that is compatible with common practice in their community, refrain from bartering, and help clients who cannot afford their fees to find other sources of help. Finally, counselors are encouraged to demonstrate beneficence by offering some services on a pro bono basis (with little or no charge).

Confidentiality

Maintenance of confidentiality has long been a hallmark of the counseling relationship and affords clients the assurance that, under most circumstances, information they disclose in counseling will not be shared with others. Counselors are responsible for clearly explaining confidentiality guidelines to clients as well as clarifying for them circumstances under which confidentiality may be broken. Client permission must be obtained for recording or observation of sessions.

In addition, counselors take effective steps to preclude violations of confidentiality. They inform their employees and assistants of the need to maintain confidentiality. They keep records in locked and secure cabinets. When counselors do provide client information, they provide only the information that is necessary to accomplish the purpose of the disclosure. If they are conducting research on their counseling or presenting case studies based on their clients, they make sure that the clients cannot be identified from the information provided.

Family counseling and group counseling, as well as supervision and case consultation, all pose risks to confidentiality. In addition, with minors, especially those under the age of 12, counselors typically do share some information about the clients' treatment with parents or guardians. Here, too, counselors take steps to safeguard confidentiality, even with minors, but they also inform clients of any obligation they have to share information, as well as the risks of disclosure in group and family counseling.

Counselors should keep in mind that confidentiality is owned by the client. Client information, even the fact that someone is a client, cannot be shared with others unless the client gives permission, is notified at the outset of the counseling relationship that information will be shared, or meets one of the exceptions discussed in the next paragraph. However, this does not mean that counselors need to turn over their records to clients at their request; if counselors believe that information may be harmful or subject to misinterpretation, they can provide clients with a summary or other substitute for the records in question.

The exceptions to confidentiality must be well understood by counselors. The landmark Tarasoff case, in which a young woman was killed by her unhappy suitor after he informed the counselor of his intent to harm her, makes clear that counselors must take effective protective action if clients present a clear and imminent danger to themselves or another. This means that when a client with a contagious and fatal disease refuses to communicate this information to an identifiable third party who is at high risk of contracting the disease, the counselor is justified in disclosing that information to the third party.

Knowledge of relevant state legal and ethical standards is essential for counselors. Many states require that counselors report abuse of children (in some states, even if the victim is no longer a minor), the elderly, and people with disabilities. In addition, counselors may receive a subpoena or court order for information on clients; state statutes and the nature of the court order determine whether counselors have the right of privileged communication, which protects them from compulsory disclosure of client information, or whether counselors need to yield the information.

Professional Responsibility

This section of the Ethical Standards addresses counselors' responsibility to present themselves accurately, to ensure competence in their areas of practice, to maintain professional development and involvement, and to establish positive and professional relationships with other mental health treatment providers. Specifically, counselors should "practice only within the boundaries of their competence" (ACA, 1995, p. 6) and should not embark on new areas of practice until they have obtained adequate training and supervision. They should constantly monitor their professional effectiveness and seek consultation or supervision if they are not performing well. If their work is impaired by their own emotional or other difficulties, they refrain from practice.

Counselors represent their credentials and services accurately and rectify situations in which others are misrepresenting the counselors' qualifications and experience. They do not mislead others as to their credentials; for example, a counselor with a doctorate in anthropology would not use the title Doctor in counseling settings.

Counselors take a proactive stance in improving their skills and safeguarding their clients. They maintain involvement in their professional associations and pursue continuing education. They address situations in their place of employment that may have a negative impact on clients and ensure that support staff are performing effectively. If a client is also being seen by another mental health treatment provider, they obtain client authorization and inform that treatment provider of the counselor's work with the client. Finally, counselors do not exploit their staff or clients, nor do they use their place of employment to recruit clients for their private practices.

Relationships with Other Professionals

This relatively brief section of the Ethical Standards gives a clear and strong message that counselors and consultants "have a responsibility both to clients and to the agency or institution within which services are performed to maintain high standards of professional conduct" (ACA, 1995, p. 9). They must limit their practice to their areas of competence, monitor the quality of their work, and seek consultation if they need assistance. Specific guidelines in this section advise counselors not to accept fees for services from people already entitled to those services through the counselors' place of employment and prohibit counselors from accepting referral fees.

Evaluation, Assessment, and Interpretation

This section of the Ethical Standards is intended to ensure that "the whole range of appraisal techniques, including test and nontest data" is used in ways that are appropriate and likely to be helpful to clients as well as in their best interests (ACA, 1995, p. 10). Particularly important to readers of this book is the statement that "Counselors take special care to provide proper diagnosis of mental disorders" (ACA, 1995, p. 11).

Counselors should only use assessment approaches that are within their range of competence and should ensure that their staff and supervisees follow the same procedures. They must select tools that are appropriate for the intended purpose and that are current. Administration, scoring, and interpretation should reflect standardized procedures, and test security should be maintained. Particular care should be exercised when using assessments with people from culturally diverse backgrounds.

Clients should be informed of the nature and purpose of any assessment tools and how the results will be used. Appropriate interpretation should accompany the release of assessment information to clients or others (e.g., family, school system, psychiatrist).

Teaching, Training, and Supervision

This section of the Code of Ethics and Standards of Practice focuses on the ethical responsibilities of students, teachers, trainers, and supervisors. Although "students and supervisees have the same obligations to clients as those required of counselors" (ACA, 1995, p. 15), some additional standards are relevant to the education of counselors.

Counselor educators and trainers are expected to be skilled as both teachers and treatment providers. They maintain professional relationships with their students and supervisees, do not engage in exploitative or sexual relationships with them, and avoid dual relationships such as close family member and professor or counselor and supervisor. When they engage in collaborative research and writing with students, they give appropriate credit to them. If counselors provide supervision, they make sure they are well trained in that process and take steps to ensure that their supervisees provide appropriate professional services.

Ethical guidelines also address the nature of counselor education and training programs. Prospective students should be oriented to the nature of such programs as well as to the program's expectations for satisfactory performance. The programs should integrate "academic study and practice" (ACA, 1995, p. 14), provide clear information on evaluation procedures, and feedback on the results of those evaluations. Students should not be graded on their nonacademic performance in personal growth experiences. Students should be presented with a range of theoretical approaches. If needed, students should be given referrals for counseling or remedial help. Programs should have clear policies for field placements and students' roles in those placements. Clients of students and supervisees should be informed of their counselor's status and qualifications. Recourse should be available to students who are dissatisfied with decisions faculty make about their education.

Research and Publication

Of course, many differences exist between the role of counselor and the role of writer/researcher. However, mental health professionals in either role are expected to act in ways that reflect respect, integrity, and appreciation for others; that advance the profession; and that do no harm.

Counselors engaged in research must ensure that they cause no emotional, physical, or social harm to their subjects. Counselor-researchers are charged with respecting the cultural diversity of their subjects, maintaining their confidentiality, and allowing them freedom of choice. Whenever possible, research studies should avoid deception and make participation voluntary, allowing people to withdraw from the study at any time if they so choose. Participants in research studies should be given full and clear information on the procedures and any risks or discomfort inherent in those procedures, have the opportunity to ask questions, and receive full information on the nature of the study after data are collected. Any commitments made to participants must be honored.

Similarly, counselor-researchers must follow ethical principles in writing up and disseminating their research. They are obligated to disclose full and accurate information about their study, including all conditions potentially having an impact on the study, and results that reflect negatively on programs, services, interests, and opinions of others. Counselor-researchers treat sponsors and institutions with respect and acknowledge their contributions to the research. In addition, they provide information that will help other qualified researchers to replicate their studies. Manuscripts are submitted for consideration to only one journal at a time, and material that has been published in one publication is not replicated in another publication without appropriate permission.

Graduate students and beginning mental health counselors are often asked to collaborate with their professors and other established writers in research and professional writing. This can provide an excellent opportunity for novice researchers to learn about writing and publishing in their field and develop their research and writing skills. Seeing one's name as author of a professional article can be very rewarding! Keep in mind that ACA's ethical standards mandate that all who contribute substantially to a research study or publication be given credit, either by an acknowledgment or by being listed as a co-author. The first author of a publication is viewed as the principal contributor. The *ACA Code of Ethics* specifically states, "For an article that is substantially based on a student's dissertation or thesis, the student is listed as the principal author" (ACA, 1995, p. 17).

Resolving Ethical Issues

Counselors are responsible for ensuring that their behavior reflects the ethical standards of their profession. In the words of the *ACA Code of Ethics* (ACA, 1995, p. 18), "Counselors are familiar with the Code of Ethics and the Standards of Practice and other applicable ethics codes from other professional organizations of which they are member, or from certification and licensure bodies. Lack of knowledge or misunderstanding of an ethical responsibility is not a defense against a charge of unethical conduct."

In addition, counselors are also responsible for taking appropriate action when they have reason to believe that another counselor may be acting unethically. In such cases, counselors should take the following steps:

1. Consult with colleagues, obtain information from an ACA representative, and review the Code of Ethics and Standards of Practice to be sure they have reason to question whether another counselor is acting ethically.
2. Attempt to resolve the issue informally with the other counselor. This gives the person the benefit of the doubt, offers an opportunity for clarification, and provides the other counselor with knowledge and resources he or she may have been lacking. This may well lead to a change in behavior or a recognition that the questionable behavior was, in fact, ethically appropriate.
3. However, if the other counselor's behavior continues to raise suspicions of unethical conduct, the counselor with awareness of this behavior should file a written ethical complaint with ACA's Ethics Committee and/or the appropriate licensure or certification boards. The counselor making the report does not need to be certain that an ethical violation has occurred,

but only have reasonable cause to suspect a violation. It is then the task of the ethics committee or appropriate board to determine whether or not an ethical violation has occurred and to take appropriate steps to rectify the situation and determine the consequences for the violator.

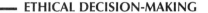

ETHICAL DECISION-MAKING

The first step in becoming an ethical counselor is reading and understanding the *ACA Code of Ethics* and *Standards of Practice*. However, counselors often encounter ethical dilemmas that are not easily resolved, perhaps because of lack of clarity and specificity in the ethical codes or because the nature of the dilemma entails a conflict in ethical standards or includes ambiguous or confusing circumstances. According to Williams and Freeman (2002), the areas of professional responsibility (knowledge, competence, credentials, advertising) and confidentiality are those that are most often reflected in ethical inquiries. Other particularly challenging ethical areas include minor children's rights to confidentiality and the use of electronic approaches to counseling (e.g., email, videoconferencing). Particularly important in both arenas is safeguarding clients' confidentiality as much as possible but being clear with the clients about possible limits to confidentiality.

Many models have been developed to help counselors deal with challenging ethical issues and make sound decisions. The following 10-step model reflects a synthesis of several of these models (Forester-Miller & Davis, 1996; Welfel, 1998):

1. Maintain knowledge of ethical codes and standards and develop ethical sensitivity.
2. Obtain information on the situation and describe it as clearly as possible.
3. Apply the ACA or another appropriate code of ethics to the situation.
4. Based on that review of the ethical standards, define the nature of the dilemma.
5. Generate potential courses of action.
6. Identify the potential consequence of each course of action, along with the risks, benefits, and likelihood of each course of action.
7. If indicated, consult with a colleague, supervisor, or representative of the organization issuing the ethical standards or do some additional reading and research.
8. Evaluate each course of action, balancing risks and benefits, and determine the best course of action.
9. Implement the decision.
10. Reflect on the experience and determine what can be learned from this and applied to future ethical issues.

Application of Ethical Decision-Making Model ————————————

Let's apply the 10-step ethical decision-making model to a case. The counselor, David Lee, has been treating a 45-year-old woman named Maureen Manly, who has been diagnosed with advanced cancer. The client's physicians have told her that she has approximately 6 months to live. In counseling, she has been addressing end-of-life issues and has recently given her counselor a copy of letters she wants to leave for her closest family members, a 20-year-old daughter and an older brother. Counselor and client planned to discuss these letters at their next session.

When Maureen fails to appear for her next session, David telephones her home. Maureen's brother answers the telephone and informs David that Maureen is in a coma and may not regain consciousness. The brother then asks who David is and how he knows Maureen. How this situation should be handled reflects an ethical dilemma, addressed in the 10 steps previously presented.

1. The counselor has knowledge of the ethical codes as well as ethical sensitivity.

2. The counselor has been seeing a client who is currently in a coma, cannot communicate with the counselor, and may not recover from the coma. The counselor has letters that the client intended to share with family members but she has not yet put these letters in their final form or shared them with family. The letters are very loving and positive. The counselor has a therapeutic relationship with the client and wants to help as much as possible but does not have the client's permission to communicate with family members. The counselor knows that Maureen's brother has her power of attorney. In addition, the counselor is saddened by learning that Maureen's death is apparently imminent and wants to say good-bye to her.

3. Three statements from the *ACA Code of Ethics* seem especially relevant:

   a. "Counselors respect their clients right to privacy and avoid illegal and unwarranted disclosures of confidential information" (ACA, 1995, p. 4).

   b. "The primary responsibility of counselors is to respect the dignity and to promote the welfare of clients" (ACA, 1995, p. 1).

   c. "When counseling ... individuals who are unable to give voluntary informed consent, parents or guardians may be included in the counseling process as appropriate ... Counselors act in the best interests of clients ... " (ACA, 1995, p. 5).

4. Ethical questions: Should the counselor identify himself to the client's brother or should he maintain her confidentiality? Should the counselor share the letters with Maureen's daughter and brother or should he maintain her confidentiality? How should the counselor address his wish to say good-bye to his client?

5. Potential courses of action:

   a. David could share no information with Maureen's family.

   b. David might inform the brother that he is Maureen's counselor but provide no other information.

   c. David might inform the brother that he is Maureen's counselor and ask permission to see her.

   d. David might inform the brother that he is Maureen's counselor, ask permission to see her, and share Maureen's letters with the family, either all at once or as separate acts.

6. Potential consequences of each course:

   a. The family would not receive the messages Maureen had intended for them, they would not be able to benefit from any help the counselor could offer, and David would not have the opportunity to say good-bye to Maureen. David's actions would not violate Maureen's confidentiality.

   b. The family would not receive the messages Maureen had intended for them, they probably would not be able to benefit from any help the counselor could offer, and David probably would not have the opportunity to say good-bye to Maureen. David's actions would violate Maureen's confidentiality and might not reflect her wishes.

   c. The family would not receive the messages Maureen had intended for them, but David could offer help to the family and might have the opportunity to say good-bye to Maureen. David's actions would violate Maureen's confidentiality and might not reflect her wishes.

   d. The family would receive the messages Maureen had intended for them, David could offer help to the family and might have the opportunity to say good-bye to Maureen. David's actions would violate Maureen's confidentiality and might not reflect her wishes.

7. David consulted with a trusted colleague and a former professor, being careful to conceal Maureen's identity when presenting the ethical dilemma.

8. David knows that Maureen was close to her brother, wanted to share her loving letters with her daughter and brother, and was comfortable about seeking counseling. Breaking confidentiality to offer the family help and the comfort of Maureen's letters seems likely to coincide with what Maureen would wish and is likely to bring benefit to the family. Although that course of action is most likely to afford David the opportunity to say good-bye to

Maureen, the client's welfare is paramount and David's decisions should not be directed by his own needs. Choosing not to break confidentiality will probably deprive the family of any help David could provide and would deny them access to Maureen's letters, potentially a great loss to them.

David decides that he will inform the family of his role and will offer some ways in which he might be helpful to them. Because Maureen may awaken from the coma, David will not initially inform the family of the letters she has written. However, if David is not able to communicate with her before her death, he will then share Maureen's letters with her daughter and brother.

9. David moves forward to implement the first part of the decision. He brother asks David to meet with him and Maureen's daughter in Maureen's hospita room to help them deal with her medical condition and probable death. David agrees and also has the opportunity to say his own good-byes to Maureen. He shares her letters with the family a few days later following Maureen's death.

10. David reflects on what he learned from this situation, particularly the importance of acting in the best interests of the client.

CASES FOR ETHICAL DECISION-MAKING

Included in this section are some cases that raise ethical challenges. Using your understanding of the ethical code and standards, as well as the model for ethical decision-making, determine the most ethical way to handle each of these situations.

Case 1. Your client is a 12-year-old girl. She tells you that recently, when she was left in her grandfather's care, he forced her to take a shower while he watched her She pleads with you not to tell her parents about this and insists that they probably will punish her for lying. In addition, she tells you that her grandfather has a heart condition and might have a heart attack if he learns she has told anyone about this

Case 2. Your client is a man in midlife who contacts you for help in making career related decisions. He has no symptoms of an emotional disorder but asks you to indicate, on his payment receipt, that he has a mental disorder so that he can obtain third-party payments for your services. He says that this is the only way he can afford your services.

Case 3. Your client is a 30-year-old man who presents with depression and marital conflict. You are seeing him for individual counseling; he and his wife are seeing another counselor for marital counseling. He tells you, with considerable pleasure, that the marital counselor has recently invited him and his wife to spend a weekend with her family at their beach house "so that he can see how a healthy family operates."

Case 4. You are the counselor for a therapy group for women with social and inter-personal difficulties. One of the women, considerably older than the others, has said almost nothing during the first three sessions of the group. During the fourth session, the youngest member of the group begins verbally attacking the quiet member and encouraging her to leave the group because she is "just dead weight and has nothing to contribute."

Case 5. Your client is a 50-year-old woman who seeks help with panic attacks. After several sessions, you discover that she consumes several bottles of wine each day. Her panic attacks only occur when she is intoxicated. Her dependence on alcohol has resulted in social and occupational impairment as well as other symptoms. Although you are well trained and experienced in helping people diagnosed with Panic Disorders, you have little training and no experience in treating people with Substance Use Disorders. The client insists that she has her alcohol use "under control" and that it is not a problem for her. In addition, she refuses a referral for assessment and treatment of her alcohol use.

Case 6. You have written an excellent paper on the use of systematic desensitization with people who have had heart attacks. Your professor tells you that your paper is so good that she is going to include it in a book she is writing on behavioral counseling. She says nothing about payment or credit for your work.

Case 7. You have been searching for an instrument to assess clients' overinvolvement with the Internet. Finally, you find such an instrument on the Internet. No information is provided on authorship of the instrument nor are any statistics included on the reliability or validity of the instrument. You would like to use it with several of your clients.

PROFESSIONAL DEVELOPMENT

Understanding and practicing according to the ethical guidelines of the counseling profession is one aspect of professional development. Other aspects include:

- Developing awareness of your strengths and limitations
- Clarifying your professional interests and goals
- Expanding your knowledge base and conceptual skills
- Earning professional degrees and certifications
- Joining and participating in professional associations
- Identifying and obtaining employment in a desired work setting where you can practice counseling

- Obtaining supervision
- Taking the relevant examinations and become licensed or certified in your profession
- Continuing your education and development as a counselor

The rest of this chapter will take a closer look at each of these steps in counselors' professional development. Keep in mind, as we review these steps, that professional development for counselors never ends. The counseling profession is an exciting and dynamic field in which new knowledge is constantly generated. Each new client brings his or her own unique history, concerns, and personality into the room. Counselors must constantly read, attend conferences and presentations, and develop their knowledge and skills to keep up with the rapid expansion and evolution of our field.

Counseling is a profession that can bring you considerable personal and professional gratification as you meet the challenges of helping others and advancing the profession. However, counseling can also bring ambiguity and unanticipated pitfalls, leading to frustration and discouragement. The rewards of this rich profession can be maximized if you give thought and planning to your professional goals and development.

DEVELOPING AWARENESS OF YOUR STRENGTHS AND LIMITATIONS ————

The skilled clinician is characterized by three broad areas of strength (Seligman, 2004)

1. *Self-Awareness*, including the capacity for introspection, self-reflection and accurate assessment of one's own personal and professional characteristics, strengths, and limitations.
2. *Self-Efficacy*, including feelings of empowerment, appropriate self-confidence, self-control, and an eagerness to address problems and challenges.
3. *Strong Knowledge Base and Sound Conceptual Skills*, including knowledge of ethics, diagnosis, treatment theories and strategies, multicultural counseling, and other important counseling skills and concepts as well as the ability to apply those skills, learn new skills, and refine existing skills

In Chapter 1 of this book is a list of 10 core areas in which it is important for counselors to have skills and knowledge. These include the following:

1. Professional orientation, identity, and ethics
2. Social and cultural foundations
3. Human growth and development
4. Life-style and career development

5. Counseling theory and helping relationships
6. Group counseling
7. Assessment and appraisal
8. Research and program evaluation
9. Diagnosis and psychopathology
10. Psychotherapy

In addition, counselors need to have competence in the following three additional areas:

11. Emotional health and self-awareness
12. Communication skills
13. Training, supervisory, and other management skills

Current writings on counselor effectiveness suggest a strong connection between personal awareness and counseling skills (Torres-Rivera et al., 2001). An instrument to assess your skills, the Counselor Skills Personal Development Rating Form, has been developed (Torres-Rivers et al., 2002). That instrument yields four factors important in counselor training:

• Emotional sensitivity, including empathy, communication skills, awareness
• Basic listening skills
• Multicultural skills
• Influencing skills

Lumadue and Duffey (1999) conclude that graduate programs in counseling should communicate to new students the importance of developing both personal characteristics and professional skills that are conducive to effective counseling. They suggest that graduate programs should teach these skills as part of the training program and should evaluate students on both personal and professional competence.

Specific skills and competencies associated with each of these 13 broad areas are delineated in Chapter 1. In order to assess your strengths and limitations in each of these areas, I suggest that you return to Chapter 1 and review the lists of specific skills and competencies. Mark your areas of strength with a plus and areas where you have not yet had much training or where you perceive your skills to be at a beginning level with a minus. Then identify those broad areas where you have many pluses and those where you have many minuses, noticing patterns of strength and weakness. List this information in the table at the end of this chapter.

CLARIFYING YOUR PROFESSIONAL INTERESTS AND GOALS

The next step is to clarify your professional interests and goals. This can be accomplished by considering several dimensions of the counselor's role and determining your preferences. Review the following options, circle the interests and goals that are most important to you, and then transfer them to the table at the end of the chapter.

1. Preferred professional activity: administration, coaching, counseling, organizational development, research and writing, supervision, teaching, other.
2. Preferred client population:

   a. Age: children, adolescents, young adults, adults in midlifc, older people.
   b. Presenting problems/diagnoses: academic problems, behavioral difficulties, career concerns, crises, depression and anxiety, disabilities, family dysfunction, medical problems that are chronic or life-threatening, personal growth and self-esteem, psychotic disorders, relationship difficulties, religious and spiritual concerns, sexual difficulties, substance abuse, trauma, other.
   c. Other client characteristics: women, veterans, multicultural, other.

3. Preferred treatment approach: Adlerian therapy, cognitive–behavioral therapy, Gestalt therapy, person-centered counseling, play therapy, psychodynamic therapy, reality therapy, solution-focused brief therapy, other.

Consider also the following intrinsic and extrinsic values and their importance to you.

1. *Intrinsic values*—helping people to overcome their difficulties and create more rewarding lives for themselves, improving services for people in an underserved group (e.g., people with disabilities, people who have immigrated to the United States from another country), conducting research that will enhance the profession, training more effective counselors, strengthening professional associations for counselors, achieving recognition for one's work, other.

2. *Extrinsic values*—becoming the director of a mental health center, developing a large private practice that is well known in the community, becoming a published author, earning a high salary, having secure employment with excellent benefits, having flexible hours to allow ample time for family needs, other.

EXPANDING YOUR KNOWLEDGE BASE AND CONCEPTUAL SKILLS

Now that you have identified your counseling strengths and limitations, as well as particular skills needing further development, and have clarified your professional goals and interests, you are ready to think about steps you need to take to expand your knowledge base and conceptual skills. You may already be in a master's or doctoral program that is helping you develop the skills you need to achieve your goals. Whether or not you are in a structured program, you will probably want to focus your reading, papers, supervision, and elective courses, as well as your participation in conferences and continuing education programs, in such a way as to meet your specific educational and professional goals.

Review the first two sections—the ones you have completed—of the form at the end of this chapter. Then list in that table three strategies for improving your professional knowledge and skills, either because you believe you are weak in those areas or because you anticipate that improvement in those areas will help you achieve your professional goals. For example, you might want to receive training in eye movement desensitization and reprocessing because you believe that will help you become skilled at helping people cope with traumatic experiences; you might want to complete additional reading on diagnosis of personality disorders because you lack the knowledge you think you need to identify and treat these common and challenging disorders; or you might want to focus the papers you write for your courses on spirituality because you ultimately want to develop a program to help people cope with religious and spiritual concerns.

EARNING PROFESSIONAL DEGREES AND CERTIFICATIONS

Throughout the United States, people who want to become licensed or certified as counselors are required to have at least a master's degree in that field, with specific coursework included in their programs of study. In addition, licensure or certification for independent practice typically requires the equivalent of 2 years of full-time supervised experience in counseling after receiving the master's or doctoral degree.

Although the Ph.D. or Ed.D. is not required for independent practice as a counselor, many counselors do continue their education beyond the master's degree. If your state requires additional credits beyond those you received as part of the master's degree, coursework taken toward the doctoral degree may count both toward fulfillment of licensure or certification requirements and toward fulfillment of the requirements for the doctorate. Consequently, if you hope to receive a doctorate, beginning a doctoral program shortly after completing the masters degree may save time and money.

Pursuing doctoral study has many advantages. It is nearly always a requirement for obtaining a full-time university position and it can facilitate your efforts to obtain research funding and supervisory positions in schools and mental health agencies. At least as important are the opportunities to further develop your counseling skills, gain expertise in a particular aspect of counseling, and benefit from the opportunities for mentoring other students, teaching courses, and collaborating with faculty on research.

Of course, continuing your education beyond the master's degree does not need to entail pursuit of a doctorate. Many post-masters certification programs are open to counselors. Examples include certification in addictions counseling, administration and supervision of school guidance programs, play therapy, and sex therapy.

Although your plans might change as you become more established in your profession and perceive a greater need for advanced credentials, think about whether pursuing licensure or certification interests you at present. Briefly describe these goals in the appropriate box in the form at the end of the chapter.

JOINING AND PARTICIPATING IN PROFESSIONAL ASSOCIATIONS ——————

Participation in professional associations brings many benefits to both the counselor and the profession. Professional associations develop ethical standards for the profession, promote legislation that is favorable to the profession, maintain the quality of the profession through national certification and encouragement of state licensure, disseminate knowledge through journals and conferences, and offer a forum for counselors to share ideas and develop personal and professional relationships. For counselors, professional associations provide a sense of community and belonging, help them keep up-to-date on the latest developments in counseling, and offer opportunities for learning and networking.

Professional associations are always in need of volunteers to serve on committees, take on leadership roles, and advance the profession in other ways. I strongly encourage you to participate actively in at least one professional association and to join professional associations at the national, state, and local levels that reflect your interests. I recommend that all counselors become members of their national professional association, the American Counseling Association. In addition, mental health counselors probably will benefit greatly from membership in the American Mental Health Counselors Association, the national professional organization focused on their special needs and interests. Divisions of ACA reflect other special interests in the field; these are listed in Chapter 1. In addition, state branches of ACA and many of its divisions, as well as local counseling organizations, enable counselors to have a direct impact on legislation and other regulations in their state and to meet other mental health professionals in their area.

Review the information on professional associations in Chapter 1 of this book as well as the information above. Then, in the form at the end of this chapter, list those professional organizations of greatest interest to you, along with at least one way in which you might volunteer to serve your profession through one of those organizations.

OBTAINING EMPLOYMENT AS A COUNSELOR

Your work as a counselor actually will begin before you receive a graduate degree in counseling. In most counselor education programs, your initial experience comes in the classroom through role-playing with other students. Then you may progress to seeing a small number of clients in an on-campus laboratory where your performance is closely monitored by your professors and often also by advanced graduate students and your fellow students. The next step is your practicum or internship, which gives you direct work experience in a school or agency while under supervision. Finally, you will be ready to enter the work force as a counselor.

Finding a rewarding and growth-promoting setting for your internship and subsequent employment is an important decision, one that is likely to determine the future direction of your professional life. Consequently, I recommend that you establish a clear set of criteria to guide you in making a wise choice of internship and employment settings. To help you identify those criteria that are important to you, review the following information as well as the next section of this chapter on supervision.

Criteria for Rewarding Internships and Employment

Consideration of the areas described below should help you determine your own criteria for rewarding internships and employment. Keeping these in mind when you review your placement options can help you make a wise choice. When you have finished reading this section, use the form at the end of this chapter to list your preferences in terms of agency focus, the theoretical orientation of its staff, agency expectations for interns and employees, and agency benefits.

Focus of the Counseling Setting

The nature and focus of the counseling setting and the clients it serves are probably the most important criteria. If you select a small agency with a limited focus, such as helping people deal with the diagnosis of Dementia in a family member, that may curtail your future employment opportunities. Unless you are certain that you want to specialize in a particular client population, you will probably be better served by selecting a counseling setting that offers you a broad range of experiences with individual, family, and group counseling, as well as with people of various ages and diagnoses. Also beneficial to most novice counselors is having the opportunity to gain experience in many counseling tasks, such as intake interviews, diagnosis and treatment planning, collaboration with other mental health professionals, training, crisis intervention, and, of course, providing direct counseling. Community mental health centers are particularly likely to offer a broad range of experiences.

If you do select a counseling setting that has a narrow focus, carefully consider whether the skills you will acquire in such an agency are easily transferable. For example, suppose you select a rape crisis counseling center for your internship. Such an agency will afford you experience in dealing with crises, trauma, and women's issues. This experience may well help you gain employment in an agency offering counseling to displaced homemakers, and your knowledge of helping people cope with trauma should appeal to an agency specializing in people who have immigrated to the United States because of war and terrorism in their own country. However, obtaining employment in a school setting where you are helping children with behavioral disorders probably will be difficult.

Theoretical Orientation

Another important consideration, when exploring the focus of a school or agency, is the theoretical orientation of that setting. Many counseling settings advocate a particular approach to counseling; clinical staff are all expected to provide counseling according to that model. Many schools, for example, have adopted Glasser's reality therapy as their standard approach to treatment. College counseling settings serving large numbers of students may encourage staff to use brief solution-focused therapy. An agency providing family therapy may emphasize the value of structural family therapy. Think carefully about whether your own theoretical orientation is compatible with that of your potential internship or place of employment and avoid a placement where you know from the outset that your preferred approach to counseling will not be well accepted.

Expectations of the Setting

Determine exactly what is required of you as an intern or employee in a particular school or agency. Ask what your duties will be and how much of your time will be devoted to each duty. Ask also how your role might evolve over time.

If your interest is primarily in providing counseling to individuals, groups, and families, be sure that will be a significant part of your role. Many schools or agencies prefer that new interns or employees initially spend considerable time in roles that do not involve direct counseling, such as staffing a hot line, conducting intake interviews, making referrals, giving presentations, and organizing assessment centers. Then, as counselors gain experience and demonstrate good clinical skills, they are gradually given a client caseload. Asking specific questions about your role can prevent disappointment.

Also be sure to determine paperwork and time requirements of your role. Nearly all counseling roles require some paperwork, but be sure that the job or placement affords enough time for you to practice and develop your clinical skills. Also ask about the hours you are expected to keep; interns and beginning counselors often are required to work evenings and weekends, while more desirable schedules are reserved for clinicians who have spent more time at the agency. Some agencies prohibit you from establishing a private practice within a specified radius of the agency during, and a year or two after, your employment at the agency. Although you may be willing to make some compromises to obtain a desirable internship or first job, think about how the requirements of the setting mesh with your professional goals and other commitments.

Benefits of the Setting

Each school or agency counseling position offers certain benefits that may include supervision, desirable salary, paid vacations, health insurance, malpractice insurance, funding, and time off for you to attend professional conferences, a private office with attractive furniture, a flexible schedule, secretarial assistance, and other benefits. Determining your priorities and making compromises are in order here too. Decide on which benefits are essential, which are desirable, and which are unimportant to you and then keep that list in mind when making employment or internship decisions.

SELECTING SUPERVISORS AND OBTAINING SUPERVISION

Many students have told me that choosing a supervisor is at least, if not more, important than choosing an agency, and yet students sometimes agree to a placement before they have even met their supervisors. Supervisors serve as mentors, teachers, role models, consultants, and even confidants. Good supervisors orient students to the agency or school, help them form connections with other mental health professionals and support staff, plan meaningful learning experiences for their students, assign them clients that are appropriate for their level of expertise, and take other steps to ensure that those they supervise have a rewarding professional experience. Good supervisors are trustworthy and ethical; they are reliable, setting aside ample time at least once a week to discuss their supervisees' clinical and other professional concerns; they suggest ideas and resources; and they also promote and respect the ideas and efforts of their supervisees. They have multicultural competence and respect and appreciate diversity and difference. They do not insist that supervisees adopt their theoretical orientation; rather, they nurture their supervisees' independence and professional development, always making sure the supervisees are moving in directions that are ethical and compatible with accepted professional practice. Good supervisors also promote counselors' development of personal skills that enhance their effectiveness as counselors. In addition, good supervisors do not become their supervisees' therapists; they respect the dividing line between counseling and supervision.

The National Board of Certified Counselors offers an Approved Supervisor credential. Although this is not a requirement of supervisors, it is an indication of experience and competence in supervision.

While an interview with your prospective supervisor will help you assess some of these dimensions, others are more difficult to discern. Talking to people who have worked under the guidance of your potential supervisor can provide helpful information. In addition, be aware of your own reactions to the supervisor. Although you might be mistaken, a close look at your initial response to the supervisor and the reasons behind that response can help guide your decision. For example, a supervisor who is interested in hearing about your education and career goals might well be a better choice than a supervisor who spends most of your meeting talking about his or her career accomplishments.

Think also about what you need from supervision to be sure that a potential supervisor can meet your needs. Typically, novice counselors profit most from supervisors who establish clear goals and learning conditions and integrate both teaching and counseling elements into their supervision. On the other hand, more experienced and confident counselors usually benefit more from supervisors who stay in the background, allowing supervisees more independence (Littrell, Lee-Borden, & Lorenz, 1979).

A good supervisor can be someone you will turn to throughout your career, whenever you have a professional dilemma; someone who can give you advice and write recommendations that will help you advance your career; and a valued colleague and friend. (Yes, it is ethical for a supervisor to become a friend once the supervisory aspect of your relationship is over.) So choose your supervisor wisely! List your criteria for a good supervisor on the form that concludes this chapter.

BECOMING CREDENTIALED IN YOUR PROFESSION

State licensure or certification and national certification as a counselor are important goals for many counselors. While many credentials attest to counselors' education, experience, and competence, state licensure is particularly important because it enables counselors to practice independently and to receive third-party payments from insurance and managed care companies.

Counselors in private practice must become credentialed in their states. In addition, many agencies encourage their counselors to become licensed as a reflection of the quality of the agency and to facilitate third-party payments and agency accreditation. Even without these incentives, many counselors seek licensure and certification as affirmation of their competence in their field. Additional information on credentials available to counselors is included in Chapter 1 of this book.

Credentials for counselors require a combination of:

1. Education (at least a master's degree, generally including 48–60 credits and specific coursework).
2. Supervised experience (generally 3,000–4,000 hours of counseling experience, often including a specified number of hours of face-to-face counseling).
3. Supervision (e.g., 200 hours or 2 hours per week for 50 weeks for 2 years).
4. Letters of recommendation.
5. Successful performance on an examination.

Credentialing Examinations

Depending on the state in which they practice and the credential they are seeking, counselors usually will take either the National Counselor Examination (NCE) or the National Clinical Mental Health Counseling Examination (NCMHCE or NCE II). Study materials are available to facilitate preparation for each of these examinations. Be sure that any study materials you obtain are geared to the examination you plan to take.

National Counselor Examination (NCE)

The NCE consists of 200 multiple-choice questions, reflecting eight important content areas: Human Growth and Development; Social and Cultural Foundations; Helping Relationships; Group Dynamics, Processes, and Counseling; Life Style and Career Development; Appraisal of Individuals; Research and Evaluation; and Professional Orientation. Study guides for the NCE include the *Preparation Guide* published by NBCC (2001) and the *Clinical Mental Health Counselor Handbook and Study Guide* (Bullard, Lawless, Williams, & Bergstrom, 1999) published under the auspices of the American Mental Health Counselors Association. The following examples are typical of the type of questions included on the NCE:

1. A counselor debated whether a client had a Social Anxiety Disorder or an Avoidant Personality Disorder. The information that is most useful in

helping the counselor determine the correct diagnosis is:

   a. the client's age when the symptoms began
   b. the presence of similar disorders in the client's family of origin
   c. the client's motivation for help
   d. the pervasiveness of the client's symptoms

2. A client tells her counselor that her father recently punched her in the face but asks the counselor not to inform anyone of this incident. Which of the following variables is most important in determining whether the counselor should report this incident?

   a. the client's age
   b. whether the father is likely to hit the client again
   c. the ethical standards for counselors in the town in which the incident occurred
   d. the client's request that the incident not be reported

3. Donald Super's theory of career development pays little attention to:

   a. gender differences between men and women
   b. age-related stages of career development
   c. multicultural differences in career development
   d. the impact of self-esteem on career development

(Correct answers are 1d, 2a, and 3c.)

National Clinical Mental Health Counselors Examination (NCMHCE)

The NCMHCE is a very different type of examination, more grounded in the clinical work of the counselor. The NCMHCE or NCE II is recognized by 21 states as well as Tricare and other managed care organizations. Increasing numbers of states are requiring this examination for licensure; it is also required to obtain the Certified Clinical Mental Health Counselor credential. This examination consists of 10 clinical mental health cases, with five to eight sections of multiple-choice questions following each case. Each section covers either Information Gathering (IG) or Decision-Making (DM). The examination includes questions on evaluation and assessment, including the mental status examination and history taking; diagnosis and treatment planning; and clinical and ethical practice. Clearly, this examination reflects much of the content of this book. In addition to carefully reviewing this text, study information for this examination includes the National Clinical Mental Health Counseling Self-Assessment Examination (NBCC, 1999) and the following web site: http://counselingexam.com/ncmhce

The following is an example of the sort of case included in the NCMHCE:

Client Simulation—Ms. Clayton

Ms. Clayton is a 57-year-old woman who seeks counseling at a community mental health center. She tells you that she "had a terrible experience with a counselor" in the past and was reluctant to seek counseling now but felt so terrible, she felt she had no choice. Ms. Clayton has recently been diagnosed with breast cancer and states that she "just can't handle this alone."

Section A—During your first session, what information would be important to obtain in order to formulate a provisional *DSM-IV-TR* Axis I diagnosis? Select as many items as you believe are indicated.

A1. Medical history
A2. Career and educational history
A3. Changes in patterns of eating and sleeping
A4. Affective symptoms
A5. Suicidal ideation
A6. Support systems
A7. Cognitive functioning
A8. History of emotional difficulties
A9. Problems in previous counseling relationship
A10. Sexual history

(Correct choices include A3, A4, A5, A7, and A8. That information tells you that Ms. Clayton has lost a great deal of weight in the 3 weeks since her medical diagnosis and has slept over 12 hours a day. She is confused and feels unable to concentrate and make decisions. She is deeply depressed, blames herself for her medical diagnosis, and has considered suicide. She had similar symptoms 5 years ago, when her mother died.)

Section B—Based on the above information, what is your provisional DSM-IV-TR Axis I diagnosis for this client? Select only one response.

B1. Adjustment Disorder with Depressed Mood
B2. Major Depressive Disorder, recurrent
B3. Dysthymic Disorder
B4. Dependent Personality Disorder.

(The correct diagnosis is B2, Major Depressive Disorder, recurrent.)

Section C—What information would be useful to you in monitoring this client's progress? Select as many as items as you believe are indicated.

C1. Score on the Beck Depression Inventory
C2. Report of medical tests
C3. Hours of sleep, amount of weight gain or loss
C4. Ability to make medical and other decisions
C5. Scores on the Strong Interest Inventory
C6. Level of cognitive functioning
C7. Level of anger toward previous therapist
C8. Results of Minnesota Multiphasic Personality Inventory
C9. Level of grief related to death of mother
C10. Amount of time spent watching television

(Correct answers are C1, C3, C4, and C6.)

Section D—Which of the following approaches seems most useful for the initial phase of counseling with Ms. Clayton? Select only one response.

D1. Psychoanalysis
D2. Reality therapy
D3. Cognitive–behavioral therapy
D4. Motivational interviewing

(Correct answer is D3, cognitive–behavioral therapy.)

Section E—Which of the following referrals should be considered as part of your initial work with Ms. Clayton? Select as many items as you believe are indicated.

E1. A psychiatrist for a medication evaluation
E2. An acupuncturist for help in dealing with postsurgery pain
E3. A support group for people diagnosed with cancer
E4. A course to enhance social skills
E5. An exercise class
E6. A support group for women in midlife
E7. A political advocacy group, promoting funding for cancer treatments
E8. Her previous therapist, so that they can work out their conflicts

(Correct answers are E1 and E3. E2 and E5 need medical approval for a person with cancer. The other choices are inappropriate at this time.)

Section F—How would you go about addressing Ms. Clayton's bad experience with her previous counselor? Select only one response.

F1. It should not be addressed because it is not relevant to the client's presenting concern.
F2. It should be addressed immediately in order to develop a sound treatment alliance with this client.

F3. It should be addressed immediately so that the current counselor can obtain a release to speak to the previous therapist about Ms. Clayton's counseling with him.

F4. It should be addressed once Ms. Clayton is out of crisis to determine whether that continues to have a negative impact on her and to assess whether any unethical behavior on the part of the counselor occurred.

(Correct answer is F4.)

Section G—After she has made considerable progress in her work with you, Ms. Clayton asks you to help her with her social discomfort. Although she has a few acquaintances at work, she has no close friends and recognizes she needs more support and socialization. You have little experience in dealing with this problem. What would be the best approach for you to take at this point?

G1. Refer the client to group therapy so she can have more exposure to people.

G2. Tell the client you do not work with social discomfort and suggest she find a therapist who specializes in this problem.

G3. Suggest that the client work on this problem by taking classes and joining clubs.

G4. Embark on psychoanalysis to help the client with this problem.

G5. Continue working with the client but get supervision and do some reading on helping people cope with social discomfort.

(Correct answer is G5.)

Section H—What will be your best indication that the client is ready to finish treatment?

H1. The client has completed her medical treatment.

H2. The client has achieved the goals you and she identified.

H3. The client's BDI score has been in the normal range for at least 6 months.

H4. The client asks if you and she can become friends.

H5. The client cancels several appointments.

(Correct answer is H2.)

Preparing for Credentialing Examinations

Preparing for licensure and certification examinations can be a lengthy process. Of course, you already know a great deal of relevant information from your coursework and experience. However, be sure to plan out your study time, gather the resources and study materials you need, and study in the way that works best for you. Some people form study groups to review the material together, others seek supervision to help them prepare for the examination, while still others find that studying on their own works best. Of course, these options can be combined. Talk to people who have recently passed the examination to find out what helped them feel prepared and what they learned about the preparation process from taking the examination. Credentialing examinations are very important to your professional development so you want to be sure that you are well prepared.

Once again, turn to the form at the end of this chapter. Make a notation of your plans to seek licensure and certification and list those examinations you expect to take.

CONTINUING YOUR EDUCATION AND DEVELOPMENT AS A COUNSELOR

Finally! You have the graduate degrees and courses you need, you have obtained supervised experience in your first job, and you have passed the examination to become licensed or certified.

However, becoming a skilled counselor means becoming a lifelong learner. Many state and national credentialing bodies require that counselors acquire continuing education units (CEUs) in order to maintain their credential. Part of maintaining the National Certified Counselor credential, for example, is obtaining a minimum of 100 clock hours of continuing education over a 5-year period. Whether or not you need to continue your education in order to maintain certification or licensure, attending professional trainings and conferences is important for counselors, as is reading about developments in the counseling field.

In addition to continuing education, self-care is an important component of counselor development. Despite its many rewards and benefits, counseling is a stressful profession, particularly for those who work with people who are severely troubled, have been through traumas and abuse, or who are likely to achieve only small gains. Figley (1995), for example, writes of compassion fatigue in mental health professionals, a sort of secondary traumatic stress disorder in those who focus their work on helping people who have been traumatized. Secondary traumatization can lead to unhealthy coping mechanisms, anger and depression, and even the decision to leave the mental health field.

Taking steps to avoid compassion fatigue and burnout are important for counselors. Achieving balance in their lives, practicing stress management, exercising on a regular basis, developing a sound support system, establishing clear priorities and realistic goals, and making good use of time management and limit setting are important in helping counselors achieve healthy personal and professional development.

Counseling is a dynamic and exciting field and counselors must make sure that their knowledge is up-to-date so that they can provide the best possible services whether they are practicing counselors, counselor educators, coaches, or other professionals in the counseling field. I hope you will enjoy the excitement and challenges of becoming a lifelong learner in counseling.

YOUR PERSONAL PROFESSIONAL DEVELOPMENT PLAN

Now that you have learned about the steps in the professional development of an effective counselor, you have the opportunity to prepare your own personal professional development plan. Use the framework below to complete that plan, giving you a road map you can follow in future years.

PROFILE OF MY PROFESSIONAL DEVELOPMENT

Awareness of My Strengths and Limitations

Three areas of greatest competence:

1.

2.

3.

Two areas where my skills need improvement:

1.

2.

Specific skills needing particular attention:

1.

2.

3.

My Professional Interests and Goals

• Preferred professional activity:

- Preferred presenting problems/diagnoses:

- Other client characteristics:

- Intrinsic values:

- Extrinsic values:

Expanding My Knowledge Base and Conceptual Skills

Three approaches to bettering my knowledge and conceptual skills:

1.

2.

3.

Plans for Earning Professional Degrees and Certifications

1.

2.

3.

Joining and Participating in Professional Associations

- Professional associations of interest to me:

- Contributions I might volunteer to make to one of my professional associations:

Obtaining Employment as a Counselor

- Focus of the agency (problems, clients, counselor roles):

- Theoretical orientation:

- Expectations of the setting (tasks, paperwork, schedule):

- Benefits of the setting (supervision, salary, training, other):

Obtaining Supervision

- Professional credentials (e.g., education, theoretical orientation, experience)

- Personal credentials (e.g., responsible and responsive, good listener, encourages your professional growth):

Becoming Credentialed

- Credentials desired:
- Schedule for obtaining credential:
- Examinations required:
- Study/preparation plan:

Continuing Your Education and Development as a Counselor

- Continuing education plans, formal and informal
- Self-care

Future Trends and Predictions in Counseling

You are currently reading the third edition of *Diagnosis and Treatment Planning in Counseling*. The first edition was published in 1986; the second, in 1996. Each of those earlier editions included a final chapter that made predictions for the future of the counseling profession. Many of those predictions have been realized while others have not. The final chapter of this book will look at those earlier predictions and discuss which ones came true, which did not, and what we can learn from that about the direction of the field. In addition, new predictions for the future of counseling are included in this book, organized according to the 12 preceding chapters.

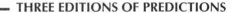 **1986 Predictions**

In the first edition of this book, published in 1986, I made the following nine predictions about the future of the counseling profession, most of which have been realized (Seligman, 1986).

1. *Changes are anticipated in counselor education programs in terms of both the students and the curriculum. Proportionately fewer students interested in school or college counseling will be enrolled while the mental health component of many programs will expand… Counselor education programs are requiring more courses to enable students to meet state licensure requirements and function effectively in mental health settings. Some professionals believe that 60 semester hours should be the standard preparation for a master's degree in counseling. These changes will increase the number of qualified mental health counselors and should increase the visibility and credibility of the profession.*

As predicted, programs to train mental health counselors, including those to prepare marriage and family counselors, have grown more rapidly than other counseling specializations. However, school counseling remains a large and strong area of specialization in counselor education programs. Sixty semester hours is now standard preparation for licensure as a counselor; master's degree programs typically require at least 48 credits, with many now requiring 60 credits. In addition, the credibility and visibility of the counseling profession have increased, although counselors have not yet achieved full parity with social workers and psychologists—professions with longer histories.

  2. *Demographic and social trends will change and expand the composition of mental health counselors' clientele, requiring counselors to develop new skills. Examples of such trends are the growing number and percentage of people over 65 in the population, the high divorce rate, the increasing number of midlife career changers, and the growth in multicultural diversity in the United States.*

  Multicultural counseling competence is essential to today's mental health counselors. Not only has the client population become more varied, it has also become more challenging. Counselors are dealing with such serious concerns as physical and sexual abuse, drug and alcohol dependence, loss of contact with reality, and criminal behavior and suicidal ideation in children and adolescents. Both the diversity and the severity of the problems people bring into counseling have increased and are expected to increase further. Approaches to counseling that emphasize multicultural competence, integration of skills and techniques, and adaptation to individual client needs have become increasingly important.

  3. *Greater emphasis will be placed on developmental and preventive approaches to counseling. This should enhance the counselors' roles in nonmedical settings and as consultants, trainers, and human resource managers.*

  Counselors have gained greater acceptance in nonmedical and nonclinical settings and are increasingly finding employment as consultants, coaches, supervisors, trainers, and employee assistance and human resource professionals. Although the professional literature has paid considerable attention to the developmental and preventive aspects of counselors' roles, a gap still exists between theory and practice. The counseling profession has not yet been fully successful in integrating preventive and developmental aspects of counseling with remedial ones. This is due to several factors, including the increasing severity of clients' concerns, the emphasis of managed care on brief treatment, and the availability of third-party payments only for treatment of mental disorders. Some progress has been made toward offering more developmental and preventive services in schools and community agencies, and new theoretical models such as feminist counseling emphasize healthy development. However, the work of most mental health counselors is still focused on ameliorating pathology, even if they pay attention to prevention of future difficulties. Counselors should continue to seek ways to integrate the preventive, developmental, and remedial elements of their work in order to provide high-quality services to their clients, and to preserve the values and qualities that distinguish mental health counselors.

4. *Increasing numbers of states will pass licensure laws for counselors. That should increase counselors' visibility and credibility and open up new opportunities.* Nearly all states now offer licensure or certification that allows counselors to practice independently. Private practice continues to be a popular career choice for counselors. In addition, counselors continue to find employment in a broad and diverse array of settings.

5. *Shortages of both psychiatrists and psychologists are predicted with the gap being filled, at least in part, by mental health counselors. Cooperation among mental health professionals should increase.* This projection, too, has come to pass. Psychiatrists today provide primarily medication management, requiring nonmedical helping professionals to assume primary responsibility for counseling and case management. Counselors are increasingly working collaboratively with psychiatrists who can provide medication to enhance the impact of counseling.

6. *Federal funds, grants, and insurance payments for mental health services all seem to be growing scarcer and more tightly controlled. In order to obtain a substantial share of those funds, counselors will have to demonstrate their effectiveness and accountability.* Funds for mental health services have, indeed, become increasingly scarce. Although this trend is unfortunate in many ways, it probably has led counselors to provide more effective and efficient services. Goal setting, treatment planning, and regular evaluation of progress have become essential to the counseling process. Client and counselors benefit from procedures that establish a clear direction to treatment and facilitate rapid improvement.

7. *Acceptance of holistic health and the relationship of physical and emotional concerns seems to be increasing and should lead to a corresponding increase in the number and frequency of counselors working with physicians to ameliorate physical illness via stress management, mental imagery, and other approaches.* Emphasis on the mind–body–spirit connection has, indeed, increased. Research has demonstrated that counseling can help people cope more successfully with serious illness and that counseling can have a beneficial impact on people's health. Counselors are increasingly employed in medical settings, working collaboratively with physicians to help people with chronic and life-threatening illnesses. In addition, counselors in other settings are making greater use of strategies such as relaxation, meditation, and imagery that reflect the mind–body–spirit connection.

8. *Improved computer technology and other developments should bring counselors more efficient systems of record keeping, better time management, and new and more precise tests and inventories.* Computerized administration and scoring of many standardized tests and inventories now are widely used. In addition, computerized systems for billing,

diagnosis and treatment planning, and writing progress reports are available. Technology has made an important contribution to counseling, although its function still is ancillary to face-to-face counseling services.

9. *The rapid change in counselors' roles and the increasing demand on counselors to work with a wide range of client groups often may be stressful and lead to frustration, apathy, cynicism, and anger. Attention will need to be paid to the professional and emotional development of counselors via peer support groups, continuing education, and the further development of support services provided by professional associations for counselors.*

Counselors today are indeed under increasing pressure, not only because of the challenges presented by their clients, but also because of the requirements of managed care, the need to market their services and obtain funding, and the threat of malpractice claims. Much has been written about burnout and compassion fatigue among mental health professionals. Counselors and agencies have sought to address this issue via peer support groups, relaxation programs, and education. However, finances and other obstacles have led the American Counseling Association and other professional organizations to offer fewer opportunities for support and continuing education. A national structure of peer support and counseling groups, to help both impaired and well-functioning counselors cope with the rigors of their profession, has not yet been put into place. Local and national professional organizations are encouraged to develop such support services. Counselors need more help in coping with stress, frustration, and burnout as they deal with the challenges of their profession.

1996 Predictions

Many future predictions were made in the previous edition of this book. Rather than addressing each one, I will present a summary of predictions that are relevant to each chapter of this book and then will discuss ways in which the predictions have and have not been realized.

The Changing Role of the Counselor

In 1996, predictions anticipated a generally accepted definition of mental health counseling, encompassing developmental, preventive, rehabilitative, and remedial aspects. A uniform definition of the profession has not emerged. Nevertheless, acceptance of and respect for counselors has greatly increased and counselors' roles and competencies have been expanded and clarified. This is due to many factors, including expansion of state licensure for counselors, CACREP's (Council for Accreditation of Counseling and Related Educational Programs) establishment of definitive standards for counselor education, the increase in CACREP-accredited graduate programs, and the identification of multicultural competencies.

Counselor education programs have become increasingly rigorous, with many requiring 60 graduate credits as predicted. In addition, as anticipated in 1996, graduate programs are now more likely to offer coursework on psychopathology and the *Diagnostic and Statistical Manual of Mental Disorders* (*DSM*), treatment planning, medication, family counseling, brief therapy, physical and sexual abuse, substance-use disorders, managed care, legal and ethical issues, supervision, consultation, and program development and evaluation. Opportunities for specialization during graduate school have increased. Counseling students now have a more realistic understanding of the challenges and rewards of their profession. Although the field may have lost some of its mystique, counselors now are better prepared and less prone to disillusionment.

Managed care organizations (MCOs) have continued to be a powerful force, but they do seem to have become more consistent and user-friendly, as well as more receptive to providing payments for the services of licensed counselors. These changes may, at least in part, be due to law suits and efforts on the part of mental health organizations to improve dealings with MCOs. MCOs will continue to play an important role in health care as long as costs escalate; only a national or international health insurance is likely to modify that.

Although licensure or certification now is available in nearly all states, reciprocity of credentials between states and uniformity of credentialing standards are still issues for the profession. Perhaps by the next issue of this book, significant headway will be made in this area. Continuing education is increasingly required to maintain one's credentials. A wide range of face-to-face courses and workshops are available along with homestudy programs and on-line courses.

Although I predicted that opportunities in private practice would decline, that has not happened, at least in part because most MCOs now make insurance payments to licensed counselors. Many private practices have become group, multidisciplinary practices, but individual private practitioners still have an important role in providing mental health services.

Opportunities for the Mental Health Counselor

All of the predictions made in this section have been realized. Counselors continue to emphasize the importance of multicultural counseling competence. They also value sensitivity to and appreciation of individual differences. Concepts of diversity have been broadened so that they focus not only on ethnic and cultural differences, but also on differences in age, gender, sexual orientation, background, abilities, and other dimensions. Broad-based models of understanding and counseling people from diverse backgrounds are widely accepted.

Especially important are models that are systemic, holistic, epistemological, and phenomenological. Greater attention now is paid to effecting change at the systemic level, reflected in counselors' increased use of marketing, grant writing, social activism, and advocacy.

Collaboration between counselors and other helping professionals has increased. Particularly strong alliances have now formed between school and mental health counselors and psychiatrists and mental health counselors.

Diagnostic Systems and Their Use

The general predictions made in 1996 about the future of diagnosis have indeed been realized. Most clinicians recognize that the *DSM* is an essential tool for counselors and that it can be integrated into any theoretical framework and successfully combined with systemic and holistic approaches to assessment and treatment. Training in diagnosis and treatment planning using the *DSM* has become a standard ingredient of counselor preparation programs, while demonstration of competence in these skills is increasingly incorporated into credentialing examinations. In addition, clinicians pay more attention to the reciprocal relationships between physical conditions and emotional functioning.

However, my prediction that a range of new diagnoses would be identified has not been realized. We have learned more about existing disorders. Clinicians and researchers continue to explore the need for additional diagnoses, especially mood, eating, and personality disorders. However, the American Psychiatric Association has not officially identified any new diagnoses since my 1996 predictions. This results from many factors, including controversy among mental health professionals, an emphasis on rigorous research to substantiate new diagnoses, and the time between editions of the *DSM*. However, advances are needed to address shortcomings in the present diagnostic system. In addition, research has not yet provided clear criteria for distinguishing between genuine and false memories of traumatic experiences, needed to facilitate diagnoses of anxiety and other disorders.

The Use of Assessment in Diagnosis

Again, all of the predictions in this section have been realized. The importance of assessment in counseling continues to grow. Particular emphasis is placed on the development of brief assessment tools, such as the Brief Symptom Inventory, that facilitate goal setting and provide a rapid measure of progress. Technology now plays an important role in the administration, scoring, and interpretation of tests and inventories, although paper-and-pencil inventories and projective tests requiring personal interpretation continue to be used.

Assessment has increasingly become multidimensional, drawing on many sources of information. It is more holistic, humanistic, and individualized, better integrated into the counseling process, and less judgmental. Greater sensitivity to and awareness of the potential for gender and cultural bias in assessment has developed, leading to more cautious use of assessment tools.

Intake Interviews

Intake interviews continue to be essential to effective diagnosis and treatment planning. Similarly, the mental status examination has become a standard ingredient of counseling. Although some tools and specific interview protocols have been developed, the intake process has not yet been standardized and varies widely from one clinician or agency to another.

The Nature and Importance of Treatment Planning

As anticipated, treatment planning now is an essential ingredient of the counseling process, although a generally accepted model for treatment planning has not emerged. Outpatient treatment has increasingly followed a brief solution-focused model, with clearly specified goals and criteria for termination. At the same time, most clinicians seem to conceptualize clients' difficulties in systemic and holistic terms, and continue to have considerable leeway in their approaches to treatment.

Clinicians also have greater appreciation for several aspects of the treatment process. Research has clearly demonstrated the profound impact on treatment outcome of the therapeutic alliance and the personal attributes of the counselor. These variables may be at least as important, if not more important, than the specific treatment strategies used. Research has also substantiated the value of combining medication and counseling in the treatment of many mental disorders such as Bipolar Disorder, Attention-Deficit/Hyperactivity Disorder, and Schizophrenia. In addition, clinicians seem to be making greater use of adjunct services and between-session tasks.

Criteria for inpatient treatment have become increasingly stringent. Inpatient treatment today is generally very brief, with clients referred out to day-treatment centers, individual therapy, or other sources of help as soon as possible.

Theories and Techniques of Individual Counseling

Most, but not all, of my predictions in this section have been realized. Research has continued to explore and identify the common elements in effective treatment, with the therapeutic alliance being paramount. Considerable attention is being paid to the empirical study of what treatments are effective in ameliorating what disorders, the study of differential therapeutics (Seligman, 1998). The development of new counseling theories has focused heavily on systematic, integrated, and eclectic approaches that facilitate prescriptive matching of interventions to diagnosis, problem, and person, while also promoting growth and development. Examples of this are Developmental Counseling and Therapy and the Stages of Change model developed by Prochaska and colleagues (1999). However, research still is needed in this area.

Mental health professionals' use of and interest in many treatment approaches also has evolved since 1996. Solution-focused treatment and other models of brief therapy have received increasing attention, as have critical-incident stress debriefing and other crisis-intervention models. I predicted that use of humanistic, psychoanalytic, existential, Gestalt, and transactional approaches to treatment would decline while use of educational, cognitive, behavioral, psychobiological, systemic, and integrated approaches would increase. While this prediction is generally correct, psychoanalysis continues to have a small but strong following. In addition, a resurgence of interest in humanistic and existential approaches has occurred, reflecting concerns that many people are struggling with, particularly in the aftermath of the events of September 11, 2001. Use of cognitive and behavioral techniques, such as skills training, *in vivo* exposure, problem solving, and cognitive restructuring, seems to have increased, while use of interpretative techniques (e.g., analysis of transference, free association) and high-risk techniques (e.g., flooding, catharsis, aversive conditioning, paradoxical intervention) do seem to have decreased. Transpersonal, Shamanic, and other spiritual approaches to counseling have received attention but have not replaced traditional models of counseling.

Assessment and Treatment of Couples and Families

All predictions in this section have been realized. Couples and family counseling has continued to grow in importance as an approach to treatment, a way of thinking, and an area of specialization. Even when counselors are providing individual therapy, they typically seek to understand and address systemic dynamics and concerns, and think in terms of complex and circular rather than linear models of change and growth. In addition, awareness of the importance of diversity has led counselors to pay more attention to clients' families, culture, and worldview. Nontraditional families have become more prevalent, and counselors seem to have become more knowledgeable and sensitive to the needs of single-parent, gay and lesbian, combined, and other nontraditional families. Treatment approaches such as narrative therapy and constructivism have received considerable attention because of their relevance to family and individual counseling.

Assessment and Treatment Planning for Groups and Organizations

Group counseling has continued to grow in use, both because it is perceived as cost-effective and because it is useful in treatment of a broad range of disorders (e.g., Eating Disorders, Posttraumatic Stress Disorder, Substance Use Disorder). In addition, the use of counseling and support groups for prevention and maintenance has increased.

However, contrary to my prediction, important new models of group counseling have not emerged. In addition, only limited attention has been paid to the use of diagnosis and treatment planning in counseling groups and to research for clarifying what disorders and clients are likely to benefit from group counseling.

Writing and Record Keeping in Counseling

Documentation of their work, via reports and progress notes, has indeed become very important for counselors. This provides a solid basis for counseling, facilitates treatment, and demonstrates effectiveness. I predicted that counselors might shorten their sessions or modify their schedules to allow time for paperwork; in fact, the 45-minute session is now replacing the 50-minute session as a standard, and many clinicians allocate part of their weekly schedule to record keeping. New tools and models, most of which are computerized, facilitate record keeping.

CURRENT PREDICTIONS

Many of the predictions I made in 1986 and 1996 have been realized, although some have not. Most of those that have not been realized are still being studied and continue to find a place in the predictions I am making in this edition. In addition, the mental health field has advanced in some unanticipated directions and this, too, is reflected in my current predictions. Here are my predictions for the future of counseling over the next 10 years, organized according to the subject matter of the preceding 12 chapters of this book.

The Evolving Role of the Counselor

1. Counselors will establish themselves even more firmly as mental health treatment providers. Indications of this will be licensure in all states, an increase in the number of CACREP-accredited counselor education programs, and increasing recognition on the part of counselors and employers of the importance of that accreditation.
2. Managed care will continue to play an important role. MCOs will slightly increase their payments and will become more user-friendly. Counselors will receive Medicare payments.
3. Parity laws will be passed in additional states, leading MCOs to authorize more mental health services.

4. Additional states will pass scope-of-practice laws to ensure that the work of the counselor, as well as the title of counselor, is protected.
5. Counselor education programs will pay increasing attention to developing and assessing students' personal qualities because of the important role they play in treatment effectiveness.
6. The role of neurophysiology in emotional development and disorders will receive increasing recognition and research support. Counselor education programs will incorporate more information on biology and neurophysiology.
7. Counselor education programs will make greater use of technology, for example, for on-line instruction, distance learning, and computer simulations.
8. Qualitative research methods will become more widely used in professional research and articles based on qualitative research will become more prevalent in the journals.
9. Some progress will be made toward reciprocity of counseling credentials from one state to another but full reciprocity will not yet be established.
10. Some progress will be made toward establishment of international health insurance, but that will not yet have a significant impact on counselors' roles.

Opportunities for the Mental Health Counselor

1. Counselors will have even more appreciation for diversity and multicultural counseling competence. Case conceptualization and treatment will increasingly become systemic, holistic, and phenomenological and will attend to the "extrapsychic forces that adversely affect the emotional and physical well being of people" (Kiselica & Robinson, 2001, p. 387).
2. Collaboration with other professionals will continue to be important. More states will follow the lead of New Mexico, allowing psychologists to obtain prescribing privileges; this will lead to greatly increased collaboration between psychologists and counselors. Partnerships between schools and mental health agencies will continue to expand.
3. Efforts to expand primary and secondary prevention programs will continue, with moderate success, notably in the schools. Efforts will focus particularly on promoting wellness and resilience (the ability to cope effectively with negative stressors). Legislation, such as the Child Healthcare Crisis Relief Act, as well as movements such as Martin Seligman's (1999) Positive Psychology, will facilitate efforts to develop both preventive and remedial programs.

4. Opportunities for counselors will continue to expand, particularly in non-clinical roles such as conducting research, grant writing, promoting social justice, advocacy, lobbying, serving as an expert witness, community organization, organizational development, and coaching.
5. Counselors will play a greater role in helping people cope with chronic and life-threatening illnesses and with grieving, dying, and death.

Diagnostic Systems and Their Use

1. The next complete revision of the *DSM* is expected to be published in 2010 (Pennington, 2002) and will contain some additional diagnoses. These might include diagnoses for mild depression, a depressive personality disorder, additional eating disorders, child and adolescent bipolar disorder, addictive use of the Internet (especially when involved in fantasy games or sexual activity linked to the Internet), premenstrual emotional dysfunction, repetitive self-mutilation, bullying, and other forms of school violence.
2. Relational Disorder, a controversial new diagnosis, defined as "persistent, painful patterns of feelings, behavior and perception involving two or more partners in personal relationships" (Pennington, 2002, p. 20) already is being debated.
3. Another diagnosis already being used, although not officially sanctioned by the *DSM*, is Executive System Dysfunction, characterized by impairment in goal setting, planning ability, abstract thinking, impulse control, problem-solving, memory, and other functions of the frontal system of the brain.
4. Increasing questions will be raised about the validity of the diagnosis of Gender Identity Disorder (GID). Perhaps, like homosexuality, GID will eventually be deleted from the *DSM* and determined not to be a mental disorder.
5. Although diagnosis will continue to be an essential tool in the counselors' repertoire of skills, the *DSM* may no longer be the one widely accepted diagnostic manual in the United States. Because of HIPAA regulations, some clinicians will find they also need to be familiar with the latest version of the *ICD Classification of Mental and Behavioural Disorders*.

The Use of Assessment in Diagnosis and Treatment Planning

1. Testing and assessment will continue to be important in counseling, particularly to help counselors make accurate diagnoses, obtain a baseline for symptom severity, and measure progress toward goal attainment.

2. Emphasis will be placed on the need for assessment procedures to reflec multicultural counseling competence.
3. New inventories will be developed, particularly those directed at assess ing specific symptoms and diagnoses and measuring emotional intelli gence (EI).
4. Computer technology will play an increasing part in the assessmen process, with many inventories administered and scored online Additional research will be done on the use, validity, and reliability o computerized assessment.
5. Assessment of suicidal ideation will continue to be very important However, counselors will see more discussion of rational suicide and physician-assisted suicide. Other states are likely to follow Oregon in passing a Death with Dignity Act.

Intake Interviews and Their Role in Diagnosis and Treatment Planning

1. Intake interviews and mental status examinations (MSEs) will continue to be important ingredients of diagnosis and treatment planning.
2. New models for intake interviews and mental status examinations will be developed and will be geared to specific client groups and settings Particularly important will be models that are comprehensive and tha view people in context, such as the biopsychosocial model and the devel opmental–contextual model.
3. Computerized versions of intake interview and MSEs will be developed and will grow in use and relevance to the process of diagnosis and treat ment planning.

The Nature and Importance of Treatment Planning

1. More information will be available on effective treatment of people with dual diagnoses.
2. The use of treatment manuals will increase.
3. Counselors will have a better understanding and appreciation of the grea importance to treatment effectiveness of the client–counselor relationship the counselor's personal characteristics, and the personal and situationa resources of the clients.
4. Counseling via telephone, email, and videoconferencing will increase In addition, national computerized databases will help people identify potential counselors and treatment programs. Additional guidelines and ethical standards will clarify the appropriate use of technology for counseling.

5. Counselors will engage in more frequent collaboration with educators and other mental health professionals.
6. Mental health professionals, as well as physicians, will become more aware of the interface between mental and physical conditions and the soft line that often exists between the two.
7. Although the use of medication, in combination with counseling, will increase, research will indicate that for some disorders, particularly those involving children and adolescents, medication has been overprescribed and insufficiently studied to determine appropriate use.
8. Clinicians will learn more about matching drug to person and problem, and will begin using studies of brain-wave activity as one way to assess the impact of a medication.

Theories and Strategies of Individual Counseling

1. Research will continue to expand the list of empirically supported (or evidence-based) treatments and clinicians will increasingly draw on that research.
2. Counseling will place more emphasis on a scientist-practitioner model in which counselors are expected to research their own practices and have a sound scientific basis for their work (Wampold, Lichtenberg, & Wachler, 2002).
3. Innovative treatment strategies will emerge, while those already established will be further studied and understood. Particular attention will be paid to filial therapy to train parents to be therapeutic agents to their own children, virtual reality for exposure treatment of Posttraumatic Stress Disorder and phobias, use of robots as adjuncts in treatment of children (Graap, September/October 2002), counseling to promote forgiveness, non-Western and holistic approaches, brief-treatment models, and others.
4. Power and energy therapies, such as Eye Movement Desensitization and Reprocessing (EMDR), Thought Field Therapy, Traumatic Incident Reduction, Visual/Kinesthetic Dissociation and others, will become better understood and researched. EMDR and perhaps others will receive clear empirical support and general acceptance.
5. Although constructivist, narrative, feminist, and male-oriented approaches will not achieve widespread use, their ideas and strategies will be increasingly integrated into well-accepted approaches to counseling because of their phenomenological and multicultural bases.
6. The resurgence of interest in phenomenological approaches such as person-centered counseling, existential therapy, and Gestalt therapy, in a modified form, will accelerate.

7. New approaches based on these approaches, such as Motivational Interviewing and Responsive Therapy based on person-centered counseling, will be developed and expanded, giving a postmodern flavor to older therapies.

Assessment, Diagnosis, and Treatment Planning for Families

1. Growing awareness of the importance of Bowlby's attachment theory will lead to shifts in how family therapy is conducted, with increased attention paid to early attachment patterns and their impact on subsequent relationships.
2. Increased attention also will be paid to patterns of relating in families such as parental-alienation syndrome, abusive father/disengaged mother, single-parent families, and others. While some research in this area will be fruitful, counselors may initially find themselves dealing with a plethora of new, confusing, and not always valid relationship syndromes.
3. Although the time is ripe for a completely new, innovative, and powerful approach to family counseling, most treatment of families will probably continue to reflect modified versions of established approaches to individual treatment.
4. However, awareness of the importance of family dynamics and subsystems, intergenerational transmission, and birth order will continue to distinguish family from individual treatment.
5. Research will continue on nontraditional families and their treatment, shedding light on how to nurture healthy, resilient families, regardless of their composition or origins.

Assessment and Treatment Planning for Groups

1. New models for group counseling will be developed. Particularly useful will be those that follow the lead of individual and family counseling and suggest integrated, brief, and systemic perspectives that have demonstrated effectiveness.
2. Group counseling will continue to be an important approach, especially in preventive work, and research will provide greater clarification of the problems, disorders, and clients for whom group counseling is most likely to be helpful.
3. Protocols will be developed for treatment of groups whose problems and clients are homogeneous, for example, children needing skills in building friendships, families who have experienced the suicide of a loved one, and young adolescent girls who are sexually active.

4. Group counseling and self-help groups will become better integrated, with more information becoming available on ways to maximize the beneficial impact of Twelve-step and other self-help groups.

Counseling for Career and Organizational Development

1. More attention will be paid to the impact of multicultural variables on career development, leading to the recognition that variables such as social values, time orientation (past–present–future), and commitment to the family are powerful determinants of career development.
2. Career and mental health counseling will become better integrated. Mental health counselors will develop greater appreciation for the place of careers in people's lives, and career counselors will develop greater appreciation for the importance of diagnosis and taking a holistic and contextual view of career development.
3. Mental health professionals working in career counseling and organizational development settings will pay greater attention to the importance of the interactions between worker personality and values and those of supervisors and colleagues.
4. Organizational development, as well as other aspects of counseling in business and industry, will grow in importance as counselors develop coaching and other relevant skills.

Documentation, Report Writing, and Record Keeping in Counseling

1. Record keeping and documentation will continue to be an essential component of counselors' role. Improved and more widely available technology will facilitate that process.
2. Use of electronic medical records will promote collaborative treatment and ease transfer of information.
3. Electronic billing will increasingly become the norm, simplifying counselors' interactions with MCOs.
4. Counselors and their clients will increasingly use the Internet for communication, scheduling, transmitting forms, assessment, follow-up, research via search engines, discussion and support groups, distance learning, and participation in listservs and online communities.
5. Increasing numbers of counselors will have their own web pages, making information on mental health services more widely available.
6. Counselors will make greater use of computerized packages for diagnosis, treatment planning, assessment, and other counseling-related activities.

7. Counseling via the Internet will increase the availability of mental health services to people who do not have proximity to such services or who do not have the physical mobility they need to get to a mental health facility.

8. Even counselors who are not strong advocates of the integration of technology into mental health services will find they need some knowledge of word processing and email to meet the basic requirements of their work.

9. HIPAA guidelines will become clarified and widely accepted, necessitating additional documentation but further safeguarding clients' rights and adding to the growing importance of making clients aware of their rights and responsibilities as clients.

10. Counselors will increasingly make use of between-session tasks as an integral part of their treatment plans.

The Importance of Ethical and Professional Development

1. Counselors will increasingly serve as expert witnesses in helping the courts determine mental competency, custody decisions, and other legal issues.

2. Ethical guidelines addressing the use of technology in counseling will be further clarified, providing counselors a greater sense of security in using electronic tools in their work.

3. Ethical standards will remain the bedrock of the profession, but will become more realistic, humanistic, and flexible.

4. Counselors will move forward in using single-subject design and less formal strategies to research their own practices and become better informed on the effectiveness of their treatment.

5. Counselors will continue to play an active role in promoting human rights.

6. Research will provide greater understanding of burnout, secondary traumatic stress, compassion fatigue, empathic strain, and other stress reactions that counselors often experience.

7. Personal, professional, and organizational changes and intervention strategies will help counselors deal with their challenging roles.

Many additional changes will emerge in the counseling field that have not been anticipated or discussed in this book. I encourage you to reflect on the information in this chapter as well as on your own knowledge and experience to generate additional predictions for changes that you expect to see in the mental health field over the next 10 years.

CONCLUSION

This chapter has reviewed the predictions made in the first and second editions of this book and discussed whether they have actually happened. In addition, new predictions, linked to each chapter in this book, are included. This chapter, as well as the previous chapters of this book, demonstrates the rich and evolving nature of the counseling profession and reflects the rewards and challenges it offers to counselors. My work in this field has been a great source of fulfillment, education, and inspiration to me. I wish you the same experience!

References

ACA. (2003). *Mission statement*. retrieved April 26, 2004 from http://www.counseling.org.

Adler, A. (1931). *What life should mean to you*. Boston: Little, Brown.

Alberding, B., Lauver, P., & Patnoe, J. (1993). Counselor awareness of the consequences of certification and licensure. *Journal of Counseling and Development, 72*(1), 33–38.

Altekruse, M. K. (1995). What mental health counselors do: A demographic analysis. In M. K. Altekruse & T. L. Sexton (Eds.), *Mental health counseling in the 90's* (pp. 13–24). Tampa, FL: National Commission for Mental Health Counseling.

Altekruse, M. K., & Sexton, T. L. (1995). Mental health counseling in the 90's. In M. K. Altekruse & T. L. Sexton (Eds.), *Mental health counseling in the 90's* (pp. 7–12). Tampa, FL: National Commission for Mental Health Counseling.

Altman, K. P. (1992). Psychodramatic treatment of multiple personality disorder and dissociative disorders. *Dissociation Progress in the Dissociative Disorders, 5*(2), 104–108.

Amatea, E. S., & Sherrard, P. A. D. (1994). The ecosystemic view: A choice of lenses. *Journal of Mental Health Counseling, 16* (1), 6–21.

American Counseling Association. (1995). *ACA code of ethics and standards of practice*. Alexandria, VA: Author.

American Psychiatric Association. (2000). *Diagnostic and statistical manual of mental disorders* (4th ed.). Washington, DC: Author.

Amerikaner, M., Monks, G., Wolfe, P., & Thomas, S. (1994). Family interaction and individual psychological health. *Journal of Counseling and Development, 72*(6), 614–620.

Anastasi, A. (1992). What counselors should know about the use and interpretation of psychological tests. *Journal of Counseling and Development, 70*(5), 610–615.

Anderson, W. P., & Niles, S. G. (1995). Career and personal concerns expressed by career counseling clients. *The Career Development Quarterly, 43*(3), 240–245.

Anderson, W. P., & Niles, S. G. (2000). Important events in career counseling: Client and counselor descriptions. *Career Development Quarterly, 48*, 251–263.

Argyris, C. (1957). *Personality and organization*. New York: Harper & Row.

Arredondo, P., Toorek, R., Brown, S., Jones, J., Locke, D. C., Sanchez, J. et al. (1996). *Operationalization of the multicultural counseling competencies*. Alexandria, VA: Association for Multicultural Counseling and Development.

Association for Specialists in Group Work. (2000). *Professional standards for the training of group workers*. Alexandria, VA: Author.

Balgopal, P. R. (1989). Establishing employee assisstance programs: A cross-cultural perspective. *Employee Assistance Quarterly, 5*, 1–20.

Bandura, A. (1986). *Social foundations of thought and action: A social cognitive theory*. Englewood Cliffs, NJ: Prentice Hall.

Bartholomew, K., & Horowitz, L. M. (1991). Attachment styles among young adults: A test of a four-category model. *Journal of Personality and Social Psychology, 61*, 226–244.

Battegay, R. (1990). New perspectives on acting out. *Journal of Group Psychotherapy, Psychodrama and Sociometry, 42*(4), 204–212.

Beck, J. S. (1995). *Cognitive therapy: Basics and beyond*. New York: Guilford Press.

Becvar, D. S., & Becvar, R. J. (1993). *Family therapy*. Boston: Allyn & Bacon.

Benson, E. (2002, December). Thinking clinically. *Monitor on Psychology, 33*, 30–31.

Berne, E. (1961). *Transactional analysis in psychotherapy*. New York: Grove.

Betz, N. E., Fitzgerald, L. F., & Hill, R. E. (1989). Trait-factor theories: Traditional cornerstone of career theory. In M. B. Arthur, D. T. Hall, & B. S. Lawrence (Eds.), *Handbook of career theory* (pp. 25–40). New York: Cambridge University Press.

Beutler, L. E., Crago, M., & Arizmendi, T. G. (1986). Therapist variables in psychotherapy process. In S. L. Garfield & A. E. Bergin (Eds.), *Handbook of psychotherapy and behavior change* (3rd ed, pp. 257–310). New York: Wiley.

Blocher, D. H., & Biggs, D. A. (1983). *Counseling psychology in community settings*. New York: Springer.

Bloom, B. L. (1983). *Community mental health: A general introduction*. Monterey, CA: Brooks/Cole.

Blustein, D. L. (1994). "Who am I?": The question of self and identity in career development. In M. L. Savickas & R. W. Lent (Eds.), *Convergence in career development theories* (pp. 130–154). Palo Alto, CA: CPP.

Boscolo, L., Cecchin, G., Hoffman, L., & Penn, P. (1987). *Milan systemic family therapy*. New York: Basic Books.

Bowen, M. (1974). Theory in the practice of psychotherapy. In P. J. Guerin, Jr. (Ed.), *Family therapy: Theory and practice*. New York: Gardner Press.

Bowlby, J. (1988). *A secure base: Parent–child attachment and healthy human development*. New York: Basic Books.

Bowman, S. L. (1993). Career intervention strategies for ethnic minorities. *The Career Development Quarterly, 42*, 14–25.

Brill, A. A. (Ed.) (1938). *The basic writings of Sigmund Freud*. New York: Modern Library.

Brown, D. (1996). Brown's values-based, holistic model of career and life-role choices and satisfaction. In D. Brown & L. Brooks (Eds.), *Career choice and development* (3rd ed., pp. 337–372). San Francisco: Jossey-Bass.

Brown, D. (2003). *Career information, career counseling, and career development* (8th ed.). Boston: Allyn & Bacon.

Brown, N. W. (1994). *Group counseling for elementary and middle school children*. Westport, CT: Praeger.

Brown, S. D., & Lent, R. W. (2000). Handbook of Counseling Psychology (3rd ed.). New York: John Wiley & Sons.

Brown, S. L. (2002). We are, therefore I am: A multisystems approach with families in poverty. *Family Journal, 10*, 405–409.

Bubenzer, D. I., Zimpfer, D. G., & Mahrle, C. L. (1990). Standardized individual appraisal in agency and private practice: A survey. *Journal of Mental Health Counseling, 12*(1), 51–66.

Bullard, B., Lawless, L., Williams, M., & Bergstrom, D. (1999). *Clinical mental health counselor handbook & study guide*. Sudbury, MA: Professional Training Institute.

Busby, D. M., Holman, T. B., & Tamiguchi, N. (2001). RELATE: Relationship evaluation of the individual, family, cultural, and couple contexts. *Family Relations, 50*, 308–316.

Cameron, S., & Turtle-Song, I. (2002). Learning to write case notes using the SOAP format. *Journal of Counseling and Development, 80*, 286–292.

Campbell, R. E., & Cellini, J. V. (1981). A diagnostic taxonomy of adult career problems. *Journal of Vocational Behavior, 19*, 175–190.

Cantor, N., Acker, M., & Cook-Flannagan, C. (1992). Conflict and preoccupation in the intimacy life task. *Journal of Personality & Social Pscyhology, 63*(4), 644–655.

Carey, A., & Varney, G. H. (1983). Which skills spell success in OD? *Training and Development Journal, 37*, 40–48.

Carroll, L., Gilroy, P. J., & Ryan, J. (2002). Counseling transgendered, transsexual, and gender-variant clients. *Journal of Counseling and Development, 80*, 131–139.

Carter, B., & McGoldrick, M. (Eds.) (1999). *The expanded family life cycle: Individual, family, and social perspectives.* Boston: Allyn & Bacon.

Carty, L. (1993). Group counseling and the promotion of mental health. *The Journal for Specialists in Group Work, 18*(1), 29–39.

Cella, D. F., & Perry, S. W. (1986). Reliability and concurrent validity of three visual analogue mood scales. *Psychological Reports, 59*, 827–833.

Chambless, D. L., et al. (1998). Update on empirically validated therapies. *The Clinical Psychologist, 51*, 1–19.

Cochran, L. (1997). *Career counseling: A narrative approach.* Thousand Oaks, CA: Sage.

Collins, A., & Watts, A. G. (1996). The death and transfiguration of career and career guidance. *British Journal of Guidance and Counseling, 24*(3), 385–398.

Comella, P. A. (1996). A brief summary of Bowen family systems theory. In P. A. Comella, J. Bader, J. S. Ball, K. K. Wiseman, & R. R. Sagar (Eds.), *The emotional side of organizations: Applications of Bowen theory* (pp. 5–7). Washington: Georgetown Family Center.

Cominskey, P. E. (1993). Using reality therapy group training with at-risk high school freshmen. *Journal of Reality Therapy, 12*(2), 59–64.

Corry, R., & Jewell, T. C. (2001). Psychiatric rehabilitation idealized: Multi-setting uses and strategies over the course of severe mental illness. *Journal of Mental Health Counseling, 23*, 93–103.

D'Andrea, M. (1999, May). Alternative needed for the *DSM-IV* in a multicultural-postmodern society. *Counseling Today, 44*, 46.

D'Andrea, M. (2000). Postmodernism, constructivism, and multiculturalism: Three forces reshaping and expanding our thoughts about counseling. *Journal of Mental Health Counseling, 20*, 1–16.

Daniels, J. A. (2002). Assessing threats of school violence: Implications for counselors. *Journal of Counseling and Development, 80*, 215–222.

Danzinger, P. R., & Welfel, E. R. (2001). The impact of managed care on mental health counselors: A survey of perceptions, practices, and compliance with ethical standards. *Journal of Mental Health Counseling, 23*, 137–150.

Davis, J. (2002, July/August). Managed care, EAP trends are promising. *The Advocate, 25*(4), 1, 5–7.

deShazer, S. (1991). *Putting difference to work.* New York: W. W. Norton.

Diamond, G. S., Serrano, A., Dickey, M., & Sonis, W. A. (1996). Current status of family-based outcome and process research. *Journal of the American Academy of Child and Adolescent Psychiatry, 35*, 6–16.

Dinkmeyer, D., & Carlson, J. (1984). *Time for a better marriage.* Circle Pines, MN: American Guidance Service.

Duckworth, J. C., & Anderson, W. P. (1995). *MMPI & MMPI-2 interpretation manual for counselors and clinicians.* Bristol, PA: Accelerated Development.

Duffy, T. K. (1990). Psychodrama in beginning recovery: An illustration of goals and methods. *Alcoholism Treatment Quarterly, 7*(2), 97–109.

Ellis, A. E., & Dryden, W. (1997). *The practice of rational emotive behavior therapy* (2nd ed.). New York: Springer.

Epstein, N., Schlesinger, S. E., & Dryden, W. (1988). *Cognitive-behavioral therapy with families.* New York: Brunner/Mazel.

Erikson, E. H. (1963). *Childhood and society.* New York: W. W. Norton.

Eron, J., & Lund, T. (1996). *Narrative solutions in brief therapy.* New York: Guilford Press.

Espelage, D. L., Bosworth, K., & Simon, T. R. (2000). Examining the social context of bully behaviors in early adolescence. *Journal of Counseling and Development, 78*, 326–333.

Falvey, J. E. (1992). From intake to intervention: Interdisciplinary perspectives on mental health treatment planning. *Journal of Mental Health Counseling, 14*(4), 471–489.

Fauman, M. A. (2002). *Study guide to DSM-IV*. Washington, DC: American Psychiatric Association.

Figley, C. R. (1995). *Compassion fatigue: Coping with secondary traumatic stress disorder in those who treat the traumatized*. New York: Brunner/Mazel.

Foley, R. J., & Redfering, D. L. (1987). Bridging the gap between counseling psychologists and organizational development consultants. *Journal of Business and Psychology, 2*, 160–170.

Fong, M. L. (1990). Mental health counseling: The essence of professional counseling. *Counselor Education and Supervision, 30*(2), 106–113.

Forcey, L. R., & Nash, M. (1998). Rethinking feminist theory and social work therapy. *Women and Therapy, 21*, 85–99.

Forrester-Miller, H., & Davis, T. E. (1996). *A practitioner's guide to ethical decision-making*. Alexandria, VA: American Counseling Association.

Fox, L. A. (1996). Bowen family systems theory as a framework for consultants. In P. A. Comella, J. Bader, J. S. Ball, K. K. Wiseman, & R. R. Sagar (Eds.), *The emotional side of organizations: Applications of Bowen theory* (pp. 121–129). Washington: Georgetown Family Center.

Frances, A., Clarkin, J., & Perry, S. (1984). *Differential therapeutics in psychiatry*. New York: Brunner/Mazel.

French, W. L., & Bell, C. H., Jr. (1999). *Organization development: Behavioral science interventions for organization improvement* (6th ed.). Saddle River, NJ: Prentice Hall.

Friedman, R. M. (1994). Psychodynamic group therapy for male survivors of sexual abuse. *Group, 18*(4), 225–234.

Gallo, F. (2002, May/June). Thawing the pond. *Psychotherapy Networker*, 71–80.

Gardner, H. (2003). Retrieved May 19, 2003, from http://www.ed.psu.edu/insys/ESD/gardner/Mitheory.html

Gati, I., & Asher, I. (2001). The PIC model of career decision making: prescreening, in-depth exploration, and choice. In F. T. L. Leong and A. Barak (Eds.), *Contemporary models in vocational psychology* (pp. 7–54). Mahwah, NJ: Erlbaum Associates.

Gibson, J. L., Ivancevich, J. M., & Donnelly, J. H., Jr. (1982). *Organizations: Behavior, structure, processes*. Plano, TX: Business.

Gillis, H. L., & Bonney, W. C. (1989). Utilizing adventure activities with intact groups: A sociodramatic systems approach to consultation. *Journal of Mental Health Counseling, 11*, 345–358.

Ginter, G. G. (1995). *Systematic treatment planning with an overview of DSM-IV*. Workshop presented at the annual meeting of the American Counseling Association.

Ginzberg, E. (1972). Toward a theory of occupational choice: A restatement. *Vocational Guidance Quarterly. 20*(2), 169–176.

Gladding, S. T. (2003). *Group work*. Columbus, OH: Merrill/Prentice Hall.

Glasser, W. (1986). *Control theory in the classroom*. New York: Harper & Row.

Glasser, W. (1998). *Choice theory*. New York: HarperCollins.

Glauser, A. S., & Bozarth, J. D. (2001). Person-centered counseling: The culture within. *Journal of Couseling and Development, 79*, 142–147.

Glosoff, H. L. (1992, May). Accrediting and certifying professional counselors. *Guidepost, 34*(12), 6–8.

Goldenberg, H., & Goldenberg, I. (2002). *Counseling today's families*. Pacific Grove, CA: Brooks/Cole.

Goldman, E. E., & Morrison, D. S. (1984). *Psychodrama: Experience and process*. Dubuque, IA: Kendall/Hunt.

Goleman, D. (1995). *Emotional intelligence*. New York: Bantam Books.

Gottfredson, L. S. (1981). Circumscription and compromise: A developmental theory of occupational aspirations. *Journal of Counseling Psychology, 28*, 545–579.

Gottfredon, L. S. (1996). Gottfredson's theory of circumscription and compromise. In D. Brown & L. Brooks (Eds.), *Career choice and development* (3rd ed., pp. 179–232). San Francisco: Jossey-Bass.

Goulding, M. (1987). Transactional analysis and redicision therapy. In J. L. Zeig (Ed.), *The evolution of psychotherapy* (pp. 285–299). New York: Burnner/Mazel.

Graap, K. (2002, September/October). Virtual reality technology here to stay, holds significant promise for psychology. *The National Psychologist, 11*(5), 18–28.

Grant, B. (1990). Principled and instrumental nondirectiveness in person-centered therapy and client-centered therapy. *Person-Centered Review, 5,* 77–88.

Gross, D. R., & Capuzzi, D. (2001). Counseling the older adult. In D. Capuzzi & D. R. Gross (Eds.), *Introduction to the counseling profession.* Needham Heights, MA: Allyn & Bacon.

Groth-Marnat, G. (1990). *Handbook of psychological assssment.* New York: John Wiley & Sons.

Gunderson, J. G. (1988). Personality disorders. In A. M. Nicholi, Jr. (Ed.), *The new Harvard guide to psychiatry* (pp. 337–357). Cambridge, MA: Harvard University Press.

Guterman, J. T. (1994). A social constructionist position for mental health counselors. *Journal of Mental Health Counselors. 16*(2), 226–244.

Gysbers, N. C., Heppner, M. J., & Johnston, J. A. (2003). *Career counseling process, issues and techniques* (2nd ed.). Boston: Allyn & Bacon.

Hackett, G., & Betz, N. E. (1981). A self-efficacy approach to the career development of women. *Journal of Vocational Behavior, 5,* 419–441.

Haley, J. (1987). *Problem-solving therapy.* San Francisco: Jossey-Bass.

Hall, A. S. (2002). Partnerships in preventing adolescent stress: Increasing self-esteem, coping, and support through effective counseling. *Journal of Mental Health Counseling. 24,* 97–109.

Hall, A. S., & Parsons, J. (2001). Internet addiction: College student case study using best practices in cognitive behavior therapy. *Journal of Mental Health Counseling, 23,* 312–327.

Harmon, L. (2001). Opportunities for using your clinical skills to solve corporate problems. In L. VandeCreek (Ed.), *Innovations in clinical practice: A source book* (Vol. 19, pp. 329–345). Professional Resource Exchange.

Harmon, L. W. (1997). Do gender differences necessitate separate career development theories and measures? *Journal of Career Assessment, 5,* 463–470.

Hayes, L. L. (2002, September). The death of college counseling. *Counseling Today,* 12–13.

Held, B. S. (2001). The postmodern turn. In B. D. Slife, R. N. Williams, & S. H. Barlow (Eds.), *Critical issues in psychotherapy,* (pp. 241–256). Thousand Oaks, CA: Sage.

Herlihy, B., & Corey, G. (1996). *ACA ethical standards casebook.* Alexandria, VA: American Counseling Association.

Herman, K. C. (1993). Reassessing predictors of therapist competence. *Journal of Counseling and Development, 72*(1), 29–32.

Hershenson, D. B. (1993). Healthy development as the basis for mental health counseling theory. *Journal of Mental Health Counseling, 15*(4), 430–437.

Hill, L. K. (1990). The future of mental health counseling in the new era of health care. In G. Seiler (Ed.), *The mental health counselors sourcebook* (pp. 105–138). New York: Human Sciences Press.

Hinkle, J. S. (1994a). Ecosystems and mental health counseling: Reaction to Becvar and Becvar. *Journal of Mental Health Counseling, 16*(1), 33–36.

Hinkle, J. S. (1994b). The *DSM-IV:* Prognosis and implications for mental health counselors. *Journal of Mental Health Counseling, 16*(2), 174–183.

Hohenshil, T. H. (1993). Teaching the *DSM-III-R* in counselor education. *Counselor Education and Supervision, 32*(4), 267–275.

Holland, J. (1966). A psychological classification scheme for vocations and major fields. *Journal of Counseling Psychology, 13,* 278–288.

Holland, J. L. (1992). *Making vocational choices: A theory of vocational personalities and work environments.* Odessa, TX: Psychological Assessment Resources.

Holland, J. L. (1994). Separate but equal is better. In M. L. Savickas & R. W. Lent (Eds.), *Convergence in career development theories* (pp. 45–52). Palo Alto, CA: Consulting Psychologists Press.

Hollis, J. W., & Wantz, R. A. (1994). *Counselor preparation: Status, trends, and implications* (Vol. II). Muncie, IN: Accelerated Development.

Honeyman, A. (1990). Perceptual changes in addicts as a consequence of reality therapy based group treatment. *Journal of Reality Therapy, 9*(2), 53–59.

Huddleston, R. (1989). Drama with elderly people. *British Journal of Occupational Therapy, 52*(8), 298–300.

Ingersoll, R. E. (2000). Teaching a psychopharmacology course to counselors: Justification, structure, and methods. *Counselor Education and Supervision, 40*, 58–69.

Ivey, A. E. (1989). Mental health counseling: A developmental process and profession. *Journal of Mental Health Counseling, 11*(1), 26–35.

Ivey, A. E., & Ivey, M. (1999). Toward a developmental diagnostic and statistical manual: The vitality of a contextual framework. *Journal of Counseling and Development, 77*, 484–490.

Janson, G. R., & Steigerwald, F. J. (2002). Family counseling and ethical challenges with gay, lesbian, bisexual, and transgendered (GLBT) clients: More questions than answers. *Family Journal, 10*, 415–418.

Johnsen, E. (1994). Utilization management and its impact on client well-being: The next frontier for mental health counseling. *Journal of Mental Health Counseling, 16*(2), 279–284.

Johnson, D., & Johnson, S. (2003). *Real world treatment planning.* Pacific Grove, CA: Brooks/Cole-Thompson Learning.

Johnson, D. L. (1993). Toward a synthesis of theory: Adopting a new perspective to advance the field of mental health counseling. *Journal of Mental Health Counseling, 15*, 236–239.

Jones, K. D., Robinson, E. H., Minatrea, N., & Hayes, B. L. (1998). Coping with reactions to clients traumatized by child sexual abuse. *Journal of Mental Health Counseling, 20*, 332–342.

Kanas, N., Schoenfeld, F., Marmar, C. R., & Weiss, D. S. (1994). Process and content in a long-term PTSD therapy group for Vietnam veterans. *Group, 18*(2), 78–88.

Kaplan, H. I., & Sadock, B. J. (1994). *Synopsis of psychiatry* (7th ed.). Baltimore: Williams & Wilkins.

Kelly, K. R., & Hall, A. S. (1992). Toward a developmental model for counseling men. *Journal of Mental Health Counseling, 14* (3), 257–273.

Kerr, M. E. (1996). The extension of Bowen theory to nonfamily groups. In P. A. Comella, J. Bader, J. S. Ball, K. K. Wiseman, & R. R. Sagar (Eds.), *The emotional side of organizations: Applications of Bowen theory* (pp. 8–17). Washington: Georgetown Family Center.

Kessler, R. C., McGonagle, K. A., Zhao, S., Nelson, C. B., Hughes, M., Eshleman, S. et al. (1994). Lifetime and 12-month prevalence of *DSM-III-R* psychiatric disorders in the United States. *Archives of General Psychiatry, 51*, 8–19.

Kiselica, M. S., & Robinson, M. (2001). Bringing advocacy counseling to life: The history, issues, and human dramas of social justice work in counseling. *Journal of Counseling and Development, 79*, 387–397.

Kivlighan, D. M., Jr., Coleman, M. N., & Anderson, D. C. (2000). Process, outcome, and methodology in group counseling research. In S. D. Brown & R. W. Lent (Eds.), *Handbook of counseling psychology* (3rd ed., pp. 767–796). New York: John Wiley & Sons.

Klein, R. (1993). Short-term psychotherapy. In H. Kaplan & B. Sadock (Eds.), *Comprehensive group psychotherapy* (pp. 257–263). Baltimore: Williams & Wilkins.

Kobasa, S. C. (1979). Stressful life events, personality, and health. *Journal of Personality and Social Psychology, 37*(1), 1–11.

Kocarek, C. E., Talbot, D. M., Batka, J. C., & Anderson, M. Z. (2001). Reliability and validity of three measures of multicultural competency. *Journal of Counseling and Development, 79*, 486–496.

Kopta, S. M., Lueger, R. J., Sanders, S. M., & Howard, K. I. (1999). Individual psychotherapy and process research: Challenges leading to greater turmoil or a positive transition? *Annual Review of Psychology, 50*, 441–469.

Korman, A. K. (1994). *Human dilemmas in work organizations: Strategies of resolution.* New York: Guilford Press.

Kormanski, C. (1988). Using group development theory in business and industry. *Journal for Specialists in Group Work, 13*(1), 30–43.

Kottler, J. A. (1994). *Advanced group leadership.* Pacific Grove, CA: Brooks/Cole.

Krumboltz, J. D. (1979). A social learning theory of career decision-making. In A. M. Mitchell, G. B. Jones, & J. D. Krumboltz (Eds.), *Social learning and career decision-making* (pp. 19–49). Cranston, RI: Carroll Press.

Krumboltz, J. D. (1993). Integrating career counseling and personal counseling. *The Career Development Quarterly, 42*, 143–148.

Kwan, K. K. (2001). Models of racial and ethnic identity development: Delineation of practice implications. *Journal of Mental Health Counseling, 23*, 269–277.

Lawless, L. L., Ginter, E. J., & Kelly, K. R. (1999). Managed care: What mental health counselors need to know. *Journal of Mental Health Counseling, 21*, 50–65.

Lazarus, A. A., & Beutler, L. E. (1993). On technical eclecticism. *Journal of Counseling and Development, 71*(4), 381–385.

Lent, R. W., & Hackett, G. (1987). Career self-efficacy: Empirical status and future directions. *Journal of Vocational Behavior, 30*, 347–382.

Leong, F. T. L. (1996). Toward an integrative model for cross-cultural career counseling and psychotherapy. *Applied and Preventive Psychology, 5*, 189–209.

Leong, F. T. L., & Brown, M. T. (1995). Theoretical issues in cross-cultural career development: Cultural validity and cultural specificity. In W. B. Walsh & S. H. Osipow (Eds.), *Handbook of vocational psychology* (2nd ed., pp. 143–180). Mahwah, NJ: Erlbaum.

Leong, F. T. L., & Serfafica, F. C. (2001). Cross-cultural perspective on super's career development theory: Career maturity and cultural accommodation. In F. T. L. Leong and A. Barak (Eds.), *Contemporary models in vocational psychology* (pp. 167–206). Mahwah, NJ: Erlbaum.

Likert, R. (1961). *New patterns of management.* New York: McGraw-Hill.

Lewis, V. J., Blair, A. J., & Booth, D. A. (1992). Outcome of group therapy for body-image emotionality and weight control self-efficacy. *Behavioural Psychotherapy, 20*(2), 155–165.

Linehan, R. R. (1993). *Skills training manual for treating borderline personality disorder.* New York: Guilford Press.

Littrell, J. M., Lee-Borden, N., & Lorenz, J. A. (1979). A developmental framework for counseling supervision. *Counselor Education and Supervision, 19*, 119–136.

Livneh, H. (1991). Counseling clients with disabilities. In D. Capuzzi & D. R. Gross (Eds.), *Introduction to counseling: Perspectives for the 1990s* (pp. 416–443). Boston: Allyn & Bacon.

Locke, E. A., & Latham, G. P. (2002). Building a practically useful theory of goal setting and task motivation: A 35-year odyssey. *American Psychologist, 57*, 705–717.

Locke, H., & Wallace, K. (1959). Short marital adjustment and prediction tests: Their reliabiity and validity. *Marriage and Family Living, 2*, 251–255.

Lofquist, L. H., & Dawis, R. V. (1991). *Essentials of person-environment correspondence counseling.* Minneapolis: University of Minnesota.

Lumadue, C. A., & Duffey, T. H. (1999). The role of graduate programs as gatekeepers: A model for evaluating student counselor competence. *Counselor Education and Supervision, 39*(2), 101–110.

MacKay, B. (1989). Drama therapy with female victims of assault. *Arts in Psychotherapy, 16*(4), 293–300.

MacLennan, B. W., & Dies, K. R. (1992). *Group counseling and psychotherapy with adolescents.* New York: Columbia University Press.

Madanes, C. (1981). *Strategic family therapy.* San Francisco: Jossey-Bass.

Martin, I. (1996). *From couch to corporation.* New York: John Wiley & Sons.

Martin, R. B., & Stepath, S. A. (1993). Psychodrama and reminiscence for the geriatric psychiatric patient. *Journal of Group Psychotherapy, Psychodrama and Sociometry, 45*(4), 139–148.

Maxmen, J. S., & Ward, N. G. (1995). *Essential psychopathology and its treatment.* New York: W. W. Norton.

McCubbin, H. I., Patterson, J. M., Rossman, M. M., & Cooke, B. (1982). *SSI social support inventory.* Madison: University of Wisconsin.

McFarland, W. P. (1992). Counselors teaching peaceful conflict resolution. *Journal of Counseling and Development, 71*(1), 18–21.

McGoldrick, M., & Gerson, R. (1988). Genograms and the family life cycle. In B. Carter & M. McGoldrick (Eds.), *The changing family life cycle* (pp. 164–189). New York: Gardner Press.

McGoldrick, M., Pearce, J., & Giordano, J. (1999). *Ethnicity and family therapy* (2nd ed.). New York: Guilford Press.

McGregor, D. (1966). The human side of enterprise. In W. G. Bennis & E. H. Schien (Eds.), *Leadership and motivation* (pp. 3–20). Cambridge: MIT.

McNair, D. M., Lorr, M., & Droppleman, L. F. (1992). *POMS manual.* San Diego, CA: EdITS.

McLaughlin, J. E. (2002). Reducing diagnostic bias. *Journal of Mental Health Counseling, 24,* 256–259.

McWhirter, J. J., & McWhirter, B. T. (1991). A framework for theories in counseling. In D. Capuzzi & D. R. Gross (Eds.), *Introduction to counseling: Perspectives for the 1990s* (pp. 69–88). Boston: Allyn & Bacon.

Mead, M. A., Hohenshil, T. H., & Singh, K. (1997). How the *DSM* system is used by clinical counselors: A national study. *Journal of Mental Health Counseling, 19,* 383–401.

Meara, N. M. (1997). Changing the structure of work. *Journal of Career Assessment, 5,* 471–474.

Mental Health, United States. (1998). Washington, DC: Department of Health and Human Service Substance Abuse and Mental Health Services Administration.

Messina, J. J. (1995). The historical context of the Orlando Model Project and the NCMHC. In M. K. Altekruse & T. L. Sexton (Eds.), *Mental health counseling in the 90s* (pp. 1–6). Tampa, FL: National Commission for Mental Health Counseling.

Meyers, R. F., Apodaca, Flicker, & Slesnick, N. (2002). Evidence-based approaches for the treatment of substance abusers by involving family members. *Family Journal, 10,* 281–288.

Miller, S., Hubble, M., & Duncan, B. (1996). *Handbook of solution-focused brief therapy.* San Francisco: Jossey-Bass.

Miller, W. (1999). Toward a theory of motivational interviewing. *Motivational Interviewing Newsletter: Updates, Education and Training, 6*(4), 2–4.

Miller-Tiedêman, A., & Tiedman, D. V. (1990). Career decision making: An individualistic perspective. In D. Brown, L. Brooks, & Associates (Eds.), *Career choice and development* (2nd ed., pp. 308–337). San Francisco: Jossey-Bass.

Millner, V. S., & Ullery, E. K. (2002). A holistic treatment approach to male erectile disorder. *Family Journal, 10,* 443–447.

Minuchin, S., & Fishman, H. C. (1981). *Family therapy techniques.* Cambridge, MA: Harvard University Press.

Minuchin, L., Lee, W.-Y., & Simon, G. M. (1996). *Mastering family therapy: Journeys of growth and transformation,* New York: John Wiley & Sons.

Mitchell, K. E., Levin, A. S., & Krumboltz, J. D. (1999). Planned happenstance: Constructing unexpected career opportunities. *Journal of Counseling and Development, 77,* 115–124.

Montag, K. R., & Wilson, G. L. (1992). An empirical evaluation of behavioral and cognitive-behavioral group marital treatments with discordant couples. *Journal of Sex and Marital Therapy, 18*(4), 255–272.

Moorey, S., & Greer, S. (1989). *Psychological therapy for patients with cancer: A new approach.* Washington, DC: American Psychiatric Press.

Morrison, J. (1995a). *DSM-IV made easy,* New York: Guilford Press.

Morrison, J. (1995b). *The first interview,* New York: Guilford Press.

Morrissey, M. (1994, December). Counselors "helping the helpers" from becoming casualities. *Counseling Today, 37*(6), 1, 6–7, 12.

Morrissey, M. (1995, January). Executive coaching increases counselors' role in industry. *Counseling Today. 37*(7), 1–2.

Motto, J., Heilbron, D. C., & Juster, R. P. (1985). Development of a clinical instrument to estimate suicide risk. *American Journal of Psychiatry, 152,* 680–686.

Mueller, R. O., Dupuy, P. J., & Hutchins, D. E. (1994). A review of the TFA Counseling System: From theory construction to application. *Journal of Counseling and Development, 72*(6), 573–577.

Myers, J. (1989). *Adult children and aging parents.* Alexandria, VA: American Counseling Association.

Myers, J. E. (1990). Aging: An overview for mental health counselors. *Journal of Mental Health Counseling, 12*(3), 245–259.

Myers, J. E. (1992). Wellness, prevention, development: The cornerstones of the profession. *Journal of Mental Health Counseling, 12,* 245–259.

Myers, J. E., Sweeney, T. J., & Witmer, J. M. (2000). The wheel of wellness counseling for wellness: A holistic model for treatment planning. *Journal of Counseling and Development, 78,* 251–266.

Nance, D. W., & Myers, P. (1991). Continuing the eclectic journey. *Journal of Mental Health Counseling. 13*(1), 119–130.

Nash, J. M. (2002, May 6). The secrets of autism. *Time,* 45–49.

National Board for Certified Counselors, Inc. (1999). *National clinical mental health counseling self-assessment examination.* Greensboro, NC: NBCC.

National Board for Certified Counselors, Inc. and Affiliates. (2001). *Preparation guide for the National Counselor Examination for Licensure and Certification.* Greensboro, NC: NBCC.

National Standards for Clinical Mental Health Counseling. (1999). Alexandria, VA: AMHCA.

Naughton, J. (2002, July/August). The coaching boom. *Psychotherapy Networker,* 24–33.

Newman, R. (2002, October). The road to resilience. *Monitor on Psychology, 33*(19), 62.

Newstrom, J. W., & Davis, K. (1993). *Organizational behavior: Human behavior at work* (9th ed.). New York: McGraw-Hill.

Nugent, F. A. (1990). *An introduction to the profession of counseling.* Columbus, OH: Merrill.

O'Donnell, J. M. (1988). The holistic health movement: Implications for counseling theory and practice. In R. Hayes & R. Aubrey (Eds.), *New directions for counseling and human development* (pp. 365–383). Denver: Love.

Olson, D. H. (1986). Circumplex model VII: Validation studies and FACES-III. *Family Process, 25,* 337–351.

Olson, D. H., & Schaefer, M. T. (2000). *PAIR: Personal assessment of intimacy in relationships manual.* Minneapolis, MN: Life Innovations.

Osipow, S. H., Walsh, W. B., & Tosi, D. J. (1980). *A survey of counseling methods.* Homewood, IL: Dorsey Press.

Paniagua, F. A. (2001). *Diagnosis in a multicultural context.* Thousand Oaks, CA: Sage.

Parsons, F. (1909). *Choosing a vocation.* Boston: Houghton Mifflin.

Patton, W., & McMahon, M. (1999). Career development and systems theory: A new relationship. Pacific Grove, CA: Brooks/Cole.

Pedersen, P. (1990). The multicultural perspective as a fourth force in counseling. *Journal of Mental Health Counseling, 12*(1), 93–95.

Pennington, D. (2002, October). Family ties? *Counseling Today, 1,* 20.

Pennington, D. (2002, December). Breaking free. *Counseling Today,* 8–10.

Perry, J. C., & Cooper, S. H. (1989). An empirical study of defense mechanisms. *Archives of General Psychiatry, 46*, 444–452.

Peters, R. J. (2000). *Organizational stress in a selected group of male and female consulting personnel.* Ann Arbor, MI: UMI Dissertation Services.

Peterson, G. W., Sampson, J. P., Jr., & Reardon, R. C. (1996). A cognitive information processing approach to career problem solving and decision-making. In D. Brown & L. Brooks (Eds.), *Career choice and development* (3rd ed., pp. 423–476). San Francisco: Jossey-Bass.

Pfeiffer, S. M. (1995, Spring). Editor's corner. *Advance, 2*, 16.

Piaget, J. (1963). *The child's conception of the world.* Patterson, NJ: Littlefield, Adams.

Pistole, M. C., & Roberts, A. (2002). Mental health counseling: Toward resolving identity confusions. *Journal of Mental Health Counseling, 24*, 1–19.

Pollak, J., Levy, S., & Breitholtz, T. (1999). Screening for medical and neurodevelopmental disorders for the professional counselor. *Journal of Counseling and Development, 77*, 350–358.

Ponterotto, J. G. (2002). Qualitative research methods: The fifth force in psychology. *The Counseling Psychologist, 30*, 394–406.

Porras, J. I., & Berg, P. O. (1978). Evaluation methodology in organization development: An analysis and critique. *Journal of Applied Behavioral Science, 14*, 151–173.

Powell, B. (2002, October). LPCs included in child mental health workforce shortage bill. *The Advocate, 25*(6), 9.

Prieto, L. R., & Scheel, K. R. (2002). Using case documentation to strengthen counselor trainees' case conceptualization skills. *Journal of Counseling and Development, 80*, 11–21.

Prochaska, J. O., & Norcross, J. C. (1994). *Systems of psychotherapy.* Pacific Grove, CA: Brooks/Cole.

Prochaska, J. O., & Norcross, J. C. (1999). *Systems of psychotherapy.* Pacific Grove, CA: Brooks/Cole.

Prouty, A. M., Markowski, E. M., & Barnes, H. L. (2000). Using the dyadic adjustment scale in marital therapy: An exploratory study. *The Family Journal, 8*, 250–257.

Riemer-Reiss, M. L. (2002). Utilizing distance technology for mental health counseling. *Journal of Mental Health Counseling, 22*, 189–203.

Rigazio-DiGilio, S. A., Ivey, A. E., Ivey, M. B., & Simek-Morgan, L. (1997). Developmental counseling and therapy: Individual and family therapy. In A. E. Ivey, M. B. Ivey, & L. Simek-Morgan (Eds.), *Counseling and psychotherapy: A multicultural perspective* (pp. 89–129). Needham Hights, MA: Allyn & Bacon.

Rogers, C. R. (1942). *Counseling and psychotherapy.* Boston: Houghton Mifflin.

Rogers, C. R. (1970). *Carl Rogers on encounter groups.* New York: Harper & Row.

Rounds, J. B., & Tracy, T. J. (1996). Cross-cultural equivalence of RIASEC models and measures. *Journal of Counseling Psychology, 43*, 210–239.

Rutan, J. S., & Stone, W. N. (1993). *Psychodynamic group psychotherapy.* New York: Guilford Press.

Ryan, N. E., & Agresti, A. A. (1999). Gerontological training in the mental health professions: The results of a national survey. *Journal of Mental Health Counseling, 21*, 352–370.

Sampson, J. P., & Loesch, L. C. (1981). Relationships among work values and job knowledge. *Vocational Guidance Quarterly, 29*, 229–235.

Sands, T. (1998). Feminist counseling and female adolescents: Treatment strategies for depression. *Journal of Mental Health Counseling, 20*, 42–54.

Satir, V. (1967). *Conjoint family therapy.* Palo Alto, CA: Science and Behavior Books.

Satir, V. (1983). *Conjoint family therapy.* Palo Alto, CA: Science and Behavior Books.

Satir, V., Banmen, J., Gerber, J., & Gomori, M. (1991). *The Satir model.* Palo Alto, CA: Science and Behavior Books.

Savickas, M. L. (1994). Measuring career development: Current status and future directions. *Career Development Quarterly, 43*, 54–62.

Savickas, M. L. (1997). Career adaptability: An integrative construct for life-span, life-space theory. *Career Development Quarterly, 45*, 247–259.

Schein, E. (1987). *Process consultation* (Vol. 2). Reading, PA: Addison-Wesley.

Schwiebert, V. L., & Myers, J. E. (1994). Midlife care givers: Effectiveness of a psychoeducational intervention for midlife adults with parent-care responsibilities. *Journal of Counseling and Development, 72*(6), 627–639.

Seiler, G., & Messina, J. (1979). Toward professional identity: The dimensions of mental health counseling in perspective. *AMHCA Journal, 1*(1), 3–8.

Seligman, L. (1986). *Diagnosis and treatment planning in counseling.* New York: Human Sciences Press.

Seligman, L. (1990). *Selecting effective treatments.* San Francisco: Jossey-Bass.

Seligman, L. (1993). Teaching treatment planning. *Counselor Education and Supervision, 33*(4), 287–297.

Seligman, L. (1994). *Developmental career counseling and assessment* (2nd ed.). Thousand Oaks, CA: Sage.

Seligman, L. (1996). *Promoting a fighting spirit.* San Francisco: Jossey-Bass.

Seligman, L. (1998). *Selecting effective treatments.* San Francisco: Jossey-Bass.

Seligman, L. (1999, November). The *DSM-IV*—An essential tool in the hands of skilled clinicians. *Counseling Today,* 6, 37.

Seligman, L. (2001a). Diagnosis in counseling. In D. Capuzzi & D. R. Gross (Eds.), *Introduction to the counseling profession* (pp. 270–289). Needham, MA: Allyn & Bacon.

Seligman, L. (2001b). *Systems, strategies, and skills of counseling and psychotherapy.* Columbus, OH: Merrill/Prentice Hall.

Seligman, L. (2004). *Technical and conceptual skills for mental health professionals.* Columbus, OH: Pearson/Merrill/Prentice Hall.

Seligman, M. E. P. (1999). *Positive psychology: Network concept paper.* Accessed October, 1999, from: http://psych.upenn.edu/seligman/pospsy.htm

Selvini Palazzoli, M. (1988). *The work of Mara Selvini Palazzoli.* New York: Jason Aronson.

Sexton, T. L. (1995). Outcome research perspective on mental health counselor competencies. In M. K. Altekruse & T. L. Sexton (Eds.), *Mental health counseling in the the 90's* (pp. 51–60). Tampa, FL: National Commission for Mental Health Counseling.

Sexton, T. L., & Alexander, J. F. (2002). Family-based empirically supported interventions. *Counseling Psychologist, 30*, 238–261.

Sexton, T. L., & Whiston, S. C. (1991). A review of the empirical basis for counseling: Implications for practice and training. *Counselor Education and Supervision, 30*(4), 330–354.

Shaffer, J., & Galinsky, M. D. (1989). *Models of group therapy.* Englewood Cliffs, NJ: Prentice Hall.

Shechtman, Z. (2002). Child group psychotherapy in the schhol at the threshold of a new millennium. *Journal of Counseling and Development, 80*, 293–299.

Shertzer, B., & Linden, J. D. (1979). *Fundamentals of individual appraisal.* Boston: Houghton Mifflin.

Shertzer, B., & Stone, S. C. (1980). *Fundamentals of counseling.* Boston: Houghton Mifflin.

Smith, D. (2001, February). Shock and disbelief. *The Atlantic Monthly,* 79–80.

Smith, D. (2002, November). Expanding psychologists' work. *Monitor on Psychology, 33*(19), 48–49.

Smith, H. B. (1999). Managed care: A survêy of counselor educators and counselor practitioners. *Journal of Mental Health Counseling, 21*, 270–284.

Smith, M. L., Glass, G. V., & Miller, T. I. (1980). *The benefits of psychotherapy.* Baltimore: Johns Hopkins University Press.

Smither, R. D., Houston, J. M., & McIntire, S. D. (1996). *Organizational development: Strategies for changing environments.* New York: Harper Collins.

Snyder, D. K. (1997). *Marital satisfaction inventory, Revised, Manual.* Los Angeles: Western Psychological Services.

Spiegel, D. (1990). Can psychotherapy prolong cancer survival? *Psychosomatics, 31*, 361–366.

Spitzer, R. L., Gibbon, M., Skodol, A. E., Williams, J. B. W., & First, M. B. (2002). *DSM-IV-TR casebook*. Washington, DC: American Psychiatric Association.

Spruill, D. A., & Fong, M. L. (1990). Defining the domain of mental health counseling: From identity confusion to consensus. *Journal of Mental Health Counseling, 12*(1), 12–23.

Standard, R. P., Sandhu, D. S., & Painter, L. C. (2000). Assessment of spirituality in counseling. *Journal of Counseling and Development, 78*, 204–210.

Sternberg, R. Triarchic abilities test. Retrieved May 19, 2003, from http://www.newhorizons.org./future/Creating_the_Future/crfut_sternberg.html

Stoltenberg, C. D. (1993). Supervising consultants in training: An application of a model of supervision. *Journal of Counseling and Development, 72*(2), 131–138.

Stuart, R. B. (1980). *Helping couples change*. New York: Guilford Press.

Sue, D. W., Arredondo, P., & McDavis, R. J. (1992). Multicultural counseling competencies and standards: A call to the profession. *Journal of Counseling and Development, 70*(4), 477–486.

Sundel, M., & Bernstein, B. E. (1995). Legal and financial aspects of midlife review and their implications for mental health counselors. *Journal of Mental Health Counseling, 17*(1), 114–123.

Super, D. E. (1957). *The psychology of careers*. New York: Harper & Row.

Swanson, J. L. (1995). The process and outcome of career counseling. In W. B. Walsh & S. H. Osipow (Eds.), *Handbook of vocational psychology: Theory, research, and practice* (pp. 217–259). Hillsdale, NJ: Erlbaum.

Swanson, J. L., & Gore, P. A. (2000). Advances in vocational psychology theory and research. In S. D. Brown & R. W. Lent (Eds.), *Handbook of counseling psychology* (3rd ed., pp. 233–269). New York: John Wiley & Sons.

Terry, A., Burden, C. A., & Pedersen, M. M. (1991). The helping relationship. In D. Capuzzi & D. R. Gross (Eds.), *Introduction to counseling: Perspectives for the 1990s* (pp. 44–68). Boston: Allyn & Bacon.

Thomas, J. C., & Hite, J. (2002). Mental health in the workplace: Toward an integration organizational and clinical theory, research, and practice. Handbook of mental health in the workplace (pp. 3–13). Thousand Oaks, CA: Sage.

Thorngren, J. M., & Kleist, D. M. (2002). Multiple family group therapy: An interpersonal/postmodern approach. *Family Journal, 10*, 167–176.

Throckmorton, E. W. (1992, March). *State licensure and third party reimbursement: Which states permit professional counselors to provide reimbursable clinical services?* Paper presented at the national convention of the American Association for Counseling and Development, Baltimore, MD.

Tiedeman, D. V., & O'Hara, R. P. (1963). *Career development: Choice and adjustment*. New York: College Entrance Examination Board.

Torres-Rivera, E., Phan, L. T., Maddux, C., Wilbur, M. P., & Garrett, M. T. (2001). Process versus content: Integrating personal awareness and counseling skills to meet the multicultural challenge of the twenty-first century. *Counselor Education and Supervision, 41*(1), 28–37.

Torres-Rivera, E., Wilbur, M. P., Maddux, C. D., Smaby, M. H., Phan, L. T., & Roberts-Wilbur, J. (2002). Factor structure and construct validity of the Counselor Skills Personal Development Rating Form. *Counselor Education and Supervision, 41*, 268–278.

Towl, G. (1994). Anger control groupwork in practice. *Issues in Criminological and Legal Psychology, 20*, 75–77.

Twohey, D., & Ewing, M. (1995). The male voice of emotional intimacy. *Journal of Mental Health Counseling, 17*(1), 54–62.

Ullery, E. K., & Carney, J. S. (2000). Mental health counselors' training to work with persons with HIV disease. *Journal of Mental Health Counseling, 22*, 334–342.

Vaillant, G. E., Bond, M., & Vaillant, C. O. (1986). An empirically validated hierarchy of defense mechanisms. *Archives of General Psychiatry, 43*, 786–794.

Vondracek, F. W., & Porfeli, E. J. (2002). Counseling psychologists and schools: Toward a sharper conceptual focus. *The Counseling Psychologist, 30*,749–756.

Walsh, B. W., & Betz, N. E. (2001). *Tests and assessment* (4th ed.). Upper Saddle River, NJ: Merrill/Prentice Hall.

Wampold, B. E., Lichtenberg, J. W., & Wachler, C. A. (2002). Principles of empirically supported interventions in counseling psychology. *The Counseling Psychologist, 30*, 197–217.

Wantz, R. A., Scherman, A., Hollis, I. W. (1982). Trends in counselor preparation: Courses, program emphases, philosophical orientation, and experimental components. *Counselor Education and Supervision, 21*, 258–268.

Waring, E. M., & Reddon, J. (1983). The measurement of intimacy in marriage: The Waring Intimacy Questionnaire. *Journal of Clinical Psychology, 39*, 53–57.

Watson, R. J., & Stermac, L. E. (1994). Cognitive group counseling for sexual offenders. *International Journal of Offender Therapy and Comparative Criminology, 38*(3), 259–270.

Watts, R. E., & Broaddus, J. L. (2002). Improving parent–child relationships through filial therapy: An interview with Garry Landreth. *Journal of Counseling and Development, 80*, 372–379.

Welfel, E. R. (1998). *Ethics in counseling and psychotherapy: Standards, research, and emerging issues*. Pacific Grove, CA: Brooks/Cole.

Welfel, E. R., Danzinger, P. R., & Santoro, S. (2000). Mandated reporting of abuse/maltreatment of older adults: A primer for counselors. *Journal of Counseling and Development, 78*, 284–292.

White, J., Keenan, M., & Brooks, N. (1992). Stress control: A controlled comparative investigation of large group therapy for generalized anxiety disorder. *Behavioural Psychotherapy, 20*(2), 97–113.

White, M. (1995). *Re-authoring lives: Interviews and essays*. Adelaide, Australia: Dulwich Centre.

Wiger, D. E., & Solberg, K. B. (2001). *Tracking mental health outcomes*. New York: John Wiley & Sons.

Wilkinson, G. B., Taylor, P., & Holt, J. R. (2002). Bipolar disorder in adolescence: Diagnosis and treatment. *Journal of Mental Health Counseling, 24*, 348–357.

Williams, C. B., & Freeman, L. T. (2002). Report of the CAC ethics committee: 2000–2001. *Journal of Counseling and Development, 80*, 251–254.

Williamson, E. G. (1939). *How to counsel students*. New York: McGraw-Hill.

Witmer, J. M., & Sweeney, T. J. (1992). A holistic model for wellness and prevention over the life span. *Journal of Counseling and Development, 71*(2), 140–148.

Wiseman, K. K. (1996). Life at work: The view from the bleachers. In P. A. Comella, J. Bader, J. S. Ball, K. K. Wiseman, & R. R. Sagar (Eds.), *The emotional side of organizations: Applications of Bowen theory* (pp. 29–38). Washington: Georgetown Family Center.

Wolber, G. J., & Carne, W. F. (1993). *Writing psychological reports: A guide for clinicians*. Sarasota, FL: Professional Resource Press.

Wolfe, D. M., & Kolb, D. A. (1980). Career development, personal growth, and experimental learning. In J. W. Springer (Ed.), *Issues in career and human resource development* (pp. 1–11). Madison, WI: American Society for Training and Development.

World Health Organization. (1992). *ICD-10 classification of mental and behavioural disorders*. Geneva: Author.

Wubbolding, R. E. (2000). *Reality therapy for the 21st century*. Briston, PA: Accelerated Development.

Yalom, I. D. (1995). *The theory and practice of group psychotherapy*. New York: Basic Books.

Zila, I. M., & Kiselica, M. S. (2001). Understanding and counseling self-mutilation in female adolescents and young adults. *Journal of Counseling and Development, 79*, 46–52.

Zinker, J. (1991). Creative process in Gestalt therapy: The therapist as artist. *Gestalt Journal, 14*(2), 71–88.

Zunker, V. G. (2002). *Career counseling applied concept of life planning* (6th ed.). Pacific Grove, CA: Brooks/Cole.

Appendix

Table A1. Overview of Key Questions Applied to *DSM-IV-TR* Categories

Category	Duration	Severity	Precipitant	Primary symptoms
1. Adjustment disorders, conditions (see Table A3, Sections I, II, III)	Brief—usually 6 months or less	May be pervasive but almost always mild-to-moderate in severity	Usually	Problems in coping with stressful situations
2. Behavior and impulse control disorders (see Table A3, Section II)	Medium to long	At least moderate	Often for episodes but usually not for disorders	Poor impulse control in at least one area
3. Mood disorders (see Table A3, Section I)	Varies	Pervasive; severity varies	Sometimes for major depression, usually not for other forms	Depression and/or unusually elevated mood
4. Anxiety disorders (see Table A3, Section III)	Medium to long	Varies	For some types (posttraumatic stress disorder)	Anxiety, avoidance, fear, somatic symptoms
5. Somatoform disorders, factitious disorders, malingering (see Table A3, Section IV)	Varies, often long	Usually moderate	Usually not	Medically unverified physical symptoms
6. Personality disorders (see Table A3, Section VI)	Long	Pervasive, usually moderate	No	Poor coping, self-esteem, relationships
7. Cognitive, dissociative, and psychotic disorders (see Table A3, Sections V and VII)	Varies	Usually Pervasive, and severe	For some types	Loss of contact with reality, confusion

Table A2. Guide to Using the Tables to Make Diagnoses

Primary symptoms	See listed section in Table A3
Depression	I
Unusually elevated mood	I
Maladaptive behavior in children, adolescents	IIa, IIe
Sexual/gender identity issues	IIb
Eating problems	IIa, IIc
Sleeping problems	IId
Problems of impulse control, behavioral problems	IIa, IIe
Anxiety, not primarily in response to physical complaints	III
Medically unverified physical complaints	IV
Psychosis	V
Long-standing pervasive dysfunction	VI
Cognitive/memory impairment, dissociation	VII

Table A3. Using the Key Questions to Make a Diagnosis

A3.I. Disorders characterized by depressed or elevated mood

Primary symptoms	Duration	Severity	Precipitant	Diagnosis
Depression	Usually 2 weeks to 6 months	Moderately severe to severe	Often	MAJOR DEPRESSIVE DISORDER
Depression	At least 2 years for adults; 1 year for youth	Mild to moderate	Rarely	DYSTHYMIC DISORDER
Mania (may also have depressive and hypomanic episodes)	Episodes lasting weeks to months	Moderately severe to severe	Sometimes	BIPOLAR I DISORDER
Hypomania (may have depressive episodes but no manic ones)	Episodes lasting weeks to months	Moderate	Sometimes	BIPOLAR II DISORDER
Numerous, relatively brief periods of mood instability	At least 2 years for adults; 1 year for youth	Moderate	Rarely	CYCLOTHYMIC DISORDER
Depression	Brief; usually no more than 6 months	Mild to moderate	Always	ADJUSTMENT DISORDER
Depression, stemming from drug/alcohol use	Varies	Mild to severe	Substance use	SUBSTANCE-INDUCED MOOD DISORDER

A3.II. Disorders characterized by maladaptive behavior, impulsivity

A3.IIa: Disorders first evident in early years

Primary symptoms	Duration	Severity	Precipitant	Diagnosis
IQ of 70 or below, poor adaptive functioning	Potentially lifelong, begins before age 18	Varies: mild to profound	Sometimes (e.g., medical condition)	MENTAL RETARDATION
Impaired social skills, communication, and behavior	Onset prior to age 3; continuous	Usually severe; often also has mental retardation	Sometimes (e.g., associated with medical condition)	AUTISTIC DISORDER
Recurrent nonrhythmic movements or vocalizations	At least 4 weeks	Varies	Exacerbated by stress, may be related to medical problems	TIC DISORDERS
Below average academic achievement in specific area	Continuous	Mild to moderate	May be abnormalities in cognitive processing	LEARNING DISORDERS
Pervasive problems in paying attention, organization, task completion	At least 6 months	Moderate	No	ATTENTION-DEFICIT HYPERACTIVITY DISORDERS
Multiple violations of rules, norms	Generally at least 12 months	Moderate to severe	Sometimes	CONDUCT DISORDER
Defiant and negativistic behavior	At least 6 months	Mild to moderate	Sometimes	OPPOSITIONAL DEFIANT DISORDER
Persistent eating of nonnutritive substances	At least 1 month	Mild to moderate	Occasionally	PICA
Regurgitation	At least 1 month	Usually moderate	Sometimes	RUMINATION DISORDER

Table A3. (continued)

A3.IIa: Disorders first evident in early years (continued)

Primary symptoms	Duration	Severity	Precipitant	Diagnosis
Inappropriate defecation	At least 3 months	Varies	Sometimes	ENCOPRESIS
Inappropriate urination	At least 3 months	Usually mild to moderate	Occasionally	ENURESIS
Refusal to speak in some or all settings	At least 1 month	Moderate	Sometimes	SELECTIVE MUTISM
Repetitive voluntary movements	At least 1 month	Moderate	Sometimes	STEREOTYPIC MOVEMENT DISORDER

A3.IIb: Sexual problems

Primary symptoms	Duration	Severity	Precipitant	Diagnosis
Lack of interest in sexual activity and/or problems in sexual arousal and/or response	Episodic or continuous; duration varies	Marked distress	Often	SEXUAL DYSFUNCTIONS
Dysfunctional primary source of arousal	At least 6 months	Varies	Sometimes	PARAPHILIAS
Discomfort with own gender	Varies, usually prolonged	Mild to moderate	Sometimes	GENDER IDENTITY DISORDERS

Table A3. (continued)

A3.IIc: Eating problems[a]

Primary symptoms	Duration	Severity	Precipitant	Diagnosis
Dysfunctional eating; body weight below 85% of expected weight	Varies; often long	Moderate to severe	Rarely	ANOREXIA NERVOSA
Recurrent binge eating, often with purging; weight at least at expected level	Varies; often long	Moderate to severe	Rarely	BULIMIA NERVOSA

[a]See also Table IIa.

A3.IId: Sleeping problems

Primary symptoms	Duration	Severity	Precipitant	Diagnosis
Difficulty falling asleep; sustaining sleep	At least 1 month	Mild to moderate	Often	INSOMNIA
Oversleeping or feeling tired even though sleeping enough	At least 1 month	Mild to moderate	Rarely	HYPERSOMNIA or BREATHING-RELATED SLEEP DISORDER
Sudden attacks of refreshing sleep	At least 3 months	Moderate	Rarely	NARCOLEPSY
Sleepwalking	Recurrent	Mild to moderate	Sometimes	SLEEPWALKING DISORDER
Recurrent bad dreams	Varies; tends to remit with age	Mild to moderate	Sometimes	NIGHTMARE DISORDER or SLEEP TERROR DISORDER

Table A3. (continued)

A3.IIe: Problems of impulse control[a]

Primary symptoms	Duration	Severity	Precipitant	Diagnosis
Impulsive theft of objects of little value	Recurrent	Varies	Sometimes	KLEPTOMANIA
Episodic emotional/ physical outbursts	Recurrent	Moderate to severe	No justification for behavior but may report precipitants	INTERMITTENT EXPLOSIVE DISORDER
Fire setting; interest in fire-related contexts	Episodic	Moderate to severe	Often	PYROMANIA
Excessive gambling	Episodic or chronic	Moderate to severe	Incidents often stress related	PATHOLOGICAL GAMBLING
Recurrent pulling out own hairs	Recurrent	Mild to moderate	Sometimes	TRICHOTILLOMANIA
Acting out	Within 3 months of stressor; up to 6 months duration after stressor	Mild to moderate	Always	ADJUSTMENT DISORDER WITH DISTURBANCE OF CONDUCT
Acting out	Very brief	Mild	Usually	ANTISOCIAL BEHAVIOR
Dysfunctional use of drugs, alcohol	Hours to 12 months	Varies	Sometimes	SUBSTANCE USE DISORDER

[a]See also Table IIa.

A3.III. Disorders characterized by anxiety, not primarily in response to physical complaints

Primary symptoms	Duration	Severity	Precipitant	Diagnosis
Brief panic attacks with avoidance	Varies	Varies	May be internal or external	PANIC DISORDER WITH AGORAPHOBIA
Brief panic attacks without avoidance	Varies	Varies	May be internal or external	PANIC DISORDER WITHOUT AGORAPHOBIA
Avoidance of situations involving crowds, inability to escape, without panic attacks	Varies	Moderate to severe	Sometimes	AGORAPHOBIA
Excessive fear of specific stimuli	Varies	Mild to moderate	Sometimes	SPECIFIC PHOBIA
Excessive fear of social situations	Frequently long term	Mild to moderate	Sometimes	SOCIAL PHOBIA
Persistent unwanted thoughts and/or repeated behaviors	May wax and wane	Varies	Usually not, stress may exacerbate	OBSESSIVE-COMPULSIVE DISORDER
Trauma-related fear, avoidance, reexperiencing	At least 1 month; may be of long duration	Moderate	Always (trauma)	POSTTRAUMATIC STRESS DISORDER
Trauma-related fear, avoidance, reexperiencing	Less than 4 weeks	Mild to moderate	Always (trauma)	ACUTE STRESS DISORDER
Pervasive anxiety	At least 6 months	Moderate	Sometimes	GENERALIZED ANXIETY DISORDER
Anxiety stemming from drug/alcohol use	Varies	Mild to moderate	Always; use of substance	SUBSTANCE-INDUCED ANXIETY DISORDER
Anxiety, usually about specific situation	Onset within 3 months of stressor; usually maximum 6 months duration	Mild to moderate	Always	ADJUSTMENT DISORDER
Difficulty separating from caretakers; onset before age 18	At least 4 weeks	Moderate	Sometimes	SEPARATION ANXIETY DISORDER

Table A3. (continued)

A3.IV. Disorders generally characterized by medically unverified physical complaints[a]

Primary symptoms	Duration	Severity	Precipitant	Diagnosis
Multiple and diverse physical complaints	Usually long	Moderate to severe	Usually not	SOMATIZATION DISORDER
Worry about at least one physical complaint	At least 6 months	Mild to moderate	Sometimes	UNDIFFERENTIATED SOMATOFORM DISORDER
Motor or sensory dysfunction	Usually acute	Moderate to severe	Often	CONVERSION DISORDER
Experience of pain not explained medically	Persistent	Varies	Sometimes	PAIN DISORDERS
Unwarranted belief that one has serious illness	Varies	Moderate	Sometimes	HYPOCHONDRIASIS
Overfocusing on minor or nonexistent physical defect	Usually long-standing	Moderate	Sometimes	BODY DYSMORPHIC DISORDER
Deliberately feigning or inducing physical or psychological symptoms in self or others for attention, nurturance	Brief to chronic	Moderate to severe	Usually not	FACTITIOUS DISORDERS
Faking sick for external gains	Varies	Mild to moderate	Sometimes	MALINGERING
Psychological symptoms that contribute to worsening of medical condition	Varies	Mild to moderate	Sometimes	PSYCHOLOGICAL FACTORS AFFECTING MEDICAL CONDITION

[a]Not fully explained by a general medical condition or a cognitive mental disorder.

A3.V. Disorders characterized by psychosis

Primary symptoms	Duration	Severity	Precipitant	Diagnosis
Severe, pervasive loss of contact with reality	At least 6 months	Severe	Usually not	SCHIZOPHRENIA
Severe, pervasive loss of contact with reality	1–6 months	Severe	Sometimes	SCHIZOPHRENIFORM DISORDER
Loss of contact with reality plus episodes of severe depression and/or mania not always related to psychosis	Varies	Severe	Usually not	SCHIZOAFFECTIVE DISORDER
Nonbizarre delusions	At least 1 month	Moderate	Often	DELUSIONAL DISORDER
Delusions and/or hallucinations	Less than 1 month	Moderate to severe	Usually	BRIEF PSYCHOTIC DISORDER
Delusions and/or hallucinations shared with another person	Usually long term	Moderate to severe	Usually not	SHARED PSYCHOTIC DISORDER
Psychosis stemming from drug or alcohol use	Varies	Moderate to severe	Substance use	SUBSTANCE-INDUCED PSYCHOTIC DISORDER

Table A3. (continued)

A3.VI. Disorders characterized by long-standing, pervasive dysfunction

Primary symptoms	Duration	Severity	Precipitant	Diagnosis
Pervasive suspiciousness, mistrust	Many years	Moderate	Usually not	PARANOID PERSONALITY DISORDER
Lack of interest in relationships	Many years	Mild to moderate	Usually not	SCHIZOID PERSONALITY DISORDER
Odd or eccentric behavior and thinking; poor social skills	Many years	Moderate to severe	Usually not	SCHIZOTYPAL PERSONALITY DISORDER
Breaking laws, violating social norms	Many years (age 18 or older)	Moderate to severe	Usually not	ANTISOCIAL PERSONALITY DISORDER
Low self-esteem, self-destructive behavior, impulsivity	Many years	Moderate to severe	Usually not	BORDERLINE PERSONALITY DISORDER
Egocentrism, overemotionalism	Many years	Mild to moderate	Usually not	HISTRIONIC PERSONALITY DISORDER
Egocentrism, grandiosity	Many years	Mild to moderate	Usually not	NARCISSISTIC PERSONALITY DISORDER
Extreme shyness, fear of rejection	Many years	Mild to moderate	Usually not	AVOIDANT PERSONALITY DISORDER
Sense of self comes from relationship with others, overinvestment in relationships, needy	Many years	Mild to moderate	Usually not	DEPENDENT PERSONALITY DISORDER
Perfectionism, overinvested in work, underinvested in relationships	Many years	Mild to moderate	Usually not	OBSESSIVE–COMPULSIVE PERSONALITY DISORDER

A3.VII. Disorders characterized by cognitive/memory impairment or dissociation

Primary symptoms	Duration	Severity	Precipitant	Diagnosis
Memory loss of prominent aspects of life	Acute to chronic	Moderate to severe	Usually but not caused by general medical condition	DISSOCIATIVE AMNESIA
Total memory loss and relocation	Usually acute. May be chronic	Severe	Usually but not caused by general medical condition	DISSOCIATIVE FUGUE
Existence of two or more distinct identities	Chronic	Severe	Usually in childhood	DISSOCIATIVE IDENTITY DISORDER
Episodes of feeling detached	Recurrent	Moderate	May accompany panic, stress, anxiety, depression	DEPERSONALIZATION DISORDER
Disturbed consciousness, change in cognition	Hours to days	Severe		DELIRIUM
Multiple cognitive deficits	Progressive, static, or remitting	Mild to severe	Usually due to general medical condition, substances or multiple etiologies	DEMENTIA

Index